Allergy Frontiers: Future Perspectives

Volume 6

Ruby Pawankar • Stephen T. Holgate
Lanny J. Rosenwasser
Editors

Allergy Frontiers: Future Perspectives

Volume 6

Springer

Ruby Pawankar, M.D., Ph.D.
Nippon Medical School
1-1-5 Sendagi, Bunkyo-ku
Tokyo
Japan

Lanny J. Rosenwasser, M.D.
Children's Mercy Hospitals and Clinics
UMKC School of Medicine
2401 Gillham Road
Kansas City, MO 64108
USA

Stephen T. Holgate, M.D., Ph.D.
University of Southampton
Southampton General Hospital
Tremona Road
Southampton
UK

ISBN: 978-4-431-54075-5 e-ISBN: 978-4-431-99365-0
DOI 10.1007/978-4-431-99365-0
Springer Tokyo Berlin Heidelberg New York

Softcover reprint of the hardcover 1st edition 2010

Printed on acid-free paper

Springer is part of Springer Science+Business Media (www.springer.com)

Foreword

When I entered the field of allergy in the early 1970s, the standard textbook was a few hundred pages, and the specialty was so compact that texts were often authored entirely by a single individual and were never larger than one volume. Compare this with *Allergy Frontiers: Epigenetics, Allergens, and Risk Factors*, the present six-volume text with well over 150 contributors from throughout the world. This book captures the explosive growth of our specialty since the single-author textbooks referred to above.

The unprecedented format of this work lies in its meticulous attention to detail yet comprehensive scope. For example, great detail is seen in manuscripts dealing with topics such as "Exosomes, naturally occurring minimal antigen presenting units" and "Neuropeptide S receptor 1 (NPSR1), an asthma susceptibility gene." The scope is exemplified by the unique approach to disease entities normally dealt with in a single chapter in most texts. For example, anaphylaxis, a topic usually confined to one chapter in most textbooks, is given five chapters in *Allergy Frontiers*. This approach allows the text to employ multiple contributors for a single topic, giving the reader the advantage of being introduced to more than one viewpoint regarding a single disease.

This broad scope is further illustrated in the way this text deals with the more frequently encountered disorder, asthma. There are no fewer than 26 chapters dealing with various aspects of this disease. Previously, to obtain such a comprehensive approach to a single condition, one would have had to purchase a text devoted solely to that disease state.

In addition, the volume includes titles which to my knowledge have never been presented in an allergy text before. These include topics such as "NKT ligand conjugated immunotherapy," "Hypersensitivity reactions to nano medicines: causative factors and optimization," and "An environmental systems biology approach to the study of asthma."

It is not hard to see that this textbook is unique, offering the reader a means of obtaining a detailed review of a single highly focused subject, such as the neuropeptide S receptor, while also providing the ability to access a panoramic and remarkably in-depth view of a broader subject, such as asthma. Clearly it is intended primarily for the serious student of allergy and immunology, but can also serve as a resource text for those with an interest in medicine in general.

I find it most reassuring that even though we have surpassed the stage of the one-volume, single-author texts, because of the wonderful complexity of our specialty and its broadening scope that has evolved over the years, the reader can still obtain an all-inclusive and comprehensive review of allergy in a single source. It should become part of the canon of our specialty.

Phillip Lieberman, M.D.

Foreword

When I started immunology under Professor Kimishige Ishizaka in the early 1950s, allergy was a mere group of odd syndromes of almost unknown etiology. An immunological origin was only suspected but not proven. The term "atopy," originally from the Greek word *à-topòs*, represents the oddness of allergic diseases. I would call this era "stage 1," or the primitive era of allergology.

Even in the 1950s, there was some doubt as to whether the antibody that causes an allergic reaction was really an antibody, and was thus called a "reagin," and allergens were known as peculiar substances that caused allergy, differentiating them from other known antigens.

It was only in 1965 that reagin was proven to be an antibody having a light chain and a unique heavy chain, which was designated as IgE in 1967 with international consensus. The discovery of IgE opened up an entirely new era in the field of allergology, and the mechanisms of the immediate type of allergic reaction was soon evaluated and described. At that point in time we believed that the nature of allergic diseases was a mere IgE-mediated inflammation, and that these could soon be cured by studying the IgE and the various mediators that induced the inflammation. This era I would like to call "stage 2," or the classic era.

The classic belief that allergic diseases would be explained by a mere allergen-IgE antibody reaction did not last long. People were dismayed by the complexity and diversity of allergic diseases that could not be explained by mere IgE-mediated inflammation. Scientists soon realized that the mechanisms involved in allergic diseases were far more complex and that they extended beyond the conventional idea of a pure IgE-mediated inflammation. A variety of cells and their products (cytokines/chemokines and other inflammatory molecules) have been found to interact in a more complex manner; they create a network of reactions via their receptors to produce various forms of inflammatory changes that could never be categorized as a single entity of inflammation. This opened a new era, which I would like to call the modern age of allergology or "stage 3."

The modern era stage 3 coincided with the discovery that similar kinds of cytokines and cells are involved in the regulation of IgE production. When immunologists investigated the cell types and cytokines that regulate IgE production, they found that two types of helper T cells, distinguishable by the profile of cytokines they produce, play important regulatory roles in not only IgE production but also in regulating allergic inflammation. The advancement of modern molecular technologies has enabled detailed analyses of molecules and genes involved in this extremely complex regulatory mechanism. Hence, there are a number of important discoveries in this area, which are still of major interest to allergologists, as can be seen in the six volumes of this book.

We realize that allergology has rapidly progressed during the last century, but mechanisms of allergic diseases are far more complex than we had expected. New discoveries have created new questions, and new facts have reminded us of old concepts. For example, the genetic disposition of allergic diseases was suspected even in the earlier, primitive era but is still only partially proven on a molecular basis. Even the molecular mechanisms of allergic inflammation continue to be a matter of debate and there is no single answer to explain the phenomenon. There is little doubt that the etiology of allergic diseases is far more varied and complex than we had expected. An immunological origin is not the only mechanism, and there are more unknown origins of similar reactions. Although therapeutic means have also progressed, we remain far from our goal to cure and prevent allergic diseases.

We have to admit that while we have more knowledge of the many intricate mechanisms that are involved in the various forms of allergic disease, we are still at the primitive stage of allergology in this respect. We are undoubtedly proceeding into a new stage, stage 4, that may be called the postmodern age of allergology and hope this era will bring us closer to finding a true solution for the enigma of allergy and allergic diseases.

We are happy that at this turning point the editors, Ruby Pawankar, Stephen Holgate, and Lanny Rosenwasser, are able to bring out such a comprehensive book which summarizes the most current knowledge on allergic diseases, from epidemiology to mechanisms, the impact of environmental and genetic factors on allergy and asthma, clinical aspects, recent therapeutic and preventive strategies, as well as future perspectives. This comprehensive knowledge is a valuable resource and will give young investigators and clinicians new insights into modern allergology which is an ever-growing field.

Tomio Tada, M.D., Ph.D., D.Med.Sci.

Foreword

Allergic diseases represent one of the major health problems in most modern societies. The increase in prevalence over the last decades is dramatic. The reasons for this increase are only partly known. While in former times allergy was regarded as a disease of the rich industrialized countries only, it has become clear that all over the world, even in marginal societies and in all geographic areas—north and south of the equator—allergy is a major global health problem.

The complexity and the interdisciplinary character of allergology, being the science of allergic diseases, needs a concert of clinical disciplines (internal medicine, dermatology, pediatrics, pulmonology, otolaryngology, occupational medicine, etc.), basic sciences (immunology, molecular biology, botany, zoology, ecology), epidemiology, economics and social sciences, and psychology and psychosomatics, just to name a few. It is obvious that an undertaking like this book series must involve a multitude of authors; indeed, the wide spectrum of disciplines relevant to allergy is reflected by the excellent group of experts serving as authors who come from all over the world and from various fields of medicine and other sciences in a pooling of geographic, scientific, theoretical, and practical clinical diversity.

The first volume concentrates on the basics of etiology, namely, the causes of the many allergic diseases with epigenetics, allergens and risk factors. Here, the reader will find up-to-date information on the nature, distribution, and chemical structure of allergenic molecules, the genetic and epigenetic phenomena underlying the susceptibility of certain individuals to develop allergic diseases, and the manifold risk factors from the environment playing the role of modulators, both in enhancing and preventing the development of allergic reactions.

In times when economics plays an increasing role in medicine, it is important to reflect on this aspect and gather the available data which—as I modestly assume—may be yet rather scarce. The big effort needed to undertake well-controlled studies to establish the socio-economic burden of the various allergic diseases is still mainly ahead of us. The Global Allergy and Asthma European Network (GA2LEN), a group of centers of excellence in the European Union, will start an initiative regarding this topic this year.

In volume 2, the pathomechanisms of various allergic diseases and their classification are given, including such important special aspects as allergy and the bone marrow, allergy and the nervous system, and allergy and mucosal immunology.

Volume 3 deals with manifold clinical manifestations, from allergic rhinitis to drug allergy and allergic bronchopulmonary aspergillosis, as well as including other allergic reactions such as lactose and fructose intolerances.

Volume 4 deals with the practical aspects of diagnosis and differential diagnosis of allergic diseases and also reflects educational programs on asthma.

Volume 5 deals with therapy and prevention of allergies, including pharmacotherapy, as well as allergen-specific immunotherapy with novel aspects and special considerations for different groups such as children, the elderly, and pregnant women.

Volume 6 concludes the series with future perspectives, presenting a whole spectrum of exciting new approaches in allergy research possibly leading to new strategies in diagnosis, therapy, and prevention of allergic diseases.

The editors have accomplished an enormous task to first select and then motivate the many prominent authors. They and the authors have to be congratulated. The editors are masters in the field and come from different disciplines. Ruby Pawankar, from Asia, is one of the leaders in allergy who has contributed to the understanding of the cellular and immune mechanisms of allergic airway disease, in particular upper airway disease. Stephen Holgate, from the United Kingdom, has contributed enormously to the understanding of the pathophysiology of allergic airway reactions beyond the mere immune deviation, and focuses on the function of the epithelial barrier. He and Lanny Rosenwasser, who is from the United States, have contributed immensely to the elucidation of genetic factors in the susceptibility to allergy. All three editors are members of the Collegium Internationale Allergologicum (CIA) and serve on the Board of Directors of the World Allergy Organization (WAO).

I have had the pleasure of knowing them for many years and have cooperated with them at various levels in the endeavor to promote and advance clinical care, research, and education in allergy. Together with Lanny Rosenwasser as co-editor-in-chief, we have just started the new *WAO Journal* (electronic only), where the global representation in allergy research and education will be reflected on a continuous basis.

Finally, Springer, the publisher, has to be congratulated on their courage and enthusiasm with which they have launched this endeavor. Springer has a lot of experience in allergy—I think back to the series *New Trends in Allergy*, started in 1985, as well as to my own book *Allergy in Practice,* to the *Handbook of Atopic Eczema* and many other excellent publications.

I wish this book and the whole series of *Allergy Frontiers* complete success! It should be on the shelves of every physician or researcher who is interested in allergy, clinical immunology, or related fields.

Johannes Ring, M.D., Ph.D.

Preface

Allergic diseases are increasing in prevalence worldwide, in industrialized as well as industrializing countries, affecting from 10%–50% of the global population with a marked impact on the quality of life of patients and with substantial costs. Thus, allergy can be rightfully considered an epidemic of the twenty-first century, a global public health problem, and a socioeconomic burden. With the projected increase in the world's population, especially in the rapidly growing economies, it is predicted to worsen as this century moves forward.

Allergies are also becoming more complex. Patients frequently have multiple allergic disorders that involve multiple allergens and a combination of organs through which allergic diseases manifest. Thus exposure to aeroallergens or ingested allergens frequently gives rise to a combination of upper and lower airways disease, whereas direct contact or ingestion leads to atopic dermatitis with or without food allergy. Food allergy, allergic drug responses and anaphylaxis are often severe and can be life-threatening. However, even the less severe allergic diseases can have a major adverse effect on the health of hundreds of millions of patients and diminish quality of life and work productivity. The need of the hour to combat these issues is to promote a better understanding of the science of allergy and clinical immunology through research, training and dissemination of information and evidence-based better practice parameters.

Allergy Frontiers is a comprehensive series comprising six volumes, with each volume dedicated to a specific aspect of allergic disease to reflect the multidisciplinary character of the field and to capture the explosive growth of this specialty. The series summarizes the latest information about allergic diseases, ranging from epidemiology to the mechanisms and environmental and genetic factors that influence the development of allergy; clinical aspects of allergic diseases; recent therapeutic and preventive strategies; and future perspectives. The chapters of individual volumes in the series highlight the roles of eosinophils, mast cells, lymphocytes, dendritic cells, epithelial cells, neutrophils and T cells, adhesion molecules, and cytokines/chemokines in the pathomechanisms of allergic diseases. Some specific new features are the impact of infection and innate immunity on allergy, and mucosal immunology of the various target organs and allergies, and the impact of the nervous system on allergies. The most recent, emerging therapeutic strategies are discussed, including allergen-specific immunotherapy and anti-IgE treatment, while also covering future perspectives from immunostimulatory DNA-based therapies to probiotics and nanomedicine.

A unique feature of the series is that a single topic is addressed by multiple contributors from various fields and regions of the world, giving the reader the advantage of being introduced to more than one point of view and being provided with comprehensive knowledge about a single disease. The reader thus obtains a detailed review of a single, highly focused topic and at the same time has access to a panoramic, in-depth view of a broader subject such as asthma.

The chapters attest to the multidisciplinary character of component parts of the series: environmental, genetics, molecular, and cellular biology; allergy; otolaryngology; pulmonology; dermatology; and others. Representing a collection of state-of-the-art reviews by world-renowned scientists from the United Kingdom and other parts of Europe, North America, South America, Australia, Japan, and South Africa, the volumes in this comprehensive, up-to-date series contain more than 150 chapters covering virtually all aspects of basic and clinical allergy. The publication of this extensive collection of reviews is being brought out within a span of two years and with the greatest precision to keep it as updated as possible. This six-volume series will be followed up by yearly updates on the cutting-edge advances in any specific aspect of allergy.

The editors would like to sincerely thank all the authors for having agreed to contribute and who, despite their busy schedules, contributed to this monumental work. We also thank the editorial staff of Springer Japan for their assistance in the preparation of this series. We hope that the series will serve as a valuable information tool for scientists and as a practical guide for clinicians and residents working and/or interested in the field of allergy, asthma, and immunology.

Ruby Pawankar, Stephen Holgate, and Lanny Rosenwasser

Contents

Contributors

Ian M. Adcock
Airway Disease Section, National Heart and Lung Institute,
Imperial College of London, London, UK

Hardeep S. Asi
Division of Clinical Immunology and Allergy, Department of Medicine,
Faculty of Health Sciences, McMaster University, 1200 Main Street West,
Hamilton, ON, L8N 3Z5, Canada

Bengt Björkstén
Institute of Environmental Medicine, Division of Lung Fysiology,
Karolinska Institutet, 171 77 Stockholm, Sweden

Gaetano Caramori
Dipartimento di Medicina Clinica e Sperimentale, Centro di Ricerca su Asma e
BPCO, Università di Ferrara, Via Savonarola 9, 44100 Ferrara, Italy

Paolo Casolari
Dipartimento di Medicina Clinica e Sperimentale, Centro di Ricerca su Asma e
BPCO, Università di Ferrara, Via Savonarola 9, 44100 Ferrara, Italy

Fook Tim Chew
Department of Biological Sciences, National University of Singapore,
Allergy and Molecular Immunology Laboratory, Lee Hiok Kwee Functional
Genomics Laboratories, 14, Science Drive 4, 117543, Singapore

Marco Contoli
Dipartimento di Medicina Clinica e Sperimentale, Centro di Ricerca su Asma e
BPCO, Università di Ferrara, Via Savonarola 9, 44100 Ferrara, Italy

Oliver Cromwell
Allergopharma J. Ganzer KG, Hermann-Koerner-Str. 52, 21465 Reinbek,
Germany

Chitra Dinakar
Department of Pediatrics, University of Missouri-Kansas City;
Division of Allergy, Asthma and Immunology,
Children's Mercy Hospital, Kansas City,
MO 64108, USA

Deendayal Dinakarpandian
School of Computing and Engineering, University of Missouri, Kansas City,
MO 64110, USA

Struan F.A. Grant
The Center for Applied Genomics and Division of Human Genetics,
The Abramson Research Center of the Joseph Stokes Jr. Research Institute,
Department of Pediatrics, The Children's Hospital of Philadelphia
and the University of Pennsylvania School of Medicine, Philadelphia,
PA 19104, USA

Hakon Hakonarson
The Center for Applied Genomics and Division of Human Genetics,
The Abramson Research Center of the Joseph Stokes Jr. Research Institute,
Department of Pediatrics, The Children's Hospital of Philadelphia
and the University of Pennsylvania School of Medicine, Philadelphia,
PA 19104, USA

Islam Hamad
Molecular Targeting and Polymer Toxicology Group, School of Pharmacy,
University of Brighton, Brighton BN2 4GJ, UK

Tomoko Hayashi
Department of Medicine, University of California San Diego,
9500 Gilman Drive, La Jolla, CA 92093, USA

Cory M. Hogaboam
Immunology Program, Department of Pathology, University of Michigan
Medical School, Ann Arbor, MI 48109-2200, USA

Ken Igawa
Department of Dermatology, Graduate School of Medicine, Tokyo Medical
and Dental University, 1-5-45 Yushima, Bunkyo-ku, Tokyo 113-8519, Japan

Yasuyuki Ishii
Laboratory for Vaccine Design, RIKEN Research Center for Allergy
and Immunology, 1-7-22 Suehiro, Tsurumi-ku, Yokohama,
Kanagawa 230-0045, Japan

Kazuhiro Ito
Airway Disease Section, National Heart and Lung Institute,
Imperial College of London, London, UK

Ramzi Kafoury
Department of Biology, Jackson State University, Jackson, MS, USA

Ichiro Katayama
Department of Dermatology, Integrated Medicine, Graduate School of Medicine, Osaka University, 2-2 Yamada-oka, Suita-shi, Osaka 565-0871, Japan

Juha Kere
Department of Biosciences and Nutrition, Karolinska Institutet, Hälsovägen 7, 14157 Huddinge, Sweden;
Clinical Research Centre, Karolinska University Hospital Huddinge, Huddinge, Sweden;
Department of Medical Genetics, Biomedicum, University of Helsinki, Haartmaninkatu 8, 00014 Helsinki, Finland

Hiroshi Kiyono
Division of Mucosal Immunology, Department of Microbiology and Immunology, The Institute of Medical Science, The University of Tokyo, Tokyo 108-8639, Japan; Core Research for Evolutional Science and Technology (CREST), Japan Science and Technology Corporation (JST), Saitama 332-0012, Japan

Mark Larché
Division of Clinical Immunology and Allergy, Department of Medicine, Faculty of Health Sciences, McMaster University, 1200 Main Street West, Hamilton, ON, L8N 3Z5, Canada

Paolo Maria Matricardi
Department of Pediatric Pneumology and Immunology, Charité – Universitätsmedizin, Augustenburger Platz 1, D-13353 Berlin, Germany

S. Moein Moghimi
Department of Pharmaceutics and Analytical Chemistry, Faculty of Pharmaceutical Sciences, University of Copenhagen, Universitestparken 2, DK2100 Copenhagen Ø, Denmark

Hiroyuki Murota
Department of Dermatology, Integrated Medicine, Graduate School of Medicine, Osaka University, 2-2 Yamada-oka, Suita-shi, Osaka 565-0871, Japan

Hiroyuki Nagase
Division of Respiratory Medicine and Allergology, Department of Medicine, Teikyo University School of Medicine, 2-11-1 Kaga, Itabashi-ku, Tokyo 173-8665, Japan

Kiyoshi Nishioka
Department of Dermatology, Graduate School of Medicine, Tokyo Medical and Dental University, 1-5-45 Yushima, Bunkyo-ku, Tokyo 113-8519, Japan

Kristen P. Oehlke
Division of Environmental Health Sciences, University of Minnesota School of Public Health, Minneapolis, MN 55455, USA;
Minnesota Department of Health, St. Paul, MN 55410, USA

Ken Ohta
Division of Respiratory Medicine and Allergology, Department of Medicine, Teikyo University School of Medicine, 2-11-1 Kaga, Itabashi-Ku, Tokyo 173-8665, Japan

Seow Theng Ong
Department of Biological Sciences, National University of Singapore, Allergy and Molecular Immunology Laboratory, Lee Hiok Kwee Functional Genomics Laboratories, 14, Science Drive 4, 117543 Singapore

Alberto Papi
Dipartimento di Medicina Clinica e Sperimentale, Centro di Ricerca su Asma e BPCO, Università di Ferrara, Via Savonarola 9, 44100 Ferrara, Italy

Susan L. Prescott
School of Paediatrics and Child Health, University of Western Australia, Perth, Australia

Eyal Raz
Department of Medicine, University of California San Diego, 9500 Gilman Drive, La Jolla, CA 92093, USA

Hirohisa Saito
Department of Allergy and Immunology, National Research Institute for Child Health and Development, Setagaya, Tokyo, Japan

Takahiro Satoh
Department of Dermatology, Graduate School of Medicine, Tokyo Medical and Dental University, 1-5-45 Yushima, Bunkyo-ku, Tokyo 113-8519, Japan

Elodie Segura
Institut Curie, Centre de Recherche, 26 rue d'Ulm, 75245 Paris Cedex 05, France; INSERM U932, 26 rue d'Ulm, 75245 Paris Cedex 05, France

Fumio Takaiwa
Transgenic Crop Research and Development Center, National Institute of Agrobiological Sciences, Ibaraki 305-8602, Japan

Clotilde Théry
Institut Curie, Centre de Recherche, 26 rue d'Ulm, 75245 Paris Cedex 05, France; INSERM U932, 26 rue d'Ulm, 75245 Paris Cedex 05, France

Martin Thurnher
Department of Urology, Immunotherapy Unit, Innsbruck Medical University and KMT Center of Excellence in Medicine, Anichstrasse 35, 6020 Innsbruck, Austria

William A. Toscano
Division of Environmental Health Sciences, University of Minnesota School of Public Health, Minneapolis, MN 55455, USA

Naomi Yamashita
Division of Respiratory Medicine and Allergology,
Department of Medicine, Teikyo University School of Medicine,
2-11-1 Kaga, Itabashi-Ku, Tokyo 173-8665, Japan;
Department of Pharmacology, Research Institute of Pharmaceutical Science,
Musashino University, 1-1-20 Shin-machi, Nishitokyo-shi, Tokyo, Japan

Hiroo Yokozeki
Department of Dermatology, Graduate School of Medicine, Tokyo Medical
and Dental University, 1-5-45 Yushima, Bunkyo-ku, Tokyo 113-8519, Japan

Yoshikazu Yuki
Division of Mucosal Immunology, Department of Microbiology and Immunology,
The Institute of Medical Science, The University of Tokyo, Tokyo 108-8639, Japan;
Core Research for Evolutional Science and Technology (CREST)
and Creation and Support Program for Start-ups from Universities,
Japan Science and Technology Corporation (JST), Saitama 332-0012,
Japan

Functional Genomics and Proteomics in Allergy Research

Struan F.A. Grant and Hakon Hakonarson

Introduction

Asthma is a complex genetic disorder with a heterogeneous phenotype. With its rising incidence over the past three decades, asthma has emerged as an epidemic that currently affects nearly 155 million individuals worldwide [1–6]. The increase in asthma incidence encompasses all age and ethnic groups and, for reasons that remain unknown, the morbidity and mortality associated with asthma are disproportionately high among children, identifying asthma as the most common chronic disease in children in all developed countries. In the U.S., approximately 20 million people are diagnosed with asthma and, each year, the disease accounts for approximately 500,000 hospitalizations and nearly 5,000 deaths. Despite recent advances in medications used to treat the disease, the management of asthma is often complicated, and adequate control of symptoms is difficult to maintain [7,8]. Moreover, many of the drugs currently used to treat asthma (e.g., steroids, β-adrenergic agents, etc.) can have deleterious side effects and, in a number of individuals, medication overuse can actually lead to worsening of the disease. Thus, asthma represents a major health problem, particularly in children, and in order to ultimately develop more effective new strategies to treat the disease, a critical need exists to identify its underlying cause.

Although the cause of asthma is unknown, it is known to be attributed to the interactions between many genes and the environment and it has been suggested that genetics may contribute to as much as 60–80% of the inter-individual variability in therapeutic response to asthma medications. Numerous genetic studies have reported linkage or association with asthma and the asthma-associated phenotypes, atopy, elevated immunoglobulin E (IgE) levels, and bronchial hyper-responsiveness. In addition, specific alleles tagging cytokine/chemokine, remodeling or IgE regulating

S.F.A. Grant and H. Hakonarson(✉)
Center for Applied Genomics, 1216E Abramson Research Center, 3615 Civic Center Blvd., Philadelphia, PA 19104-4318, USA
e-mail: hakonarson@chop.edu

R. Pawankar et al. (eds.), *Allergy Frontiers: Future Perspectives*,
DOI 10.1007/978-4-431-99365-0_1, © Springer 2010

genes have been shown to confer risk for these phenotypes. Although many studies reporting these observations are compelling, only a handful of genes have been uncovered that confer a meaningful risk of asthma based on the candidate gene or linkage approach. Moreover, the clinical implications of the genetic variations reported within the numerous candidate asthma genes with respect to asthma therapy remain largely undetermined.

The first major breakthrough in asthma discovery came through the cloning of the *ADAM33* gene [9–11], a disintegrin that includes a metalloproteinase domain 33, now widely replicated within the asthma research community [9–12]. Discoveries of other asthma-related genes followed shortly, including that of *DPP10* which encodes a homolog of dipeptidyl peptidases (DPPs) that cleave terminal dipeptides from cytokines and chemokines [13], *PHF11,* a PHD finger protein [9–11], and G protein-coupled receptor of asthma *(GPRA)* encoding the neuropeptide S (NPS)-NPS receptor 1 *(NPSR1)* [9–11]. These discoveries were fundamental to the notion that genetic/genomic factors may play key roles in the pathogenesis and pathobiology of complex disorders, such as asthma and atopy. These discoveries also stimulated interest in the study of gene–gene and gene–environment interactions as well as interest in re-sequencing these genes to pinpoint the actual functional/causative mutations involved. In addition, these variants may also influence treatment response.

It is widely accepted that common diseases, such as asthma, that have a strong but complex genetic component, together with variable drug response, are ideal targets for pharmacogenomic research [14–17]. Drugs that are in current use are not effective in all individuals, with relapse and severe adverse effects common in a high percentage of patients. The ability to analyze SNP patterns and expression levels of thousands of genes using oligonucleotide microarrays allows for a powerful screen of multiple molecular pathways simultaneously that may elucidate genes that determine drug response [18,19]. Generally, several genes are involved which, in conjunction with specific environmental factors, influence the efficacy of the drug response in some individuals and the potential for adverse events in others. In addition, the allelic interactions of the respective variants (i.e., SNP pattern) of the genes or gene pathways involved are highly complex and the resulting gene–gene and gene–environment interactions remain for the most part unexplained. Thus, it is no surprise that as many as two-third of patients with asthma may not attain full control of their symptoms despite modern therapies [20,21]. It also appears that about one-third of patients treated with inhaled corticosteroids (ICSs) may not achieve objective improvements in airway function or measures of airway reactivity [22]. A similar number of patients using oral corticosteroids develop osteoporosis [23–25]; cataracts and glaucoma are also reported side effects from ICS use [26–28]. In addition, approximately 5,000 asthma deaths occur in the US every year, which in large part is due to the use of long-acting β-agonists [29].

Drug responses vary widely between different populations and are also highly variable among individuals within the same population. A representative example is the observed response variability between asthma patients to β_2-agonist therapy, where up to three quarters of the variability is genetically based, albeit different among different ethnic groups [30]. Homozygosity for arginine at position 16 (the Arg/Arg genotype) of the β-adrenergic receptor predicts therapeutic response to β_2-agonists in Puerto Ricans but not in Mexicans [31]. There is also evidence suggesting that variants in the β_2-adrenergic receptor may explain differences in airway responsiveness in smokers versus nonsmokers [32]; this phenomenon is also evident in subjects using both ICSs and cigarettes [33]. Numerous candidate gene studies have been conducted in an attempt to unravel this mystery; however, the hunt for polymorphisms in candidate genes has not been productive thus far and the results from ongoing GWA studies in asthma are likely to fuel the interest of asthma investigators in the near future.

Polymorphisms can occur in coding and non-coding regions of genes, with their mechanism of action with respect to altered gene function generally remaining poorly understood. SNPs are by far the most commonly studied variants in pharmacogenetic/genomic studies [34]. Most disease associated variants are not expected to be directly functional themselves but instead are more likely to be in LD with the functional "smoking gun" mutations. Approximately 10 million SNPs are known to exist in the human genome, and they are stable over time [35,36]. A different set of variants, known as "microsatellites," constitute variable numbers of tandem repeats that may also produce functional changes or serve as markers for other changes in the genome. The potential effect of examining haplotypes, defined as varying combinations (similar to a barcode) of SNPs and/or variable numbers of tandem repeats over a linked region on a single chromosome, is also considered an informative way of studying disease susceptibility or drug response in pharmacogenomic association studies.

Genetic/Genomic and Proteomic Studies in Asthma and Atopy

Based on genetic, clinical, and epidemiological studies, asthma is well recognized as a common complex disorder with variable phenotype that is triggered by various environmental factors such as allergens, infectious agents, irritants, etc. [37–39]. As for other complex diseases, the genetics of asthma and atopy (its commonly related disorder) has been investigated using genome-wide linkage studies, with some followed by positional cloning, and candidate gene association studies. Many case-control studies have examined the association between one or more polymorphisms of a particular candidate gene and asthma/atopy phenotypes, with the candidate gene selected on the basis of its suspected role in the pathobiology of asthma or atopy. Such studies have included genes involved in innate immunity (e.g., toll-like receptors [TLRs], *CD14*, *CARD15*, etc.), inflammation (e.g., various cytokines, chemokines, etc.), lung function, growth and development (e.g., *TGFB1*, *ADRB2*, *NOS1* and *3*, *SPINK5*, etc.), and genes implicated as modifiers of responses to environmental exposures such as pollutants and tobacco smoke (e.g., *GSTM1*, *GSTP1*, and *GSTT1*) (see reviews [40–42]). Several studies have been consistent in demonstrating an association of asthma/atopy phenotypes with polymorphisms in various candidate genes including the β2-adrenergic receptor gene *(ADRβ2)* [43–45] and genes involved in the IL-4/IL-13 cytokine signaling pathway [46–49], which is importantly implicated in IgE switching and other immunoregulatory functions regulating atopic inflammation and asthma. Overall, however, the findings from the majority of these studies vary strikingly, and associations reported in some populations fail to be replicated in others. This discordance is not surprising given the phenotypic complexities of asthma and atopy, genetic background differences between the study populations, and the impact of the uncontrolled effects of environmental influences. Additionally, the findings in a number of studies may be complicated by type 1 errors and false positive results due to other differences between the study cases and controls (age, sex, race, etc.), genotyping errors, or insufficient control of multiple testing.

To date, approximately 20 genome-wide screens have been performed in different study populations to identify chromosomal regions that are linked to asthma/atopy and one or more of the related phenotypes of airway hyperresponsiveness (AHR), elevated IgE levels, and other allergy-associated phenotypic features. The findings from these studies (reviewed in refs [19,41,42,50,51]) also vary markedly, and are marred by inconsistencies due to such complicating factors as lack of sufficient statistical power, differences in study design, and inherent differences in the study populations. Overall, however, a number of these studies have been generally consistent in demonstrating linkage to certain chromosomal regions, identifying these loci as containing major genes influencing asthma and its associated phenotypes. These regions include genes whose transcripts are known to be biologically relevant in asthma, including the cytokine gene cluster on chromosome 5q, 11q (containing *FcεRI-β*), 12q (containing *IFNγ* and *STAT6*), and 16p (containing *IL-4Rα*). Moreover, in a study involving extended families with asthma in Iceland, significant linkage with an allele sharing lod score of 4.0 was demonstrated for an asthma susceptibility gene on chromosome 14q24 [52]. In other studies, suggestive linkage to asthma-related phenotypes also includes regions on 2q, 13q, and 6p (near the major histocompatibility complex [MHC]), and a genome screen of American families from different racial groups demonstrated weak linkage to broad regions on chromosomes 2q, 5q, 6p, 12q, 13q and 14q [19,40–42,50–53].

Linkage studies followed by positional cloning have recently identified some genes that had previously not been associated with asthma or atopy, including *ADAM33, DPP10, PHF11,* and *GPRA*. Two of these candidate genes, *ADAM33* and *GPRA*, have generated considerable interest based on their potential roles in the pathobiology of asthma. *ADAM33* encodes a disintegrin and metalloproteinase protein that mediates adhesion and proteolysis, and its detection in bronchial smooth muscle cells and in fibroblasts suggested its possible involvement in airway remodeling. In the original study, 19 SNPs in *ADAM33* were found to have associations with asthma and AHR in affected sibling-pair families from the US and UK [9]. A series of replication studies that focused on a varying number of these SNPs were subsequently conducted in different study populations, including those from ethnically diverse backgrounds. The results for single SNPs and haplotypes have, in some studies, demonstrated impressive statistical significance. However, the SNPs used in many of these linkage studies have varied between the studies and, overall, the results have been inconsistent. Recently, a meta-analysis of all published studies demonstrated that, although the ST+7 variant of *ADAM33* is significantly associated with asthma, the contribution of this locus to the risk of the population developing the disease is small [12]. The other candidate gene (for "*GPRA*") was cloned following linkage association of asthma/atopy and elevated total serum IgE levels in Canadian and Finnish cohorts to seven common haplotypes spanning a 133-kb region on chromosome 7p15-p14 [11]. *GPRA* transcripts were subsequently detected in smooth muscle cells and in epithelial cells, with relatively enhanced expression in epithelial cells of asthmatic individuals [11]. Contrasting the original report, however, a subsequent study that genotyped a haplotype tagging SNP in a Korean population failed to find a significant association with the risk of asthma, atopy, total serum IgE, or AHR [54]. This failure of replication may be due to a variety of reasons that include differences in ethnic genetic background and environmental interaction, as well as the fact that only one haplotype tagging SNP was used in the latter study rather than a broader array of SNPs or haplotypes. As for *ADAM33* and *GPRA*, further replication studies examining associations of the other candidate genes identified by positional cloning with asthma/atopy are ongoing, in addition to studies investigating the potential functional roles for these genes.

Recently, there has been a revolution occurring in SNP genotyping technology, with high-throughput genotyping methods allowing large volumes of SNPs (10^5–10^6) to be genotyped in large cohorts of patients and controls, therefore enabling large-scale GWA studies in complex diseases. Already with this technology, compelling evidence for genetic variants involved in type 1 diabetes [55–57], type 2 diabetes [57–61], age-related macular degeneration [62], inflammatory bowel disease [63], heart disease [64,65], and breast cancer [66] has been described. Even more recently, Moffat and colleagues reported the first GWA discovery in asthma [67]. In their study, they examined over 317,000 SNPs in 994 patients with childhood onset asthma and 1,243 non-asthmatics controls. They identified several markers on chromosome 17q21 that were reproducibly associated with childhood onset asthma in family and case-referent panels with a combined P value $< 10^{-12}$. In independent replication studies the 17q21 locus showed strong association with diagnosis of childhood asthma in 2,320 subjects from a cohort of German children ($P = 0.0003$) and in 3,301 subjects from the British 1958 Birth Cohort ($P = 0.0005$). They subsequently examined the relationships between markers at the 17q21 locus and transcript levels of genes in Epstein–Barr virus (EBV)-transformed lymphoblastoid cell lines from children who were being studied. The SNPs associated with childhood asthma were consistently and strongly associated ($P < 10^{-22}$) in cis with transcript levels of *ORMDL3*, a member of a gene family that encodes transmembrane proteins anchored in the endoplasmic reticulum. Accordingly, the study concluded that genetic variants regulating *ORMDL3* expression are determinants of susceptibility to childhood asthma. Although these results need to be replicated by independent investigators, they present the first GWA results in asthma, with

Table 1 Asthma susceptibility genes established by replication and/or rigid-analysis

Gene	Location	Variation	Phenotype	Odds ratios (95% Cl)	Original study or meta-analysis
ADAM33	20p	ST+7allele	Asthma	1.46(1.21–1.76)	Van Eerdewegh et al. [9]
		F+1allele	Asthma	1.20(1.00–1.45)	Van Eerdewegh et al. [9]
GPRA	7p15	GPRA-SNP 522363g>c	Asthma	2.25(2.00–3.10)	Laitinen et al. [11]
CD14	5q31	T-159allele	Asthma	1.16(0.98–1.39)	Kedda et al. [112]
TNF	6p21	TNF-308A	Asthma	1.31(0.99–1.74)	Aoki T et al. [113]
B2AR	5q31	Gly16	Noct. Asthma	2.20(1.56–3.11)	Thakkinstian et al. [111]
ORMDL3	17q21	rs3894194	Asthma	1.68(1.25–2.26)	Moffatt et al. [67]

significance level far exceeding any previous asthma gene study. It will be challenging but interesting to watch the translation work forthcoming on *ORMDL3* in the near future [68]. Taken together, genes that have been associated with asthma and have been replicated in independent studies are shown in Table 1.

A Pharmacogenomic/Proteomic Perspective in Asthma and Atopy

The classes of anti-asthma medications that are available to patients include the bronchodilators, such as β_2-adrenergic agonists, and the anti-inflammatory agents, glucocorticoids (GCs) and leukotriene modifiers, with other drugs being rarely used. **Pharmacogenomic** studies on asthma are typically designed to determine whether the variations under study influence function with respect to these drugs. Most of these studies have been hypothesis driven and are based on a relatively small number of patients, thereby lacking power to assess factors that can confound genetic associations. A more broad-based non-hypothesis driven genome wide approach requires many more patients and is more costly; but is more likely to uncover novel variants in genes that influence or modify drug response. Thus, the GWA approach extends beyond the gene or pathway of interest and is used to screen for unknown disease or drug response variants. While these studies are in their infancy, it should be noted that a somewhat comparable approach was used to identify the association between the metalloproteinase gene, *ADAM 33*, and asthma [9]. To the extent that drug response is heritable, pharmacogenomics seeks to define the relationship between variability in the human genetic code and variability in response to pharmacologic interventions. Most studies to date have dealt with the signaling pathway from the receptor drug targets themselves, to the drug transporters and metabolizing enzyme cascades, focusing on the pharmacokinetic and pharmacodynamic characteristics of the drug in terms of clinical response measures (Fig. 1). The following section addresses the genetic diversity among individuals as it pertains to the receptor signaling pathways of the major drug classes used in asthma therapy.

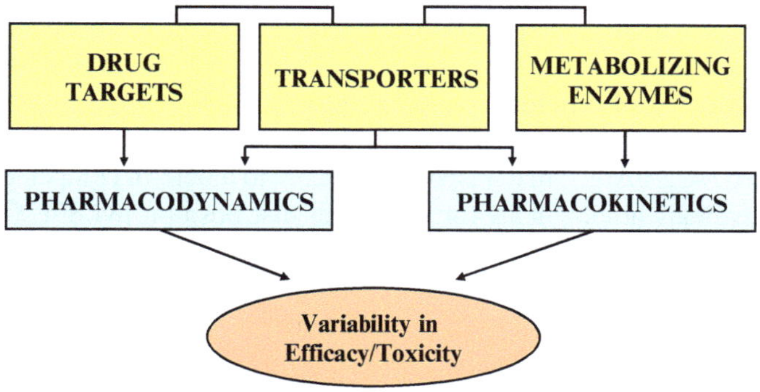

Fig. 1 Schematic overview of the key molecular pathways underlying variability in drug response

β_2-Agonists

β_2-agonists are considered the first line therapy for bronchodilation and rapid relief from asthma symptoms [69]. β_2AR is also considered a putative candidate gene in the pathogenesis of asthma and related traits. Numerous studies have highlighted the important role of the airway smooth muscle in asthma [70,71]. The sequence of β_2-AR has been known for many years and the effect of gene polymorphisms on the receptor functions has been thoroughly investigated [44,72–77]. At least nine different point mutations have been found in the gene at nucleotide positions 46, 79, 100, 252, 491, 523, 1,053, 1,098 and 1,239 [73]. Four of these were found to cause changes in the encoded amino acids at residues at positions 16, 27, 34 and 164 with Arg16Gly and Gln27Glu being most frequent and showing most effect. Several studies have suggest a role for the β_2-AR in asthma pathogenesis [44,74,75]. Asthmatic children who are homozygous for Arg-16 have significantly greater (>fivefold) bronchodilator response to albuterol than homozygous Gly-16 individuals [44]. Similar results have been reported in multiple other populations suggesting they are real [74–77]. However, replication attempted in the Indian population reported exactly the opposite effect of these genotypes [78] and others have found either no difference between Gly-16 and Arg-16 receptor variants [70] or decrease in response in mild asthmatics carrying the homozygous Arg-16 genotype [79].

Regular use of β-agonist drugs has been reported to have detrimental effects on symptoms and lung function in double-blinded placebo-controlled studies [80]. Asthma patients carrying the Arg/Arg form may benefit by minimizing the use of both short-acting and long-acting β_2-agonists and Arg/Arg patients do not get benefit from the use of salmeterol, even when used concurrently with ICSs, and may develop worse airway function with chronic use of long-acting β_2-agonists [81]. Salmeterol may even provoke pro-inflammatory effect in Arg/Arg patients [81,82]. Genotype–phenotype correlations may differ significantly across different ethnic groups as demonstrated by the association of the SNP at position 47 (Arg-19Cys) with bronchodilator drug responsiveness in certain groups and not others [83]. Replication studies are needed to validate the differential role of this SNP on drug response in subjects of different ethnic background.

Reports suggest that 60% of asthma children who are homozygous for arginine at position 16 (Arg^{16}/Arg^{16}) may respond favorably to albuterol compared with only 13% in individuals homozygous for glycine at that position [84,85]. Others have not found such a striking difference, in studies including both pediatric [78] and adult patients [31]. In a study addressing haplotype diversity based on 13 SNPs in the β_2-AR gene, different haplotypes were detected at the 5-prime end that differed significantly among different ethnic populations [72]. Interestingly, a relatively common haplotype that captured the Arg16 variant that was found to associate with decreased response to β_2-agonists, showed the opposite effect in other cohorts [31,85], illustrating the important differences among subjects of different ethnic backgrounds. It is important to test for these variants in subjects who do not respond well to standard therapies, particularly if patients are using high doses of β_2-agonists and controller medications and their asthma remains poorly controlled. The genetics of drug response traits is complex [86,87] and broader genomics approaches are needed to provide new insights into the molecular mechanisms of complex diseases and on how to optimize therapy for the individual patient.

Leukotriene Modifiers

The cysteinyl-leukotrienes, LTC_4, LTD_4 and LTE_4, are lipoxygenase-derived eicosanoids and potent proinflammatory mediators that regulate contractile and inflammatory responses through G protein-coupled receptors. Cysteinyl-LTs have been causatively implicated in asthma and allergic rhinitis, and have also been shown to play a role in other inflammatory conditions, such as cardiovascular diseases, cancer and dermatitis. Variations of the promoter region of the 5-lipoxygenase (*ALOX5*) gene and the leukotriene C_4 (LTC_4) synthase gene have been well characterized and both have been associated with functional changes of these genes that affect drug response. Genetic variants have also been identified for the *CysLT1* and *CysLT2* receptors and are being examined in the context of asthma and atopy. Although several studies addressing the effects of variations in the LT pathway genes on responses to leukotriene modifier therapy have reported effects on drug response that may have clinical relevance, there are as many studies that have reported negative findings. Better powered studies are needed since meta-analysis on existing data is unlikely to sort this out.

ALOX5

The first committed enzyme in the leukotriene biosynthetic pathway is ALOX5. Several naturally occurring mutations are known to exist in the *ALOX5* gene, including a variable number of tandem repeats in the promoter region of the gene that can modify transcription factor binding and reporter gene transcription. These microsatellites have been shown to code for the binding motif of the Sp1 and Egr1 transcription factors, thereby affecting the transcription rate of the gene [88]. Alterations in the number of tandem repeats have been shown to alter the efficiency of gene transcription such that any variation from the wild type decreased gene transcription at least in subjects with asthma [30]. Patients with mild-to-moderate asthma who were treated with a ALOX5 inhibitor and who carried at least one wild-type allele of the *ALOX5* promoter locus were shown to have greater improvement in FEV_1 than those without any wild-type alleles [89]. These data suggest that the absence of at least one copy of the wild-type allele creates a phenotype that is less responsive to leukotriene modifiers. While these results may sound intriguing with respect to pharmacogenetic applications, these variations account for only about 5% of the variability in response to leukotriene modifier therapy.

Leukotriene C_4 *(LTC_4)* synthase

The LTC_4 synthase enzyme converts LTA_4 to LTC_4. The latter molecule is a critical mediator of the adverse reactions in aspirin-sensitive patients with asthma [90]. Substitution of A to C at the −444 site of the promoter of the gene is associated with three times the eosinophil-mediated LTC_4 production in individuals with the wild-type genotype [91]. Asthma patients with variant *LTC_4* synthase genotypes receiving the leukotriene receptor antagonist zafirlukast for 2 weeks were found to have approximately 10% increase in FEV_1, whereas patients with the wild-type genotype had a 12% reduction compared to the placebo group [91]. In contrast, no genotype effects were shown on AHR in patients on leukotriene modifier therapy [92]. As such, the observed differential response in FEV_1 to leukotriene modifier therapy with respect to *LTC_4* synthase polymorphisms, suggests that this locus may help identify those who may benefit more from this therapy. Because variant *LTC_4* synthase genotypes are prevalent in patients with both aspirin-tolerant and -intolerant asthma [93], if the effects of this polymorphism are confirmed, its high prevalence may make it a useful predictor of response to this class of agents. Leukotriene-modifer drugs are widely used to treat asthma; however, there is growing evidence that the vast majority of asthma patients may not benefit from leukotriene antagonists when administered in combination with other therapies [94,95]. LTC_4 receptor antagonist drugs have been found to be safe and well tolerated. In contrast, up to 5% of patients using *ALOX5* inhibitors develop increases in liver function enzymes [96].

Corticosteroids

GCs are the most effective drugs available in asthma therapy [97]. In sensitive individuals, inhalation of GCs at doses <1,000 μg per day has been shown to have relatively little capacity to activate transcription within peripheral blood mononuclear cells (PBMC) at concentrations found in plasma, and their action is thought to occur mainly within the lung [98]. This finding is in keeping with their relatively restricted systemic side effects at low or intermittent doses, whereas the repression of transcription factor activities, such as AP-1 and NF-B, in the airways concurs with their clinical efficacy in glucocorticoid sensitive (GC-S) patients [98]. In contrast, glucocorticoid resistant (GC-R) patients may suffer serious side effects because of escalation of drug doses caused by hypo-responsiveness. GC resistance has been defined as the lack of a response to a prolonged course of high-dose (0.5–1.0 mg/kg per day) oral GC [99,100]. Two forms of GC-R asthma have been reported, primary and acquired types [101–103]. The acquired form (type I) has been associated with abnormally reduced GC receptor ligand and DNA binding affinity, whereas type II GC-R asthma has been associated with primary GC receptor binding abnormality. In both forms, there is lack of GC-mediated inhibition of expression and release of molecules in PBMC, including the cytokines, interleukin (IL)-13, and IL-4 [101–103].

Modern asthma therapy is largely centered on ICSs with vast majority of patients demonstrating favorable response to therapy [104]. ICSs have been shown to mediate multiple beneficial effects in individuals with asthma but are also associated with multiple adverse effects. The mechanisms of action of ICSs are complex and remain incompletely characterized and only few pharmacogenomic studies have been reported. A candidate gene study in three study populations suggested a relationship between the response to ICSs and a polymorphism in the corticotropin-releasing hormone receptor 1 (*CRHR1*) gene [105]. Polymorphisms in *CRHR1* were positively associated with significantly improved lung function after 8 weeks of ICS therapy. A haplotype in 27% frequency (GAT) showed modest increase in FEV_1 in response to ICSs in homozygous subjects in two out of the three populations· whereas a single SNP correlated with similar improvement in the third population. The association of different SNPs in the same gene with changes in lung function suggests that the actual causal variant in *CRHR1* remains to be discovered but that the three variants studied are imperfectly correlated markers in LD with a causal polymorphism. However, it is too early to tell whether the *CRHR1* polymorphisms will be useful clinical predictors of response to ICSs.

A functional variant in the gene coding for transcription factor T-bet (T-box expressed in T cells) was recently reported by the same group [105], a finding that may be able to predict responsiveness to ICSs. A variant in the *TBX21* gene associates with significant improvement in methacholine responsiveness in children with asthma who are being treated with ICSs. However, the minor allele frequency for this mutation (H33Q) is only 4.5%, suggesting that although the effect of the mutation may be large, it may only affect a small number of individuals.

In a study applying a high-density oligonucleotide microarray approach to search for differences in mRNA expression profiles in PBMC, from GC-S and GC-R asthma patients, gene expression was examined at baseline (resting PBMCs) and following treatment with a combination of IL-1β and TNFα [106]. In an attempt to further unveil genes that contribute to responsiveness of GC, in vitro effects of GC treatment on gene expression were compared in cells that were activated with IL-1β and TNFα. The rationale for this strategy was based on the concepts, that the manifestations of asthma are, at least in part, channeled through the actions of IL-1β and TNFα [107,108], and that the efficacy of GCs in asthma is, at least in part, through its effect on the expression of genes that are modulated by proinflammatory cytokines [107]. The authors showed that GC responders could be separated from nonresponders with over 80% accuracy, by using the expression levels of only a few genes. The gene encoding the NFκB DNA binding subunit (*NFKB1*) was shown to confer the best predictive ability. A large number of genes are being translated after NFκB activation, including cytokines, chemokines, growth factors, cellular ligands, and adhesion molecules, many of which have been strongly associated with asthma and most of which react briskly to glucocorticoid therapy in sensitive individuals. Indeed, the efficacy of GC drugs in asthma is, at least in part, related to their efficacy in inhibiting transcription factors such as NFκB. Thus, NFκB is an exciting pharmacogenetic candidate and a growing body of evidence suggest it may be among the key culprit candidates in asthma [109,110].

Genomics/Proteomics Efforts in Pediatric Asthma and Atopy

Several Universities and Institutes have put together efforts to sample and store biological specimens for future genomic/proteomic research of complex medical disorders. At the Children's Hospital of Philadelphia (CHOP), we recently launched a high-throughput pediatric genomic center, the Center for Applied Genomics (CAG), which is directed at high-throughput genetic/genomic analyses in children, with genotyping throughput of hundreds of DNA samples per day, on the high-resolution SNP genotyping platforms. The program was established with the aim of genotyping over 100,000 children in a couple of years, with major emphasis on asthma and other inflammatory disorders. The facility is coupled to electronic medical records with the health care network at CHOP for those patients who volunteer to participate. All personal information and data, including both phenotypes and genotypes, are thoroughly encrypted to ensure de-identification of the research. Over 40,000 subjects have been genotyped in the past 15 months at a SNP density of 550,000 per sample or higher. The diseases that are being examined include some of the most common complex pediatric disorders, including the inflammatory diseases, asthma, IBD, T1D, SLE, JIA and atopic dermatitis, in addition to obesity, attention deficit hyperactivity disorder and autism to name a few. In addition, extensive effort has been devoted towards high-resolution mapping of copy number variations (CNVs) in "healthy" individuals, wherein several thousand subjects and family trios have been examined, in order to better define "normal" CNVs of the genome, rendering it easier to assess both *de novo* alterations, as well as novel heritable CNVs, based on the family trios analysis, and addressing the role these variations play in disease. Finally, PBMCs from all patients are being harvested for future proteomic biomarker research that will be guided by the genomic results, including through EBV cell lines that are genotyped at high-density and have a wealth of phenotypic information.

Since several of the diseases under study manifest themselves as inflammatory disorders (i.e., Asthma, IBD, JIA, T1D, SLE, AD) where the same underlying cell type may be involved in the pathogenesis, albeit in different organ systems, the notion that there may be a final common pathway involved that underlies the cellular perturbation in these disorders is highly compelling. Thus, an effort is underway directed at addressing the genetic/genomic/proteomic factors involved in these disorders "collectively." This is likely to bear fruit, given the recent advances in the technology platforms that have made gene discovery highly robust. Thus, by applying a GWA approach to address the causes of some of these most common and complex diseases that we are challenged with every day, and we currently treat empirically, discovery can be made not only on those genetic factors that are specific for diseases such as asthma, but more importantly also on those factors that are common among many related genetic/inflammatory disorders. Moreover, apart from unveiling the mechanisms of these diseases themselves, a project of this size and scope is also in a position to dissect out the environmental factors that interact with the disease genes and constitute a gene-environment network that may underlie complex diseases and also address the pharmacogenomic and proteomic opportunities for those subjects who harbor these variants, through which we will establish biomarkers that will identify those who are most likely to benefit from a given therapy.

Summary

Asthma is a complex disorder with multiple phenotypes where multiple genes and environmental factors act together to cause the disease. Several genes have been associated with asthma, albeit, only a handful have been replicated in independent studies. The recent advances in genotyping technology, coupled with the fundamental information provided by the Human Genome and International HapMap Projects have revolutionized our abilities to search for disease genes. Although multiple laboratories are using the new genotyping approach, only one such study has already delivered significant findings [67].

Pharmacogenomics is a developing field with the principal objective of dissecting the effects of genetic variations on human drug responses. Until recently, pharmacogenetic studies were usually limited to investigations of a single polymorphism/gene (such as the *B2AR* gene) in small groups of individuals. With the development of GWA studies taking over the candidate gene and family-based linkage approaches, the results are expected to unveil the inter-individual variations that underlie differential drug response. It is anticipated that the new generation of drugs and diagnostics resulting from these efforts will lead to a major paradigm shift from conventional medicine to efficient predictive medicine.

The powerful combination of GWA coupled with ultra-high-throughput microarray genotyping platforms, gene expression technologies, innovative bioinformatics, and computational biology approaches is bringing such knowledge closer to reality as these integrative strategies enable scientists to pinpoint disease-causing gene pathways that may also influence differential responses to drugs. With optimal use of the HapMap dataset, future GWA studies conducted on large cohorts and replicated in different populations will uncover most major genes that confer disease susceptibility. The incorporation of pharmacogenetic data into clinical practice will guide risk assessment and treatment decision, and thereby revolutionize the practice of medicine for complex medical disorders such as asthma.

Future Perspective

With the successful completion of genome wide association (GWA) studies, numerous loci have been identified that associate with complex medical disorders. In order to pinpoint a disease mutation, resequencing of the genomic loci presents a natural extension. Ultra high throughput bi-directional resequencing of the corresponding linkage disequilibrium (LD) blocks (averaging 50 kb in Caucasians) for all candidate loci in genomic DNA derived from both cases and controls harboring the key SNP alleles and/or haplotypes that associate with the disease phenotype under study will enhance the chances that causal variants are identified and provide unprecedented information to fully understand and interpret the regions under study, unveiling the underlying causative mutations. Validation of SNP genotypes via direct sequencing will verify any newly discovered sequence variants directly by sequencing in both directions. New single nucleotide insertion or deletion alterations discovered during resequencing need to be analyzed in the context of the existing SNP data. The high-throughput sequencing systems available from Illumina, Roche and ABI allow for the sequencing of billion(s) of bases (1 Gb) per run in a matter of days. This represents a major advance in sequencing technologies as more established methodologies, such as capillary-based platforms, require many years to generate the same amount of data. No doubt, the whole genome sequencing approach will have a stunning impact on the practice of medicine within the next 5 years.

References

1. Mannino DM, Homa DM, Akinbami LJ et al. Surveillance for asthma – United States, 1980–1999. MMWR Surveillance Summaries, 51(1), 1–13 (2002).
2. Weiss KB, Sullivan SD, Lyttle CS. Trends in the cost of illness for asthma in the United States, 1985–1994. The Journal of Allergy and Clinical Immunology, 106(3), 493–499 (2000).
3. Barnes PJ, Jonsson B, Klim JB. The costs of asthma. The European Respiratory Journal, 9(4), 636–642 (1996).
4. Smith DH, Malone DC, Lawson KA et al. A national estimate of the economic costs of asthma. American Journal of Respiratory and Critical Care Medicine, 156(3 Pt 1), 787–793 (1997).

5. Worldwide variations in the prevalence of asthma symptoms: the International Study of Asthma and Allergies in Childhood (ISAAC). The European Respiratory Journal, 12(2), 315–335 (1998).
6. Eder W, Ege MJ, von Mutius E. The asthma epidemic. The New England Journal of Medicine, 355(21), 2226–2235 (2006).
7. Lozano P, Finkelstein JA, Hecht J, Shulruff R, Weiss KB. Asthma medication use and disease burden in children in a primary care population. Archives of Pediatrics & Adolescent Medicine, 157(1), 81–88 (2003).
8. Rabe KF, Vermeire PA, Soriano JB, Maier WC. Clinical management of asthma in 1999: the Asthma Insights and Reality in Europe (AIRE) study. The European Respiratory Journal, 16(5), 802–807 (2000).
9. Van Eerdewegh P, Little RD, Dupuis J et al. Association of the ADAM33 gene with asthma and bronchial hyperresponsiveness. Nature, 418(6896), 426–430 (2002).
10. Zhang Y, Leaves NI, Anderson GG et al. Positional cloning of a quantitative trait locus on chromosome 13q14 that influences immunoglobulin E levels and asthma. Nature Genetics, 34(2), 181–186 (2003).
11. Laitinen T, Polvi A, Rydman P et al. Characterization of a common susceptibility locus for asthma-related traits. Science, 304(5668), 300–304 (2004).
12. Blakey J, Halapi E, Bjornsdottir US et al. Contribution of ADAM33 polymorphisms to the population risk of asthma. Thorax, 60(4), 274–276 (2005).
13. Allen M, Heinzmann A, Noguchi E et al. Positional cloning of a novel gene influencing asthma from chromosome 2q14. Nature Genetics, 35(3), 258–263 (2003).
14. Hakonarson H, Gulcher JR, Stefansson K. deCODE genetics, Inc. Pharmacogenomics, 4(2), 209–215 (2003).
15. McLeod HL. Pharmacogenetics: more than skin deep. Nature Genetics, 29(3), 247–248 (2001).
16. Fenech A, Hall IP. Pharmacogenetics of asthma. British Journal of Clinical Pharmacology, 53(1), 3–15 (2002).
17. Hall IP. Pharmacogenetics, pharmacogenomics and airway disease. Respiratory Research, 3, 10 (2002).
18. Roses AD. Pharmacogenetics and future drug development and delivery. Lancet, 355(9212), 1358–1361 (2000).
19. Hakonarson H, Wjst M. Current concepts on the genetics of asthma. Current Opinion in Pediatrics, 13(3), 267–277 (2001).
20. Bateman ED. Measuring asthma control. Current Opinion in Allergy and Clinical Immunology, 1(3), 211–216 (2001).
21. Bateman ED, Boushey HA, Bousquet J et al. Can guideline-defined asthma control be achieved? The Gaining Optimal Asthma Control study. American Journal of Respiratory and Critical Care Medicine, 170(8), 836–844 (2004).
22. Szefler SJ, Martin RJ, King TS et al. Significant variability in response to inhaled corticosteroids for persistent asthma. The Journal of Allergy and Clinical Immunology, 109(3), 410–418 (2002).
23. Ledford D, Apter A, Brenner AM et al. Osteoporosis in the corticosteroid-treated patient with asthma. The Journal of Allergy and Clinical Immunology, 102(3), 353–362 (1998).
24. Wong CA, Walsh LJ, Smith CJ et al. Inhaled corticosteroid use and bone-mineral density in patients with asthma. Lancet, 355(9213), 1399–1403 (2000).
25. Baylink DJ. Glucocorticoid-induced osteoporosis. The New England Journal of Medicine, 309(5), 306–308 (1983).
26. Garbe E, LeLorier J, Boivin JF, Suissa S. Inhaled and nasal glucocorticoids and the risks of ocular hypertension or open-angle glaucoma. The Journal of the American Medical Association, 277(9), 722–727 (1997).
27. Garbe E, Boivin JF, LeLorier J, Suissa S. Selection of controls in database case-control studies: glucocorticoids and the risk of glaucoma. Journal of Clinical Epidemiology, 51(2), 129–135 (1998).

28. Cumming RG, Mitchell P, Leeder SR. Use of inhaled corticosteroids and the risk of cataracts. The New England Journal of Medicine, 337(1), 8–14 (1997).
29. Chinchilli VM. General principles for systematic reviews and meta-analyses and a critique of a recent systematic review of long-acting beta-agonists. The Journal of Allergy and Clinical Immunology, 119(2), 303–306 (2007).
30. Drazen JM, Silverman EK, Lee TH. Heterogeneity of therapeutic responses in asthma. British Medical Bulletin, 56(4), 1054–1070 (2000).
31. Choudhry S, Ung N, Avila PC et al. Pharmacogenetic differences in response to albuterol between Puerto Ricans and Mexicans with asthma. American Journal of Respiratory and Critical Care Medicine, 171(6), 563–570 (2005).
32. Litonjua AA, Silverman EK, Tantisira KG et al. Beta 2-adrenergic receptor polymorphisms and haplotypes are associated with airways hyperresponsiveness among nonsmoking men. Chest, 126(1), 66–74 (2004).
33. Chalmers GW, Macleod KJ, Little SA et al. Influence of cigarette smoking on inhaled corticosteroid treatment in mild asthma. Thorax, 57(3), 226–230 (2002).
34. Palmer LJ, Cookson WO. Using single nucleotide polymorphisms as a means to understanding the pathophysiology of asthma. Respiratory Research, 2(2), 102–112 (2001).
35. Gray IC, Campbell DA, Spurr NK. Single nucleotide polymorphisms as tools in human genetics. Human Molecular Genetics, 9(16), 2403–2408 (2000).
36. Schork NJ, Fallin D, Lanchbury JS. Single nucleotide polymorphisms and the future of genetic epidemiology. Clinical Genetics, 58(4), 250–264 (2000).
37. Kauffmann F. Post-genome respiratory epidemiology: a multidisciplinary challenge. The European Respiratory Journal, 24(3), 471–480 (2004).
38. Vercelli D. Genetics, epigenetics, and the environment: switching, buffering, releasing. The Journal of Allergy and Clinical Immunology, 113(3), 381–386; quiz 387 (2004).
39. Bleecker ER, Postma DS, Meyers DA. Genetic susceptibility to asthma in a changing environment. Ciba Foundation symposium, 206, 90–99; discussion 99–105, 106–110 (1997).
40. Kabesch M. Candidate gene association studies and evidence for gene-by-gene interactions. Immunology and Allergy Clinics of North America, 25(4), 681–708 (2005).
41. Hoffjan S, Nicolae D, Ober C. Association studies for asthma and atopic diseases: a comprehensive review of the literature. Respiratory Research, 4, 14 (2003).
42. Halapi E, Hakonarson H. Recent development in genomic and proteomic research for asthma. Current Opinion in Pulmonary Medicine, 10(1), 22–30 (2004).
43. Liggett SB. Genetics of beta 2-adrenergic receptor variants in asthma. Clinical and Experimental Allergy , 25 Suppl 2, 89–94; discussion 95–96 (1995).
44. Martinez FD, Graves PE, Baldini M, Solomon S, Erickson R. Association between genetic polymorphisms of the beta2-adrenoceptor and response to albuterol in children with and without a history of wheezing. The Journal of Clinical Investigation, 100(12), 3184–3188 (1997).
45. Potter PC, Van Wyk L, Martin M, Lentes KU, Dowdle EB. Genetic polymorphism of the beta-2 adrenergic receptor in atopic and non-atopic subjects. Clinical and Experimental Allergy , 23(10), 874–877 (1993).
46. Rosenwasser LJ, Klemm DJ, Dresback JK et al. Promoter polymorphisms in the chromosome 5 gene cluster in asthma and atopy. Clinical and Experimental Allergy, 25 Suppl 2, 74–78; discussion 95–96 (1995).
47. Shirakawa I, Deichmann KA, Izuhara I et al. Atopy and asthma: genetic variants of IL-4 and IL-13 signalling. Immunology Today, 21(2), 60–64 (2000).
48. Howard TD, Whittaker PA, Zaiman AL et al. Identification and association of polymorphisms in the interleukin-13 gene with asthma and atopy in a Dutch population. American Journal of Respiratory Cell and Molecular Biology, 25(3), 377–384 (2001).
49. Heinzmann A, Mao XQ, Akaiwa M et al. Genetic variants of IL-13 signalling and human asthma and atopy. Human Molecular Genetics, 9(4), 549–559 (2000).
50. Hoffjan S, Ober C. Present status on the genetic studies of asthma. Current Opinion in Immunology, 14(6), 709–717 (2002).

51. Steinke JW, Borish L. Genetics of allergic disease. The Medical Clinics of North America, 90(1), 1–15 (2006).
52. Hakonarson H, Bjornsdottir US, Halapi E et al. A major susceptibility gene for asthma maps to chromosome 14q24. American Journal of Human Genetics, 71(3), 483–491 (2002).
53. Smith AK, Meyers DA. Family studies and positional cloning of genes for asthma and related phenotypes. Immunology and Allergy Clinics of North America, 25(4), 641–654 (2005).
54. Shin HD, Park KS, Park CS. Lack of association of GPRA (G protein-coupled receptor for asthma susceptibility) haplotypes with high serum IgE or asthma in a Korean population. The Journal of Allergy and Clinical Immunology, 114(5), 1226–1227 (2004).
55. Hakonarson H, Grant SFA, Bradfield JP et al. A genome-wide association study identifies KIAA0350 as a type 1 diabetes gene. Nature, 448(7153), 591–594 (2007).
56. Todd JA, Walker NM, Cooper JD et al. Robust associations of four new chromosome regions from genome-wide analyses of type 1 diabetes. Nature Genetics, 39(7), 857–864 (2007).
57. Wellcome Trust Case Control Consortium. Genome-wide association study of 14,000 cases of seven common diseases and 3,000 shared controls. Nature, 447(7145), 661–678 (2007).
58. Sladek R, Rocheleau G, Rung J et al. A genome-wide association study identifies novel risk loci for type 2 diabetes. Nature, 445(7130), 881–885 (2007).
59. Saxena R, Voight BF, Lyssenko V et al. Genome-wide association analysis identifies loci for type 2 diabetes and triglyceride levels. Science, 316(5829), 1331–1336 (2007).
60. Zeggini E, Weedon MN, Lindgren CM et al. Replication of genome-wide association signals in UK samples reveals risk loci for type 2 diabetes. Science, 316(5829), 1336–1341 (2007).
61. Scott LJ, Mohlke KL, Bonnycastle LL et al. A genome-wide association study of type 2 diabetes in Finns detects multiple susceptibility variants. Science, 316(5829), 1341–1345 (2007).
62. Klein RJ, Zeiss C, Chew EY et al. Complement factor H polymorphism in age-related macular degeneration. Science, 308(5720), 385–389 (2005).
63. Duerr RH, Taylor KD, Brant SR et al. A genome-wide association study identifies IL23R as an inflammatory bowel disease gene. Science, 314(5804), 1461–1463 (2006).
64. Helgadottir A, Thorleifsson G, Manolescu A et al. A common variant on chromosome 9p21 affects the risk of myocardial infarction. Science, 316(5830), 1491–1493 (2007).
65. McPherson R, Pertsemlidis A, Kavaslar N et al. A common allele on chromosome 9 associated with coronary heart disease. Science, 316(5830), 1488–1491 (2007).
66. Easton DF, Pooley KA, Dunning AM et al. Genome-wide association study identifies novel breast cancer susceptibility loci. Nature, 447(7148), 1087–1093(2007).
67. Moffatt MF, Kabesch M, Liang L et al. Genetic variants regulating ORMDL3 expression contribute to the risk of childhood asthma. Nature, 448(7152), 470–473 (2007).
68. Dixon AL, Liang L, Moffatt MF et al. A genome-wide association study of global gene expression. Nature Genetics, 39(10), 1202–1207 (2007).
69. Sears MR. Asthma treatment: inhaled beta-agonists. Canadian Respiratory Journal, 5 Suppl A, 54A–59A (1998).
70. Hancox RJ, Sears MR, Taylor DR. Polymorphism of the beta2-adrenoceptor and the response to long-term beta2-agonist therapy in asthma. The European Respiratory Journal, 11(3), 589–593 (1998).
71. Billington CK, Penn RB. Signaling and regulation of G protein-coupled receptors in airway smooth muscle. Respiratory Research, 4, 2 (2003).
72. Drysdale CM, McGraw DW, Stack CB et al. Complex promoter and coding region beta 2-adrenergic receptor haplotypes alter receptor expression and predict in vivo responsiveness. Proceedings of the National Academy of Sciences of the United States of America, 97(19), 10483–10488 (2000).
73. Reihsaus E, Innis M, MacIntyre N, Liggett SB. Mutations in the gene encoding for the beta 2-adrenergic receptor in normal and asthmatic subjects. American Journal of Respiratory Cell and Molecular Biology, 8(3), 334–339 (1993).
74. Kotani Y, Nishimura Y, Maeda H, Yokoyama M. Beta2-adrenergic receptor polymorphisms affect airway responsiveness to salbutamol in asthmatics. The Journal of Asthma, 36(7), 583–590 (1999).

75. Lima JJ, Thomason DB, Mohamed MH et al. Impact of genetic polymorphisms of the beta2-adrenergic receptor on albuterol bronchodilator pharmacodynamics. Clinical Pharmacology and Therapeutics, 65(5), 519–525 (1999).
76. Tan S, Hall IP, Dewar J, Dow E, Lipworth B. Association between beta 2-adrenoceptor polymorphism and susceptibility to bronchodilator desensitisation in moderately severe stable asthmatics. Lancet, 350(9083), 995–999 (1997).
77. Cho SH, Oh SY, Bahn JW et al. Association between bronchodilating response to short-acting beta-agonist and non-synonymous single-nucleotide polymorphisms of beta-adrenoceptor gene. Clinical and Experimental Allergy, 35(9), 1162–1167 (2005).
78. Kukreti R, Bhatnagar P, C BR et al. Beta(2)-adrenergic receptor polymorphisms and response to salbutamol among Indian asthmatics*. Pharmacogenomics, 6(4), 399–410 (2005).
79. Israel E. Assessment of therapeutic index of inhaled steroids. Lancet, 356(9229), 527–528 (2000).
80. Israel E, Chinchilli VM, Ford JG et al. Use of regularly scheduled albuterol treatment in asthma: genotype-stratified, randomised, placebo-controlled cross-over trial. Lancet, 364(9444), 1505–1512 (2004).
81. Jackson CM, Lipworth B. Benefit-risk assessment of long-acting beta2-agonists in asthma. Drug Safety, 27(4), 243–270 (2004).
82. Abramson MJ, Walters J, Walters EH. Adverse effects of beta-agonists: are they clinically relevant? American Journal of Respiratory Medicine, 2(4), 287–297 (2003).
83. Tsai HJ, Shaikh N, Kho JY et al. Beta 2-adrenergic receptor polymorphisms: pharmacogenetic response to bronchodilator among African American asthmatics. Human Genetics, 119(5), 547–557 (2006).
84. Snyder EM, Beck KC, Dietz NM et al. Influence of beta2-adrenergic receptor genotype on airway function during exercise in healthy adults. Chest, 129(3), 762–770 (2006).
85. Silverman EK, Kwiatkowski DJ, Sylvia JS et al. Family-based association analysis of beta2-adrenergic receptor polymorphisms in the childhood asthma management program. The Journal of Allergy and Clinical Immunology, 112(5), 870–876 (2003).
86. Shah RR. Pharmacogenetics in drug regulation: promise, potential and pitfalls. Philosophical Transactions of the Royal Society of London, 360(1460), 1617–1638 (2005).
87. Goldstein DB. The genetics of human drug response. Philosophical Transactions of the Royal Society of London, 360(1460), 1571–1572 (2005).
88. Silverman ES, Du J, De Sanctis GT et al. Egr-1 and Sp1 interact functionally with the 5-lipoxygenase promoter and its naturally occurring mutants. American Journal of Respiratory Cell and Molecular Biology, 19(2), 316–323 (1998).
89. Drazen JM, Silverman ES. Genetic determinants of 5-lipoxygenase transcription. International Archives of Allergy and Immunology, 118(2–4), 275–278 (1999).
90. Sampson AP, Cowburn AS, Sladek K et al. Profound overexpression of leukotriene C4 synthase in bronchial biopsies from aspirin-intolerant asthmatic patients. International Archives of Allergy and Immunology, 113(1–3), 355–357 (1997).
91. Sampson AP, Siddiqui S, Buchanan D et al. Variant LTC(4) synthase allele modifies cysteinyl leukotriene synthesis in eosinophils and predicts clinical response to zafirlukast. Thorax, 55 Suppl 2, S28–S31 (2000).
92. Currie GP, Lima JJ, Sylvester JE et al. Leukotriene C4 synthase polymorphisms and responsiveness to leukotriene antagonists in asthma. British Journal of Clinical Pharmacology, 56(4), 422–426 (2003).
93. Sanak M, Simon HU, Szczeklik A. Leukotriene C4 synthase promoter polymorphism and risk of aspirin-induced asthma. Lancet, 350(9091), 1599–1600 (1997).
94. Deykin A, Wechsler ME, Boushey HA et al. Combination therapy with a long-acting beta-agonist and a leukotriene antagonist in moderate asthma. American Journal of Respiratory and Critical Care Medicine, 175(3), 228–234 (2007).
95. American Lung Association Asthma Clinical Research Centers.Clinical trial of low-dose theophylline and montelukast in patients with poorly controlled asthma. American Journal of Respiratory and Critical Care Medicine, 175(3), 235–242 (2007).

96. Lazarus SC, Lee T, Kemp JP et al. Safety and clinical efficacy of zileuton in patients with chronic asthma. The American Journal of Managed Care, 4(6), 841–848 (1998).
97. Barnes PJ. Efficacy of inhaled corticosteroids in asthma. The Journal of Allergy and Clinical Immunology, 102(4 Pt 1), 531–538 (1998).
98. Gagliardo R, Chanez P, Vignola AM et al. Glucocorticoid receptor alpha and beta in glucocorticoid dependent asthma. American Journal of Respiratory and Critical Care Medicine, 162(1), 7–13 (2000).
99. Sher ER, Leung DY, Surs W et al. Steroid-resistant asthma. Cellular mechanisms contributing to inadequate response to glucocorticoid therapy. The Journal of Clinical Investigation, 93(1), 33–39 (1994).
100. Chan MT, Leung DY, Szefler SJ, Spahn JD. Difficult-to-control asthma: clinical characteristics of steroid-insensitive asthma. The Journal of Allergy and Clinical Immunology, 101(5), 594–601 (1998).
101. Chikanza LC, Panayi GS. The effects of hydrocortisone on in vitro lymphocyte proliferation and interleukin-2 and -4 production in corticosteroid sensitive and resistant subjects. European Journal of Clinical Investigation, 23(12), 845–850 (1993).
102. Sousa AR, Lane SJ, Cidlowski JA, Staynov DZ, Lee TH. Glucocorticoid resistance in asthma is associated with elevated in vivo expression of the glucocorticoid receptor beta-isoform. The Journal of Allergy and Clinical Immunology, 105(5), 943–950 (2000).
103. Lane SJ, Lee TH. Mechanisms of corticosteroid resistance in asthmatic patients. International Archives of Allergy and Immunology, 113(1–3), 193–195 (1997).
104. Leung DY, Chrousos GP. Is there a role for glucocorticoid receptor beta in glucocorticoid-dependent asthmatics? American Journal of Respiratory and Critical Care Medicine, 162(1), 1–3 (2000).
105. Tantisira KG, Lake S, Silverman ES et al. Corticosteroid pharmacogenetics: association of sequence variants in CRHR1 with improved lung function in asthmatics treated with inhaled corticosteroids. Human Molecular Genetics, 13(13), 1353–1359 (2004).
106. Hakonarson H, Bjornsdottir US, Halapi E et al. Profiling of genes expressed in peripheral blood mononuclear cells predicts glucocorticoid sensitivity in asthma patients. Proceedings of the National Academy of Sciences of the United States of America, 102(41), 14789–14794 (2005).
107. Hakonarson H, Halapi E, Whelan R et al. Association between IL-1beta/TNF-alpha-induced glucocorticoid-sensitive changes in multiple gene expression and altered responsiveness in airway smooth muscle. American Journal of Respiratory Cell and Molecular Biology, 25(6), 761–771 (2001).
108. Kim MH, Agrawal DK. Effect of interleukin-1beta and tumor necrosis factor-alpha on the expression of G-proteins in CD4+ T-cells of atopic asthmatic subjects. The Journal of Asthma, 39(5), 441–448 (2002).
109. Roth M, Black JL. Transcription factors in asthma: are transcription factors a new target for asthma therapy? Current Drug Targets, 7(5), 589–595 (2006).
110. D'Acquisto F, Ianaro A. From willow bark to peptides: the ever widening spectrum of NF-kappaB inhibitors. Current Opinion in Pharmacology, 6(4), 387–392 (2006).
111. Thakkinstian A, McEvoy M, Minelli C et al. Systematic review and meta-analysis of the association between {beta}2-adrenoceptor polymorphisms and asthma: a HuGE review. American Journal of Epidemiology, 162(3), 201–211 (2005).
112. Kedda MA, Shi J, Duffy D et al. Characterization of two polymorphisms in the leukotriene C4 synthase gene in an Australian population of subjects with mild, moderate, and severe asthma. The Journal of Allergy and Clinical Immunology, 113(5), 889–895 (2004).
113. Aoki T, Hirota T, Tamari M et al. An association between asthma and TNF-308G/A polymorphism: meta-analysis. Journal of Human Genetics, 51(8), 677–685 (2006).

Bioinformatics in Allergy: A Powerful Tool Joining Science and Clinical Applications

Deendayal Dinakarpandian and Chitra Dinakar

Introduction

In the words of Elias Zerhouni, director of the National Institutes of Health (NIH), "at no other time has there been a need for a robust, bidirectional information flow between basic and translational scientists so necessary [1]." As an example, in the last few decades, advances in molecular biology have resulted in the sequencing of large portions of the genomes of several species such as bacterial genomes, simple eukaryotes and eventually humans as a part of the Human Genome Project. Popular sequence databases, such as GenBank [2] and the European Molecular Biology Laboratory (EMBL) [3], have been growing at exponential rates. Recent advances in Biotechnology have added to the growth in the form of microarray [4,5] and proteomic [6,7] data. This deluge of information has necessitated the careful storage, organization, indexing and analysis of sequence information. This application of information science to biology has produced the field called *Bioinformatics*. While the initial visibility of Bioinformatics was based on its role in working with DNA and protein sequences, a broader definition is the following one drafted by an NIH committee in 2000:

"Research, development, or application of computational tools and approaches for expanding the use of biological, medical, behavioral or health data, including those to acquire, store, organize, archive, analyze, or visualize such data [8]." The committee wisely concluded that this was just a working definition and an inclusive, rather than a restrictive, definition. From a clinical viewpoint, it represents any and all approaches that assist clinical decision-making based on the capacity to deal

D. Dinakarpandian
Department of Computer Science and Electrical Engineering, School of Computing and Engineering, University of Missouri-Kansas City, MO 64110, USA

C. Dinakar (✉)
Department of Pediatrics, University of Missouri-Kansas City;
Division of Allergy, Asthma and Immunology, Children's Mercy Hospital, 2401, Gillham Road, Kansas City, MO 64108, USA
e-mail: cdinakar@cmh.edu

R. Pawankar et al. (eds.), *Allergy Frontiers: Future Perspectives*,
DOI 10.1007/978-4-431-99365-0_2, © Springer 2010

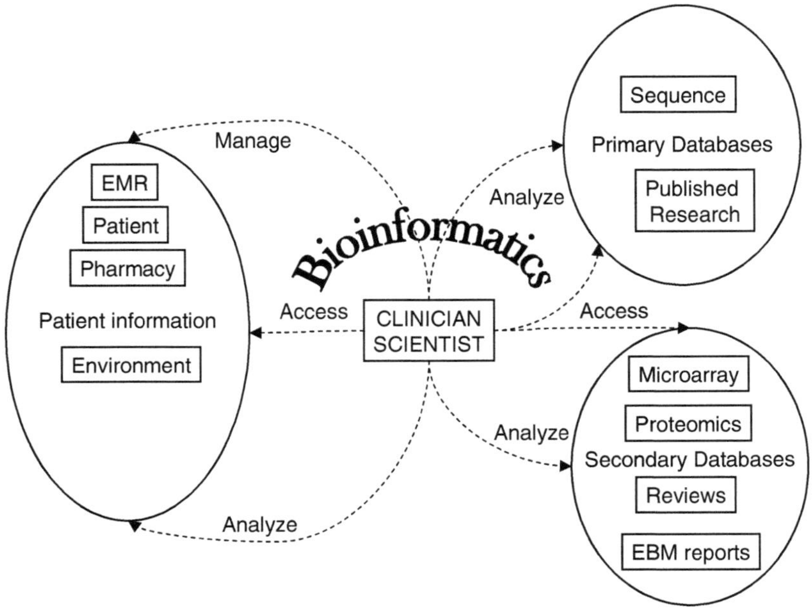

Fig. 1 Scope of bioinformatics. The figure illustrates approaches to manage, access and analyze different kinds of information including integration of the approaches and optimization of overall workflow

with, and learn from, large volumes of diverse biomedical data. This chapter focuses on the current and emerging clinical role of Bioinformatics, with emphasis on material pertaining to Allergy/Immunology (A/I).

As shown in Fig. 1, the clinician or clinical scientist typically interacts with three broad groups of information. The first major class of information is data that is specific to the patient. The second major class of information pertains to data that a clinician or researcher may access or use. This may be conceptually divided into two broad subclasses: one consisting of primary information (sequences and original papers), and the second based on either evaluation of or additional research based on the primary information. From a pragmatic perspective, Bioinformatics is concerned with the management, access to and analysis of such information. This is discussed in detail below.

Bioinformatic Applications

Patient Information

Arguably, the electronic medical or health record [(EMR) or (EHR)] is one of the most important types of health information technology. The EMR electronically collects, stores, and organizes health information about individual patients, facilitates communication between clinicians about patient issues, supports improved clinical decision-making, and aids the management of groups of patients by health care organizations. Computer programs can automate a lot of the steps involved by using special vocabularies that have been developed specifically for use in EMR. While some of these were originally developed to standardize medical codes for billing, many of them have been adapted to document patient care as part of the EMR. A couple of examples are *HL7* [9,10] and *SNOMED-CT* [11,12]. HL7 stands for "*Health Level Seven*," an American National Standards Institute (ANSI) -accredited Standards Developing Organization that develops coding methodology for clinical and administrative data. Its responsibilities include the EHR, the Health Insurance Portability and Accountability Act (HIPAA) and the Reference Information Model (RIM) that standardizes the exchange of clinical information in the form of computer-readable codes. SNOMED-CT stands for *Systemized Nomenclature of Medicine–Clinical Terms*, originally developed by the College of American Pathologists. Comprised of several hundred thousand terms, it is arguably the most comprehensive list of medical terms.

A limitation of the EMR, in spite of the large size of controlled vocabularies that are available, is that a large proportion of the information is still recorded in the form of natural language or free text. Several computational approaches [13,14] are being used to get around this problem. An important development that is likely in the near future is the inclusion of various types of genomic information specific to the patient that may indicate unique susceptibilities to disease or differential sensitivity to drugs [15].

Geographical information systems [16] have the potential to provide additional information that may help to identify environmental exacerbating factors. The integration of prescription with dispensation data (pharmacy records) may be of prognostic value. For example, pharmacy records have been used as a predictor of emergency hospital visits for persistent asthma [17]. Pharmacy record computerization has also been used to increase patient safety [18,19] and bring down costs [20]. Ideally, compliance data should also be part of the EMR, for lack of it is a major barrier to controlling asthma.

Facilitating Clinician–Patient Communication

One promising use of computer technology is the use of *Telemedicine* to bridge the challenges of physical separation between clinicians and patients by creating a virtual connection. An example of telemonitoring in asthma is the use of mobile phones with feedback screens for electronic peak flow monitoring in self-management plans [21]. About 75% of participating patients reported that the system helped them to better manage their symptoms. Another study evaluated the effectiveness of spirometry self-testing combined with internet-based home-telemonitoring [22]. Patients were asked to carry out 3 weeks of self-monitoring followed by a supervised monitoring session. No statistically significant difference was observed between unsupervised and supervised home spirometry self-testing. Despite the fact that the majority of participating patients had no computer experience, they found it easy to carry out self-testing, and more than 85% expressed strong interest in continuing such home-based monitoring. Potential advantages of telemonitoring include closer follow-up, ability to provide health-care services without using hospital beds, decreased patient travel, time off from work, and overall costs [23]. Disadvantages include the initial costs of the systems and issues such as physician licensing in multiple states and reimbursement. A recent review of telemedicine studied the use of computers to deliver education to children with respiratory illness and to their parents [24]. It concluded that the quality of material was highly variable and recommended that educational computer interventions need to be evidence-based and rigorously evaluated to maximize their benefit. Use of asthma websites for patient and parent education is another potentially promising application of telemedicine, though a recent evaluation concluded that there is a lot of room for improvement, as there are significant accessibility barriers and most approaches are not very innovative [25]. Another report claimed that an interactive website for patients helped them learn to interact more fruitfully with their physician, resulting in a better level of perceived care [26].

Primary Databases

Research Literature

The MEDLINE database is the largest publicly available repository of biomedical research literature. The commonest interface that provides access to abstracts of publications is *Pubmed (*http://www.ncbi.nlm.nih.gov/Pubmed*).* An increasing subset is freely available as full-length publications through PubMed Central [27]. The *Medical Subject Headings* (MeSH) [28], developed by the National Library of Medicine (NLM) [29] is an example of a standard vocabulary of commonly used terms in the medical field arranged in the form of a hierarchical classification. Catalogers at the NLM use this predefined vocabulary to unambiguously label each new publication added to *Pubmed.* Out of the 23 major types of diseases included in MeSH, the most relevant ones to A/I are grouped under "Respiratory Tract Diseases" and "Immune System Diseases." One can use the MeSH Browser [28] or the drop down box on the PubMed interface to select specific terms to use in literature searches. For example, if "Delayed Hypersensitivity" is specified as a MeSH search term, the system also searches for synonyms like "Type IV Hypersensitivity" and sub-concepts (i.e., types) of delayed hypersensitivity like "Allergic Contact Dermatitis" and "Photo-allergic Dermatitis." MeSH is only one of several terminologies that constitute The *Unified Medical Languages System* (UMLS) [30] developed at the NLM. Translational mappings that connect similar concepts in different vocabularies are also provided, referred to as the UMLS Meta-Thesaurus.

Analogous to MeSH, which is mainly focused on representing concepts in the medical field, the *Gene Ontology* (GO) [31] aims to be a common vocabulary for describing gene products. In effect, it serves as a detailed list of adjectives to describe the properties of naturally occurring biological molecules. For example, this allows a search query to distinguish between proteins that are involved in "active evasion of host immune response via regulation of host cytokine network" versus proteins that are involved in "active evasion of immune response *of other organism via modification* of cytokine network *of other organism during symbiotic interaction.*" An important distinction to appreciate is that the GO vocabulary is restricted to normal biology/physiology; it is not designed to include any pathological or clinical terms. MeSH, on the other hand, covers both health and disease, though the individual terms are less expressive than GO. *GO-Pubmed* [32] is an attempt to reclassify the literature in Pubmed based on the occurrence of terms from the Gene Ontology. In principle, it is meant to enable distinctions like those between articles on "nitric oxide transport" and "nitric oxide synthase activity." Pubmed also offers preformed queries called *Clinical queries* [33–35] that are composed of "MeSH terms" to limit searches to articles about Diagnosis, Prognosis, Therapy, Etiology, or Clinical Prediction.

The use of "MeSH terms" cannot help to distinguish between articles that have coincidental occurrence of two terms (e.g., mention of azathioprine and asthma in the same article, but in different contexts) versus those about a direct relationship between the two terms (e.g., explicit study about the effectiveness of azathioprine in asthma). This is one of the main reasons for the false positive and false negative document retrievals that one has to deal with in Pubmed searches. MachineProse is an experimental system that attempts to mitigate this problem by proposing an indexing mechanism that facilitates highly specific searches [35]. A study on the use of information retrieval (IR) systems by physicians showed that overall use of IR systems occurs just 0.3–9 times per physician per month, with physicians having two unanswered questions for every three patients. Most searches retrieved only one fourth to one half of the relevant articles on a given topic. Bibliographic rather than full-text databases tended to be used more [36].

The use of MeSH and "GO terms" in searches may be somewhat helpful in making searches more efficient and accurate. However, further research and development is needed to improve the situation. There are alternative interfaces to the MEDLINE database. *PubCrawler* [37] is a program that can retrieve updated results for a set of custom queries from MEDLINE via the Pubmed interface on a regular basis. Alternative user-friendly interfaces to MEDLINE are *Pubmed Assistant* [38], the *Community of Science (COS)* interface [32] and one that incorporates phrase-based searches [13]. *Ovid* [39] is a commercial alternative to Pubmed.

Sequence Data

The other kind of primary data is biological sequence data, consisting of sets of protein, DNA and RNA sequences found in different species. The archives are housed redundantly at multiple locations in the world in the US [40], Europe [3] and Japan [41]. These are being annotated with valuable functional information based on the collective effort of the world-wide research community. Since the Gene Ontology has become the *de facto* standard for describing biological sequences, it has become easier to find relevant information using automated methods (http://www.geneontology.org). In its wake, several ontologies for use in the biomedical field are being developed under the umbrella of the Open Biomedical Ontologies [42].

Secondary Databases

Review articles represent the second wave of publications, often providing useful updates to busy clinicians. Since its inception [43,44], *Evidence Based Medicine* (EBM) has come to play an indispensable role in linking research to medical practice [45]. Typically, the existing literature on a topic constitutes the data that is analyzed with respect to a specific clinical question. Meta-analysis is used to summarize opinion based on available current evidence. The *Cochrane Collaboration* [2,46] has carried out more than 100 systematic reviews on topics that are relevant to Allergy, Asthma, & Immunology. A framework to facilitate searches of EBM content has been proposed [39]. Journals that are exclusively dedicated to EBM are beginning to emerge (http://ebm.bmj.com/).

The raw sequence data mentioned in the previous section have additionally spawned a wide variety of secondary databases. These are either specialized subsets of information relevant to a particular field or experimental information based on studies of the sequence. The journal *Nucleic Acids Research* publishes a representative list and a short abstract of these databases each year. However, this represents only the tip of the iceberg.

The following are examples of secondary databases relevant to Allergy/Immunology:

Allergen Databases

One of the earliest attempts at compiling allergenic molecules is the list of allergens compiled by *SWISS-PROT* [17,47] that currently includes 327 allergenic molecules. The *Biotechnology Information for Food Safety Database* maintained by the National Center for Food Safety and Technology [26,48] organizes allergens into food, nonfood and gluten sequences. The definitive list of allergens organized according to species of origin is maintained by the International Union of Immunological Societies [42] with allergens named after the guidelines of the Allergen Nomenclature sub-committee [49]. The *Allergome* database [50] is a superset of this list culled from about 6,000 publications and contains around 1,500 allergens. In contrast to the above resources that mainly focus on the sequences of allergenic molecules, the *Structural Database of Allergenic Proteins* (SDAP) [51] highlights the structural biology aspects of allergens, and includes information on about 50 allergens whose 3D structure is known.

Immunology Databases

The international *ImMunoGeneTics* (IMGT) information system [52] is perhaps the most comprehensive resource for molecules of the immune system. It is comprised of data on molecules belonging to the immunoglobulin or the major histocompatibility complex superfamily. A notable feature of this resource is the effort taken to use a consistent and standardized way, i.e., an *Ontology*, to represent information. A more recent development is the establishment of the *Immune Epitope Database and Analysis Resource* (IEDB) [53,54] that contains over 16,000 distinct epitopes. SuperHapten is a database of small immunogenic compounds [55].

Genetic Susceptibility

The *Asthma database* [56] represents a notable attempt to catalog putative genetic markers for susceptibility to asthma. It contains data on 72 mutations in 24 genes based on 88 research studies. More recently, the *HapMap project* [57,58] is an attempt to catalog a representative sample of human genetic variation by the analysis of more than a million Single Nucleotide Polymorphisms (SNPs) in 270 different individuals drawn from different populations.

The following approaches are examples of sequence analysis relevant to Allergy and Immunology.

Predicting Allergenicity

The simplest method to predict allergenicity of a protein is to look for evidence of similarity by comparing it to known allergens. *Allermatch* [59] is an online resource that performs this comparison. Two of the criteria that have been recommended as being suggestive of allergenicity are a minimum of 35% sequence similarity in a stretch of 80 amino acids or contiguous identity of at least six amino acids [60]. Raising the threshold for match length to eight amino acids has been reported to have fewer false positive errors. A unique feature of SDAP mentioned earlier is the use of physicochemical properties of amino acids to calculate the similarity between two protein sequences [61]. A recent analysis of sequence similarity of fungal allergenic molecules concluded that while allergens like *Asp f 1* were highly species specific, several others were found to be ubiquitous across diverse fungi [62].

Epitope Analysis

The IEDB [53,54] offers several online analysis tools for the prediction of epitope candidates. For example, given a protein sequence, it can be analyzed to determine if it contains a T-cell epitope (binding to Class I or Class II MHC molecules) or a B-cell epitope. Other tools can predict the fraction of the population likely to react to a given set of epitopes, how conserved a given epitope is, and what its 3D structure is likely to be.

Clinical Trials Data

Another kind of secondary data is to provide access to clinical trials data that may be interpreted or reused by other researchers. A notable effort to standardize clinical trials data representation is *Trialbank* [63]. It attempts to use 219 concepts to store the details of a clinical trial in a structured format. The goal is to facilitate evidence-based analysis. However, the initial version contains data on only 14 clinical trials, none of which are relevant to A/I. Efforts are ongoing to expand this to a *Global Trial Bank* [64]. An alternative resource is the *Clinical Trials* [41] website sponsored by NIH. It offers a summary of ongoing clinical trials, more as a qualitative informative resource rather than being suited to meta-analysis. As such, it is meant to serve more as a public source of information than a source of data for researches and clinicians. Since 2005, it has been possible to find corresponding publications in Pubmed by using the query term "clinicaltrials.gov[si]." Over 300 papers are available, with about 5% being relevant to A/I.

Modeling Clinical Workflow and Outcomes

An aspect of informatics that is often overlooked is the need to analyze and optimize work flow. The average clinician has to cope with a wide variety of tasks in a finite period of time. This section highlights just a few aspects of this issue. The Institute of Medicine of the National Academy of Sciences has identified the critical need to accurately measure, manage, and improve the quality of medical care. A robust healthcare quality information system (HQIS) has the potential to address this need by gathering, coding and analyzing data about patient treatments and related outcomes [65]. Small-scale attempts have been made to develop patient-centered technology that promotes capture of critical information necessary to drive guideline-based care. An example is the *asthma kiosk* which was able to capture patient-specific data during real-time care in the emergency department (with a mean completion time of 11 min) and successfully link the data to guideline recommendations [66]. Other endeavors include the *Breathmobile program* that uses portable clinical workstations equipped with advanced information technology to facilitate asthma disease management in inner city children [67]. A modeling exercise to estimate whether the addition of a *decision-support system to medications order-entry* [20] concluded that this would reduce adverse drug events by 4–8% and result in substantial economic savings as well. Using patients as experts in a collaborative *performance support system* [68] for pediatric asthma has been proposed as a new form of *consumer informatics*. A report that compared integrated medical groups to individual practice associations concluded that the latter had better health outcomes [69].

Conclusion

We conclude by considering a hypothetical (and partly futuristic) example of a clinical encounter in an "informatics" context. Corresponding informatics resources that might potentially be useful in optimizing the management of this case are indicated within square brackets.

A 35-year-old bartender wants to know how to better manage his asthma and allergies. He finds himself in the emergency room at least four times a year with a couple of visits ending up as hospitalizations. Since he has missed a lot of work he would like to have some kind of home-monitoring device and be in communication with his provider [Telemedicine: peak flow monitoring, telemetry, EMR] and would also like to be actively involved in decision-making regarding his asthma management [consumer informatics]. He is concerned about potential side effects of the medicine [EBM] and wants to know if there is a way of finding out which medicine would suit him best [Pharmacogenomics]. Being brought up in a developing country which he frequently visits, he wants to know if some of the foods and environmental inhalants back home and not studied in the USA are allergenic [Allergen databases]. His wife is pregnant and he wants to know if there is a genetic test to know if the unborn child will have allergies and how to prevent the development of allergies [Asthma Gene Database]. Are there any ongoing clinical trials he can be enrolled in [http://www.clinicaltrials.gov]? The scenario pictured above assumes the existence of the required information and infrastructure, and enough time on the part of the physician to obtain the information. Admittedly, there are limitations in the current process of retrieval of information, some of which were mentioned earlier. There is considerable interest in recent developments that facilitate the development of informatics [35]. However, it is clear that much more needs to be done. The immediate future is challenging, but heralds the inevitable and promising era of better informed care.

Bibliography

1. Zerhouni EA. Translational and clinical science – time for a new vision. *N Engl J Med.* Oct 2005;353(15):1621–1623.
2. Benson DA, Karsch-Mizrachi I, Lipman DJ, Ostell J, Wheeler DL. GenBank. *Nucleic Acids Res.* Jan 2007;35(Database issue):D21–25.
3. Kulikova T, Akhtar R, Aldebert P, et al. EMBL Nucleotide Sequence Database in 2006. *Nucleic Acids Res.* Jan 2007;35(Database issue):D16–20.
4. Ball CA, Awad IA, Demeter J, et al. The Stanford Microarray Database accommodates additional microarray platforms and data formats. *Nucleic Acids Res.* Jan 2005;33(Database issue):D580–582.

5. Barrett T, Troup DB, Wilhite SE, et al. NCBI GEO: mining tens of millions of expression profiles – database and tools update. *Nucleic Acids Res.* Jan 2007;35(Database issue): D760–765.
6. Crameri R. The potential of proteomics and peptidomics for allergy and asthma research. *Allergy.* Oct 2005;60(10):1227–1237.
7. Martens L, Hermjakob H, Jones P, et al. PRIDE: the proteomics identifications database. *Proteomics.* Aug 2005;5(13):3537–3545.
8. Huerta M, Haseltine F, Liu Y, Downing G, Belinda S. NIH working definition of bioinformatics and computational biology. http://www.bisti.nih.gov/CompuBioDef.pdf.
9. Jones TM, Mead CN. The architecture of sharing. An HL7 Version 3 framework offers semantically interoperable healthcare information. *Healthc Inform.* Nov 2005;22(11):35–36, 38.
10. Dolin RH, Alschuler L, Boyer S, et al. HL7 Clinical Document Architecture, Release 2. *J Am Med Inform Assoc.* Jan-Feb 2006;13(1):30–39.
11. Fung KW, Hole WT, Nelson SJ, Srinivasan S, Powell T, Roth L. Integrating SNOMED CT into the UMLS: an exploration of different views of synonymy and quality of editing. *J Am Med Inform Assoc.* Jul-Aug 2005;12(4):486–494.
12. Spackman KA. SNOMED CT milestones: endorsements are added to already-impressive standards credentials. *Healthc Inform.* Sep 2004;21(9):54, 56.
13. Rebholz-Schuhman D, Cameron G, Clark D, et al. SYMBIOmatics: synergies in Medical Informatics and Bioinformatics – exploring current scientific literature for emerging topics. *BMC Bioinformatics.* 2007;8(Suppl 1):S18.
14. Jensen LJ, Saric J, Bork P. Literature mining for the biologist: from information retrieval to biological discovery. *Nat Rev Genet.* Feb 2006;7(2):119–129.
15. Hoffman MA. The genome-enabled electronic medical record. *J Biomed Inform.* Feb 2007;40(1):44–46.
16. Tatalovich Z, Wilson JP, Milam JE, Jerrett ML, McConnell R. Competing definitions of contextual environments. *Int J Health Geogr.* 2006 Dec;5:55.
17. Schatz M, Zeiger RS, Vollmer WM, et al. Development and validation of a medication intensity scale derived from computerized pharmacy data that predicts emergency hospital utilization for persistent asthma. *Am J Manag Care.* Aug 2006;12(8):478–484.
18. Tamblyn R. Improving patient safety through computerized drug management: the devil is in the details. *Healthc Pap.* 2004;5(3):52–68; discussion 82–54.
19. Kuperman GJ, Teich JM, Gandhi TK, Bates DW. Patient safety and computerized medication ordering at Brigham and Women's Hospital. *Jt Comm J Qual Improv.* Oct 2001;27(10):509–521.
20. Fung KW, Vogel LH. Will decision support in medications order entry save money? A return on investment analysis of the case of the Hong Kong hospital authority. *AMIA Annu Symp Proc.* 2003:244–254.
21. Ryan D, Cobern W, Wheeler J, Price D, Tarassenko L. Mobile phone technology in the management of asthma. *J Telemed Telecare.* 2005;11(Suppl 1):43–46.
22. Finkelstein J, Cabrera MR, Hripcsak G. Internet-based home asthma telemonitoring: can patients handle the technology? *Chest.* Jan 2000;117(1):148–155.
23. Meystre S. The current state of telemonitoring: a comment on the literature. *Telemed J E Health.* Feb 2005;11(1):63–69.
24. McPherson AC, Glazebrook C, Smyth AR. Educational interventions – computers for delivering education to children with respiratory illness and to their parents. *Paediatr Respir Rev.* Sep 2005;6(3):215–226.
25. Croft DR, Peterson MW. An evaluation of the quality and contents of asthma education on the World Wide Web. *Chest.* Apr 2002;121(4):1301–1307.
26. Hartmann CW, Sciamanna CN, Blanch DC, et al. A website to improve asthma care by suggesting patient questions for physicians: qualitative analysis of user experiences. *J Med Internet Res.* 2007;9(1):e3.
27. Eisen MB, Brown PO, Varmus HE. Public-access group supports PubMed Central. *Nature.* Sep 2002;419(6903):111.

28. Nelson SJ, Schopen M, Savage AG, Schulman J, Arluk N. The MeSH translation maintenance system: structure, interface design, and implementation. *Medinfo.* 2004;2004:67–69.
29. Aronson AR, Bodenreider O, Chang HF, et al. The NLM Indexing Initiative. *Proc AMIA Symp.* 2000:17–21.
30. Browne AC, Divita G, Aronson AR, McCray AT. UMLS language and vocabulary tools. *AMIA Annu Symp Proc.* 2003:798.
31. Ashburner M, Ball CA, Blake JA, et al. Gene ontology: tool for the unification of biology. The Gene Ontology Consortium. *Nat Genet.* May 2000;25(1):25–29.
32. Doms A, Schroeder M. GoPubMed: exploring PubMed with the Gene Ontology. *Nucleic Acids Res.* Jul 2005;33(Web Server issue):W783–786.
33. Haynes RB, McKibbon KA, Wilczynski NL, Walter SD, Werre SR. Optimal search strategies for retrieving scientifically strong studies of treatment from Medline: analytical survey. *BMJ.* May 2005;330(7501):1179.
34. Haynes RB, Wilczynski NL. Optimal search strategies for retrieving scientifically strong studies of diagnosis from Medline: analytical survey. *BMJ.* May 2004;328(7447):1040.
35. Dinakarpandian D, Lee Y, Vishwanath K, Lingambhotla R. MachineProse: an ontological framework for scientific assertions. *J Am Med Inform Assoc.* Mar-Apr 2006;13(2): 220–232.
36. Hersh WR, Hickam DH. How well do physicians use electronic information retrieval systems? A framework for investigation and systematic review. *JAMA.* Oct 1998;280(15):1347–1352.
37. Hokamp K, Wolfe KH. PubCrawler: keeping up comfortably with PubMed and GenBank. *Nucleic Acids Res.* Jul 2004;32(Web Server issue):W16–19.
38. Ding J, Hughes LM, Berleant D, Fulmer AW, Wurtele ES. PubMed Assistant: a biologist-friendly interface for enhanced PubMed search. *Bioinformatics.* Feb 2006;22(3):378–380.
39. Dinakarpandian D, Tong T, Lee Y. Modeling biomedical assertions in the Semantic Web. Paper presented at: Proceedings of the 2007 ACM Symposium on Applied Computing (SAC); Mar 11–15, 2007, 2007; Seoul, Korea.
40. Wheeler DL, Barrett T, Benson DA, et al. Database resources of the National Center for Biotechnology Information. *Nucleic Acids Res.* Jan 2007;35(Database issue):D5–12.
41. Miyazaki S, Sugawara H, Ikeo K, Gojobori T, Tateno Y. DDBJ in the stream of various biological data. *Nucleic Acids Res.* Jan 2004;32(Database issue):D31–34.
42. Rubin DL, Lewis SE, Mungall CJ, et al. National Center for Biomedical Ontology: advancing biomedicine through structured organization of scientific knowledge. *OMICS.* Summer 2006;10(2):185–198.
43. Rosenberg WM, Sackett DL. On the need for evidence-based medicine. *Therapie.* May-Jun 1996;51(3):212–217.
44. Sackett DL, Rosenberg WM, Gray JA, Haynes RB, Richardson WS. Evidence based medicine: what it is and what it isn't. *BMJ.* Jan 1996;312(7023):71–72.
45. Guyatt G, Cook D, Haynes B. Evidence based medicine has come a long way. *BMJ.* Oct 2004;329(7473):990–991.
46. The Cochrane Collaboration at 10: kudos and challenges. *CMAJ.* Sep 2004;171(7):701, 703.
47. Boeckmann B, Bairoch A, Apweiler R, et al. The SWISS-PROT protein knowledgebase and its supplement TrEMBL in 2003. *Nucleic Acids Res.* Jan 2003;31(1):365–370.
48. Nakamura R, Teshima R, Takagi K, Sawada J. [Development of Allergen Database for Food Safety (ADFS): an integrated database to search allergens and predict allergenicity]. *Kokuritsu Iyakuhin Shokuhin Eisei Kenkyusho Hokoku.* 2005;(123):32–36.
49. King TP, Hoffman D, Lowenstein H, Marsh DG, Platts-Mills TA, Thomas W. Allergen nomenclature. WHO/IUIS Allergen Nomenclature Subcommittee. *Int Arch Allergy Immunol.* Nov 1994;105(3):224–233.
50. Mari A. Importance of databases in experimental and clinical allergology. *Int Arch Allergy Immunol.* Sep 2005;138(1):88–96.
51. Ivanciuc O, Schein CH, Braun W. SDAP: database and computational tools for allergenic proteins. *Nucleic Acids Res.* Jan 2003;31(1):359–362.

52. Lefranc MP. IMGT, the international ImMunoGeneTics information system(R): a standardized approach for immunogenetics and immunoinformatics. *Immunome Res.* Sep 2005;1(1):3.
53. Peters B, Sidney J, Bourne P, et al. The design and implementation of the immune epitope database and analysis resource. *Immunogenetics.* Jun 2005;57(5):326–336.
54. Peters B, Sidney J, Bourne P, et al. The immune epitope database and analysis resource: from vision to blueprint. *PLoS Biol.* Mar 2005;3(3):e91.
55. Gunther S, Hempel D, Dunkel M, Rother K, Preissner R. SuperHapten: a comprehensive database for small immunogenic compounds. *Nucleic Acids Res.* Jan 2007;35(Database issue):D906–910.
56. Immervoll T, Wjst M. Current status of the Asthma and Allergy Database. *Nucleic Acids Res.* Jan 1999;27(1):213–214.
57. Phimister EG. Genomic cartography – presenting the HapMap. *N Engl J Med.* Oct 2005; 353(17):1766–1768.
58. Thorisson GA, Smith AV, Krishnan L, Stein LD. The International HapMap Project Web site. *Genome Res.* Nov 2005;15(11):1592–1593.
59. Fiers MW, Kleter GA, Nijland H, Peijnenburg AA, Nap JP, van Ham RC. Allermatch, a webtool for the prediction of potential allergenicity according to current FAO/WHO Codex alimentarius guidelines. *BMC Bioinformatics.* Sep 2004;5:133.
60. Hileman RE, Silvanovich A, Goodman RE, et al. Bioinformatic methods for allergenicity assessment using a comprehensive allergen database. *Int Arch Allergy Immunol.* Aug 2002; 128(4):280–291.
61. Ivanciuc O, Schein CH, Braun W. Data mining of sequences and 3D structures of allergenic proteins. *Bioinformatics.* Oct 2002;18(10):1358–1364.
62. Bowyer P, Fraczek M, Denning DW. Comparative genomics of fungal allergens and epitopes shows widespread distribution of closely related allergen and epitope orthologues. *BMC Genomics.* 2006;7:251.
63. Carini S, Sim I. SysBank: a knowledge base for systematic reviews of randomized clinical trials. *AMIA Annu Symp Proc.* 2003:804.
64. Sim I, Detmer DE. Beyond trial registration: a global trial bank for clinical trial reporting. *PLoS Med.* Nov 2005;2(11):e365.
65. Niland JC, Rouse L, Stahl DC. An Informatics Blueprint for Healthcare Quality Information Systems. *J Am Med Inform Assoc.* Apr 2006;13(4):402–417.
66. Porter SC, Cai Z, Gribbons W, Goldmann DA, Kohane IS. The asthma kiosk: a patient-centered technology for collaborative decision support in the emergency department. *J Am Med Inform Assoc.* Nov-Dec 2004;11(6):458–467.
67. Jones CA, Clement LT, Hanley-Lopez J, et al. The Breathmobile Program: structure, implementation, and evolution of a large-scale, urban, pediatric asthma disease management program. *Dis Manag.* Aug 2005;8(4):205–222.
68. Porter SC. Patients as experts: a collaborative performance support system. *Proc AMIA Symp.* 2001:548–552.
69. Mehrotra A, Epstein AM, Rosenthal MB. Do integrated medical groups provide higher-quality medical care than individual practice associations? *Ann Intern Med.* Dec 2006;145(11): 826–833.

Engineering Allergy Vaccines: Approaches Towards Engineered Allergy Vaccines

Oliver Cromwell

Introduction

The basic principle of allergen specific immunotherapy conducted by subcutaneous injection is the administration of increasing doses of allergen up to a maintenance dose or a maximum tolerated dose to ameliorate IgE antibody mediated allergic inflammation and associated symptoms, and reduce the need for symptomatic medication. The magnitude of the dose is apparently important in ensuring the success of treatment. Whereas low allergen doses favor a Th2 cytokine response and a switch to IgE, high allergen doses favor induction of regulatory T-cells and modification or down-regulation of the Th2 phenotype [1]. However the administration of high doses in man carries an increased risk for the induction of undesirable side-effects, and at worst life-threatening anaphylactic reactions which are a logical risk with a causal treatment.

One of the few major developments made in allergen specific immunotherapy since the first scientific reports in the early 1900s has been the introduction of allergoids, hypoallergenic derivatives produced by chemical modification of the allergen extracts [2]. These preparations are intended to minimize the risk of inducing IgE-mediated reactions while ensuring an adequate dose to favor a therapeutic effect. The reduced IgE-reactivity also minimizes IgE-dependent uptake by antigen presenting cells, which would normally favor promotion of the allergic phenotype with production of Th2 cytokines and allergen specific IgE [3]. The methods of chemical modification most commonly used involve treatment of natural allergen extracts with either formaldehyde or glutaraldehyde, although various other strategies including the use of acid anhydrides [4] and carbamylation with potassium cyanate are also applicable [5]. Formaldehyde interacts initially with amino groups and in a second step cross-linking can occur between the reaction product and

O. Cromwell
Allergopharma J. Ganzer KG, Hermann-Koerner-Str. 52, 21465 Reinbek, Germany
e-mail: oliver.cromwell@allergopharma.de

R. Pawankar et al. (eds.), *Allergy Frontiers: Future Perspectives*,
DOI 10.1007/978-4-431-99365-0_3, © Springer 2010

tyrosine, arginine, and acid amine residues with formation of stable methylene bridges leading to intra- and inter-molecular cross-linking with consequent changes in the 3-dimensional structure of the allergens. Glutaraldehyde is a bi-functional reagent and gives rise to larger molecular weight aggregates. Reaction conditions can be manipulated with both aldehydes to influence the extent of aggregation, for example by inclusion of an amino acid with competing amino groups. Potassium cyanate and acid anhydrides both react with the primary amino groups of lysine thereby changing the net charges on the proteins without causing any cross-linking. It has been suggested that these low molecular weight allergoids are particularly suitable for uptake at mucosal surfaces. In the case of all these chemical treatments it is not possible to exercise precise control over the sites of modification, and therefore the possibility to develop methods to produce tailor-made hypoallergenic molecules may present some advantages. Recombinant DNA-technology provides the opportunity to use genetic engineering techniques to create hypoallergenic variants as well as molecular constructs in the form of fusion proteins designed to influence the processing of an allergen by the immune system and thereby favor a non-allergic scenario.

Engineered hypoallergenic variants can be precisely defined and the design features validated with respect to the intended specific immunotherapeutic application. The vaccine field has already seen such developments with genetic detoxification of bacterial toxins by gene mutations at sites coding for the amino acids involved in the enzymatic sites and thus the toxic effects [6]. In such cases the choice of mutation site may be seen as relatively straight-forward, but this is often not so with allergens in which the IgE-binding epitopes rely principally on the conformation of the protein. It may prove difficult to predict how to achieve a change in the conformation of an allergen that is sufficient to impart hypoallergenic characteristics without compromising the immunomodulatory potential of the protein or giving rise to problems such as insolubility.

The use of recombinant allergens per se offers many advantages over natural allergen extracts. For example, vaccine constituents can be restricted to relevant proteins, avoiding the many non-allergenic proteins present in natural extracts; the proteins are produced in high purity to exacting pharmaceutical standards; the dosage of all active pharmaceutical ingredients is defined thus eliminating the difficulties of standardization associated with native allergen extracts in which the composition is determined largely by the raw material from which they are derived.

Considerations for the Design of Hypoallergenic Variants

Various strategies for the generation of hypoallergenic recombinant allergen variants have been tried and tested. Many factors need to be taken into account when designing such molecules, and experience has shown that the application of theoretical considerations often fails to lead to the anticipated reduction in IgE-reactivity. Therefore the development of hypoallergenic variants remains very much an empirical exercise. Even the application of the same strategy to structurally homologous allergens does not necessarily achieve a similar result. Therefore it is necessary to consider each allergen in turn and optimize the design of a hypoallergenic variant on the basis of the results of extensive immunological tests using sera and cells obtained from representative panels of allergic subjects. Reduced IgE-reactivity can be demonstrated using in vitro techniques, such as immunoassays to assess inhibition of IgE-binding, basophil activation, and basophil mediator release, and in vivo methods including skin testing and nasal provocation. The antigenicity of the preparations can be demonstrated by their ability to activate allergen specific T-cells and immunogenicity by the induction of allergen specific IgG-antibody responses

The unique primary amino acid sequence of a protein ultimately determines how the molecule folds under the influence of the solvent, salt concentration, temperature, and molecular chaperones. The latter apparently safeguard a protein and prevent it from aggregating with other molecules before it has achieved its correct tertiary conformation. This native structure is characterized by a minimum free energy, and if the protein is to be stable this energy state must not be susceptible to small changes in the immediate environment and must be sufficiently different from the free energy states of other potential conformations so as to avoid switching between one and the other. These considerations also apply to engineered proteins, and any changes that are introduced should not unduly affect the biochemical properties of the molecule and give rise to poor stability, insolubility, or aggregation.

The principal objective for the engineering of hypoallergenic variants is the removal of a substantial part of the IgE-binding reactivity of an allergen, while at the same time retaining T-cell reactivity and immunogenicity. Therefore a detailed knowledge of the locations of the respective epitopes is particularly important. The availability of 3-dimensional molecular models based on data from nuclear magnetic resonance (NMR) spectroscopy of solutions of the allergen and X-ray diffraction studies with crystals of the allergen and allergen–antibody complexes, together with theoretical considerations in respect of charge and polarity of surface amino acid residues, are helpful in identifying potential antibody binding sites. This in turn suggests candidate sites for introducing mutations and provides a basis for assessing the consequences of those mutations, particularly in respect of changes in surface topography and charge distribution. Allergen fragments and overlapping synthetic peptides spanning the whole sequence of the allergen can be used in IgE-antibody binding assays to identify binding regions. Introduction of point mutations into those peptides to compromise their recognition by the antibody can provide more precise information as to the involvement of specific amino acids. Such peptides representing linear sequences do however have their limitations for the identification of conformational epitopes [7]. Whereas mutation of specific amino acids directly in an IgE-binding epitope may influence reactivity, it is also possible that mutations outside the epitope may influence the secondary and tertiary structure of the protein such that conformational epitopes are compromised.

Libraries of overlapping synthetic peptides for the full sequence of the allergen, typically 12–20 amino acids in length, also fulfill an important role in the identification of T-cell epitopes. Screening of these libraries using allergen specific T-cell lines and clones identifies those peptides with the capacity to activate T-cells. Selected peptides can then be tested with cells from large numbers of sensitized subjects in order to confirm the location of epitopes and establish their relative importance in the allergic population. In a few cases a single T-cell epitope may be dominant, but usually more epitopes are scattered over the whole sequence of a protein, possibly grouped in immunodominant regions.

Various attempts have been made to identify characteristics that define an allergen, and strong associations between allergenicity and particular protein families have been established [8,9]. The choice of sites for introducing structural modifications may be facilitated by comparisons of the primary structure of the allergen in question with isoforms or homologues from the same protein family. The house dust mite allergen Der p 1 is a cysteine protease. Through the use of comparative molecular modeling focused on a recognized IgE-binding epitope in the allergen it was possible to identify corresponding epitopes in other cysteine proteases, albeit with varying shapes and degree of accessibility, and a conserved central tyrosine residue was a common feature [10].While the isoform Bet v 1.0101 from birch pollen was identified on the basis of high IgE-reactivity, the Bet v 1.0401 isoform, which differs by seven amino acid residues, was found to be fully T-cell reactive but to have little IgE-reactivity [11]. A Bet v 1.0101 variant including five substitutions based on the Bet v 1.0401 isoform, together with the replacement of a proline residue at position ten in the amino acid sequence, chosen on the basis of characteristics of a homologous hazel allergen, proved to be hypoallergenic in both in vitro and in vivo tests and fully T-cell reactive [12]. A strategy based on targeting surface residues identified from crystal structure data focused on nine totally different residues, but nevertheless resulted in a hypoallergenic T-cell reactive molecule [13].

Single amino acids can have a substantial effect on the folding of a protein. Glycine imparts flexibility into local peptide structure as a consequence of the small volume occupied by the two protons attached to the α-carbon. Proline is frequently found in turns, where it introduces a 30° kink, and at the ends of α-helices. It lacks a backbone –NH group that would be available to contribute to hydrogen-bonding and therefore is not at home in either α-helix or β-sheet structures. Removal or introduction of proline can have a substantial effect on conformation. Cysteine pairs can form disulphide bridges which constitute the only covalent linkages that depart from the linear backbone structure of a protein. Polar positively charged lysine and arginine residues are mostly found on the surface of a protein where they are in a position to contribute to solubility. Alteration of surface charge in antigenic regions, for example by substitution of aspartic acid (negative charge) for alanine (non-polar) or vice versa, will modify folding and thus the ability to react with the antibody. The guanidinium moiety of arginine provides five H-bond donors and forms ion-pairs with carboxyl residues in aspartate and glutamate as well as C-terminal ends. Serine frequently occurs in turns and threonine is often found in amphipathic anti-parallel β-sheets. The knowledge of such properties can often be used to advantage when deciding on a modification strategy.

When is a Hypoallergenic Variant Truly Hypoallergenic?

Before embarking on the development of hypoallergenic variants it is important to decide which levels of reactivity are acceptable. Allergic subjects differ widely in the amounts of specific IgE directed against a particular allergen. Furthermore affinity for individual epitopes may differ and the number of epitopes recognized may vary. Consequently it is not sufficient to compromise reactivity of only one of several IgE-binding epitopes in an allergen. For these reasons it is always important to screen new variants with a library of sera from allergic subjects and then to select the most promising candidates for further characterization. A molecule that goes forward to clinical development must have advantages for a very large majority of potential recipients, that is to say it must have obvious hypoallergenic characteristics for all those patients. A variant with only 50% reduced reactivity compared with the wild-type allergen is unlikely to be a useful candidate for immunotherapy.

Some of these problems are exemplified by experience with various allergens. PCR-mutagenesis was used to target IgE-binding epitopes of the peanut allergen Ara h 2, but the resulting mutant only showed a substantial decrease in reactivity with 12 of 16 subjects tested. Point mutations were introduced into each of the four IgE-binding epitopes of the peanut allergen Ara h 3 with substitution of critical amino acids by alanine. Investigation of only five peanut sensitive patients showed that activity was reduced by 35–85% as assessed by only one method, namely nitrocellulose immunoblotting. Pooling the sera for an IgE-inhibition assay suggested that modified Ara h 3 was approximately 28-fold less reactive than the native allergen [14]. Five patients cannot be seen as representative for all peanut allergic subjects and a reduction in IgE-reactivity of only 35% offers a minimal safety advantage. Similar reservations can be expressed in respect of a hypoallergenic variant of fish parvalbumin made by introducing point mutations into each of the two calcium-binding loops of the allergen so as to prevent calcium binding and thereby influence conformation [15]. Mean IgE-reactivity of sera from 21 fish allergic patients was calculated to be 4.4% of that of the wild-type molecule. However, the individual data showed two sera with approximately 50% reactivity, two in excess of 25% reactivity and a further two with more that 10% reactivity.

Therefore it is important to take account of the heterogeneous nature of the response to allergen derivatives and to use an adequate panel of methods to assess hypoallergenicity. First, it is usually not appropriate to use pool sera to assess hypoallergenic characteristics. If only a small number of sera in the pool react strongly with a variant their contribution would be masked by a large number of weak reactors. Second, as large a number of subjects as possible should be screened to come as close as possible to a representative population. Third, various methods should be used to assess the derivatives, including solid-phase and liquid-phase immunoassays and cellular assays such as basophil activation or histamine release. Skin or provocation testing may then be used to confirm hypoallergenic characteristics in vivo. Ideally hypoallergenic characteristics should be observed consistently with all test methods. Finally, the reduction in IgE-reactivity should be sufficient to confer a meaningful advantage. As the primary objective is to improve safety of allergen specific immunotherapy, and considering the large variation in reactivity that can be seen between patients, it seems both reasonable and realistic to suggest a minimum tenfold reduction in IgE-reactivity, particularly for dangerous and aggressive allergens such as those from peanut.

Chemical Modification

The chemical modification methods used to produce allergoids, e.g., treatment with formaldehyde and glutaraldehyde, can also be applied to purified natural or biotechnologically produced allergens, but they have the disadvantage that the end product cannot be defined in molecular terms because it is not possible to dictate the exact sites of chemical reaction. Therefore many of the advantages provided by recombinant allergens in terms of quality and purity would be sacrificed.

Peptides and Allergen Fragments

Peptide mixtures derived by proteolytic digestion of allergen extracts were considered for immunotherapy, but dismissed because of problems of consistent production and standardization. Availability of detailed information on protein structure now allows a designer approach. Allergen derived peptides representing continuous, discontinuous or portions of T or B cell epitopes have been expressed or synthesized either singly or in combination to create new molecular forms. In the case of the major cat allergen Fel d 1, a mixture of overlapping 16–17 amino acid peptides, spanning most of the sequence of the two chains, were selected on the basis of T-cell reactivity and ability to bind to MHC molecules [16]. The peptides were shown to be effective in influencing surrogate markers of allergy, reducing cutaneous responses to allergen challenge, as well as modifying T-cell responses with increased IL-10 production, decreased IFN-γ and Th2 cytokines, and induction of allergen specific regulatory T-cells [17,18]. Although the peptides are not IgE-reactive, dosage is critical, because dose-dependent isolated late asthmatic reactions have been observed after intradermal administration.

The IgE-binding reactivity of allergens such as Bet v 1 from birch pollen is very dependent on the 3-dimensional structure. Cleavage of the gene to enable the allergen to be expressed as two peptide fragments (amino acid residues 1–73 and 74–159) results in random-coil conformations with minimal allergenicity [19].

The cleavage point does not compromise recognized T-cell epitopes. The hypoallergenic characteristics were also manifest in skin tests in which 18/23 and 8/23 birch pollen allergic subjects failed to respond in skin prick and intradermal tests respectively [20]. Positive reactions showed a clear dose response effect. It has been proposed that a similar result can be achieved by cleaving the grass pollen allergen Phl p 6 [21], but experience has shown that the approach is not generally applicable.

It seems that it may be realistic to extend the peptide concept through the use of altered peptide ligands (APL) as suggested by Kinnunen et al [22] with an immunodominant epitope of the lipocalin allergen Bos d 2 from cow dander. A single amino acid substitution of asparagine for aspartic acid in peptide 127-142 resulted in an approximately 100-fold enhancement of its ability to stimulate a human Bos d 2 specific T-cell clone. It was subsequently shown that both the native and altered peptides induced T-cell lines from peripheral blood, but whereas peptide 127-142 induced a Th2/Th0 response, the APL induced Th1/Th0 deviated T-cell lines that were highly cross-reactive with those to the native peptide in subjects with a similar MHC genotype [23]. The APL also appeared to invoke usage of a broader repertoire of T-cell receptor Vβ-subtypes. If this approach proves to be more generally applicable it may serve to enhance the efficacy of peptide immunotherapy.

Schuffled Molecules and Allergen Hybrids

Rather than administering single peptides, there may be advantages in recombining them in a different sequence. This approach was used to create so-called mosaic antigens and, provided the break-points are chosen carefully, it should be possible to abolish most of the IgE-reactivity while retaining the repertoire of T-cell epitopes [24].

An alternative strategy is to create a gene-construct encoding several T-cell determinants to produce a large hybrid peptide as has been achieved for the two major allergens of Japanese cedar, Cry j 1 and Cry j 2 [25]. Three dominant T-cell epitopes from Cry j 1 and four from Cry j 2 were identified by screening cells from 113 sensitized individuals. The order in which gene sequences encoding the peptides were subsequently linked together and the presence or absence of linker sequences did not influence the ability to induce T-cell proliferation. This is perhaps surprising since the processing of the hybrid peptide by antigen presenting cells will be influenced by its new sequence which would not necessarily be expected to favor recovery of the same T-cell determinants. A similar approach was used to create a chimeric protein of the three major bee venom allergens, phospholipase A2, hyaluronidase and melittin. In this case a gene construct was produced encoding overlapping peptides covering the full sequences of the allergens [26].

Hybrids can be generated by a random approach using "gene-shuffling," also referred to as molecular breeding or directed molecular evolution, which gives rise to a large number of new protein sequences which are then screened to identify candidate molecules that fulfill criteria for hypoallergenic character and T-cell reactivity, and possibly enhanced immunogenicity [27–29]. Random fragmentation of two or more homologous genes is followed by reassembly of the fragments into full-length genes in a self-priming polymerase chain reaction, with DNA fragments acting as both primers and templates. Homology between the genes means that fragments from different genes are able to hybridize and create chimeras with component peptides derived from related allergens. The technique requires no prior knowledge of structure and immunological reactivity of the allergens and may give rise to molecular derivatives that would not have been conceived of on the basis of such knowledge. Screening for hypoallergenic candidate molecules has to identify full-length proteins and exclude variants arising from shifts in the codon reading-frame, protein fragments, truncations, gross mutations etc. that exhibit low IgE-reactivity. An example of the application of gene-schuffling technology concerns the allergen Gly d 2 and two isoforms of Lep d 2 from the dust mites *Glycyphagus domesticus* and *Lepidoglyphus destructor* respectively [29]. Lep d 2 isoforms show 89.6% identity and share nearly 80% identity with Gly d 2. A chimeric construct comprised of the first 20 codons of Gly d 2 and codons 21 to 125 of Lep d 2.01 was schuffled with full-length genes of Gly d 2 and Lep d 2.02. Subsequent cloning, expression, and screening identified two hypoallergenic derivatives showing intact T-cell reactivity. The genes encoding such chimeras may also be candidates for the development of DNA vaccines.

Patients who are polysensitized are often treated either with allergen mixtures or more than one preparation simultaneously. It has been suggested that it may be realistic to simplify treatment by using allergen chimers produced from allergens from different sources. The feasibility of this approach was tested by producing an expression plasmid encoding the birch pollen allergen Bet v 1 with immunodominant peptide epitopes of Timothy grass allergens Phl p 1 and Phl p 5 linked to the N- and C-terminal ends. A chimeric protein was recovered with Bet v 1 in a conformation comparable to that of the native allergen [30]. The usefulness of this approach is questionable as it offers no obvious advantages over a mixture of allergens.

Oligomers

Recombinant oligomers can be produced by linking several copies of one gene in sequence. The birch pollen allergen Bet v 1 has been used as a model system, and either two or three copies of the Bet v 1 gene linked by short oligonucleotide spacers were expressed in *E. coli* [31]. The resulting dimmer and trimer retain the primary structure of the allergen, and therefore T-cell epitopes and T-cell reactivity remain intact. The oligomers exhibit similar circular dichroism spectra to the monomer, consistent with a mixed α-helical / β-sheet secondary structure, and are able to bind IgE antibodies in in vitro immunoblot and ELISA test systems. However, human basophil mediator release was reduced 100-fold or more, albeit with cells from only three subjects, but the observations were supported by skin test data showing that the trimer was significantly less active than the dimer, and that in turn less active than the monomer. The hypoallergenic characteristics of the trimer were confirmed in more extensive skin test studies [20,32] and in terms of reduced basophil activation [33]. The fact that the hypoallergenic characteristics are only manifest in vivo and in basophil activation suggests that the ability of the trimer to cross-link receptor-bound IgE antibodies is impaired, possibly as a result of steric hindrance of IgE-binding sites. The strong immunogenic character of the trimer was clearly manifest in a clinical study, and this may be seen as one advantage of the oligomerization strategy [34].

Application of the same strategy to the Bet v 1 homologue Dau c 1 from carrot [35] resulted in dimers and trimers that appeared to retain the native conformation of the monomer as judged by circular dichroism spectroscopy. Both molecules showed enhanced IgE-binding in a solid-phase in vitro assay compared with the monomer, the effect being statistically significant in the case of the trimer with increases between 20 and 193% with 24 sera tested. Histamine release studies were conducted with cells from only two donors, but in both cases the dimer and trimer were at least as active as the monomer. These results clearly indicate that the oligomerization strategy is not generally applicable, even for homologues, although enhanced immunogenicity was again seen as an attribute.

Combining the genes encoding two different grass pollen allergens, as in the cases of Phl p 2 – Phl p 6, Phl p 6 – Phl p 2 and Phl p 5 – Phl p 1, resulted in hybrids which retained IgE reactivity, whilst immunogenicity was enhanced as a consequence of the larger molecular size [36]. Such constructs may find application for diagnosis.

Point Mutations

Polymerase chain reaction amplification, in conjunction with oligonucleotide primers, can give rise to allergen variants with little or no IgE-binding activity as a result of chance mutations. However point mutations will normally be introduced by site-directed mutagenesis either directly in IgE-binding epitopes, or at sites outside the epitopes in positions such that they influence the conformation of the molecule and thereby IgE-binding activity.

One of the first reports on the application of site-directed mutagenesis to create hypoallergenic variants implicated six amino acid residues of the birch pollen allergen Bet v 1.0101 with the IgE-reactivity of the allergen [12]. Mutations at all six positions were necessary to reduce IgE-reactivity with all sera tested, without influencing T-cell reactivity. The same strategy was applied to the apple allergen Mal d 1, which shows 55% sequence identity with Bet v 1.0101, in the expectation of achieving a similar result [37]. Introduction of mutations at the same six positions resulted in 88–30% reductions of IgE-binding compared with the wild-type molecule with 10 of 14 sera tested, while a further three sera showed only a 13% reduction and one no effect. In contrast to this multiple point mutation strategy, a single point mutation at position 112 with introduction of proline can also achieve a substantial hypoallergenic effect [38]. The results clearly point to the heterogeneity of the IgE response and endorse the view that the design of hypoallergenic variants is highly empirical.

Several allergens belong to classes of ligand binding proteins, and IgE-reactivity is associated with conformation of the protein when associated with the ligand. Introduction of mutations into the binding site in order to deny ligand-interaction can prevent the protein from adopting the correct 3-dimensional structure and thus confer hypoallergenic characteristics. This strategy has been used with some degree of success with calcium-binding proteins such as parvalbumin from fish and pollen allergens with two calcium-binding domains, including Phl p 7 from Timothy grass and Bet v 4 from birch [15,39]. In the case of parvalbumin, cation-coordinating aspartate and asparagine residues in the calcium-binding loops were replaced by non-polar alanine residues.

Intra-molecular disulphide bonds can be destroyed by replacing one or both cysteine residues resulting in degeneration of tertiary structure and conformational changes, an approach used successfully to produce hypoallergenic variants of the group 2 allergens of house dust mites and the storage mite *Lepidoglyphus destructor*, as well as the group 1 allergen of *Parietaria* and the major latex allergen Hev b 6.01 [40–44]. Der f 2 is comprised of 129 amino acid residues and with a single-domain of Ig fold with a β-sheet structure. Three intra-molecular disulphide bonds at C8-119, C21-27 and C73-78 stabilize the 3-dimensional structure. Substitution with serine residues at positions 8 and 119 eradicates the disulphide bond linking the C-terminal and N-terminal ends of the molecule and which is crucial for the Ig-fold [45]. IgE-reactivity of the resulting variant is reduced, but T-cell reactivity is retained or indeed enhanced. The same strategy has been applied successfully to the 139 amino acid mature Par j 1 allergen of *Parietaria judaica* by substituting serine for cysteine in the four disulphide bonds. Two bonds were shown to have a particular influence on IgE-binding [43]. This allergen is a member of the non-specific lipid transfer protein family, members of which have been identified as allergens in various pollens and plant derived foods. The proteins show extensive homology and this suggests that the same strategy may be applicable to other family members. Another allergen family in which disulphide-bridging has considerable influence on IgE-binding is that of the lipocalins. Substitution of a cysteine residue close to the C-terminal end of bovine lipocalin, Bos d 2, excludes linking to an internal cysteine with a consequent influence on molecular conformation and IgE-binding [46]. Limited data with sera from Bos d 2 sensitive subjects suggest that activity may be reduced by 15- to 24-fold.

The inclusion or removal of proline residues can have a considerable influence on protein architecture. The 129 amino acid Der f 2 contains six proline residues and substitution of various of these by alanine influences the structure and IgE-reactivity of the allergen [47]. Prolines 95, 99 and 34 lie close together and are located in loop regions between β-strands. Substitution by alanine confirms that they are involved in an IgE-binding epitope. The fact that the wild-type Der f 2 and all proline/analine mutants with the exception of that at position 79 showed IgE binding activity on immunoblots from SDS–PAGE under reducing conditions suggests that proline 79 is important for correct refolding.

Point mutations were introduced into highly conserved sequence domains of IgE-binding regions of the major ryegrass pollen allergen Lol p 5. The various resulting mutants showed hypoallergenic characteristics, but not to the extent achieved when a more radical deletion mutation strategy was adopted (see below) [48].

Deletion Mutations

The deletion of short sequences can also be used to good effect, provided that T-cell epitopes are left undisturbed [49]. The Timothy grass pollen allergen Phl p 5a is comprised of 285 amino acids and two four-helix bundles in the N- and C-terminal halves of the molecule. The introduction of two deletion mutations encompassing the amino acid residues 94–113 and 175–198, outside previously mapped T-cell epitopes and spanning predominantly α-helical regions in each of the two bundles, resulted in a hypoallergenic variant [50]. Reduced IgE-binding was shown in all 43 sera tested by immunoblotting and less than 10% of the activity of the wild-type molecule was detected by basophil activation using cells from 12 grass pollen allergic subjects. Remarkably, despite the deletion of 20 and 24 amino acids respectively, the molecule folded to a stable soluble structure retaining substantially the α-helical structure, as judged by circular dichroism measurements, and with no tendency to aggregate or degrade. The T-cell reactivity was undiminished when tested on a range of T-cell lines.

The deletion mutation strategy was also applied to the 145 amino acid allergen Ole e 1 from olive pollen, removal of the ten C-terminal amino acids accounting for the immunodominant IgE-binding epitope. However, reactivity varied considerably between olive pollen allergic patients, with a mean reduction of only 37% (SD ± 12%) with 13 sera tested in an indirect ELISA [51]. Furthermore, basophil degranulation studies showed considerable variation and the absence of dose response experiments makes it impossible to draw meaningful conclusions. Deletion of 16 amino acids in the N-terminal region of the 145-amino acid *Aspergillus fumigatus* allergen Asp f 1 removed a prominent β-hairpin structure together with the cytotoxic activity of this ribonuclease, while also causing some reduction in IgE-reactivity. However the reduction only amounted to more than 50% in half of the cystic fibrosis subjects tested, and in even fewer asthma and allergic bronchopulmonary aspergillosis patients [52].

Clinical Experience of Immunotherapy with Hypoallergenic Allergen Preparations

The first study of allergen specific immunotherapy with recombinant preparations investigated the clinical effects, immunological activity, and tolerance of a mixture of two Bet v 1 fragments and a Bet v 1 trimer in comparison to placebo.

The proteins were adsorbed to aluminium hydroxide suspensions, and immunotherapy conducted with a course of eight pre-seasonal injections of increasing concentrations from 1 to 80 μg protein, with further 80 μg injections up until the beginning of the pollen season [34].

Results for 71 patients from one of the three study centers showed that both active preparations were highly immunogenic, inducing Bet v 1 specific IgG and IgA antibody responses. The serum antibodies inhibited allergen induced basophil histamine release in vitro. Sera from trimer treated subjects were more effective, reflecting higher IgG antibody titers. IgG1 antibody titers correlated with both improvement in clinical symptoms, as judged by a ten-point interval scale, and reduction in skin test reactivity to Bet v 1. Bet v 1 specific IgE responses showed a threefold increase in the placebo group as a consequence of seasonal pollen exposure, whereas the responses in the two treatment groups were blunted. Nasal lavage fluid collected from a randomly selected subgroup showed significantly raised IgG1 levels at the end of the pollen season and again at 12 months in treated subjects (ten trimer; three fragment mixture) by comparison with ten placebo subjects [53]. Levels of IgG2 and IgG4 were also raised, but not significantly, and there were no apparent differences in IgA. Allergen specific nasal IgG4 correlated with reduced specific nasal sensitivity at the end of the birch pollen season. Perhaps not surprisingly, the nasal antibody levels mirrored those in serum. It was concluded that reduced nasal sensitivity reflected the inhibitory effect of antibodies on basophil and mast cell mediator release. Cytokine responses investigated in one of the other two study centers showed that treatment with trimer resulted in significant reductions in IL-5 and IL-13 producing cells, indicative of a suppression of the Th2 response [54]. There were also trends for decreased numbers of IL-4 producing cells and increased numbers of IL-12 producing cells, but the differences were not significant, very probably because of the small number of subjects. The results from the measurements of immunological parameters provide an encouraging basis for pursuing the further development of hypoallergenic derivatives, but emphasis has to be placed on the generation of data to provide evidence of clinical efficacy.

A second clinical study in birch pollen rhinitis investigated a recombinant folding-variant of the allergen Bet v 1 which has a stable random-coil structure that can be clearly distinguished from the secondary structure of the native molecule by circular dichroism spectroscopy. The variant exhibits hypoallergenic properties as judged by immunoassay inhibition tests and basophil activation [33,55]. An open, randomized comparative study with the folding variant and a natural birch pollen extract, together with a parallel reference group to compare symptoms and medication usage, involved pre-seasonal courses of injections over 4 months prior to the pollen seasons in two successive years, achieving a maximum dose of 80 μg of the folding variant, fourfold higher than the Bet v 1 content of the natural allergen preparation. A median combined symptom-medication score showed a substantial improvement in the first year of treatment with the recombinant protein by comparison with the natural preparation and the reference group, with values of 5.90, 12.48 and 14.67 respectively. In the second year the benefit from the two preparations was similar, suggesting that the higher dose with the hypoallergenic variant achieved a more rapid effect apparent in the first year of treatment [56]. Clinical efficacy of both preparations was supported by data showing increased allergen tolerance in nasal provocation tests, and allergen specific IgG1 and IgG4 antibody responses. These results have since been substantiated in a larger double-blind placebo controlled study [57].

Constructs to Facilitate Allergen Presentation or Achieve an Adjuvant Effect

CpG-oligonucleotides (CPGs) belong to a group of immune response modifiers that exert their influence through binding to Toll-like receptors (TLR) expressed on cells of the innate immune system. CPGs bind to TLR-9, particularly on dendritic cells, resulting in the expression of cytokines which counteract the Th2 response that is characteristic of the allergic phenotype, and therefore have a potential as adjuvants for immunotherapy. When chemically coupled to an allergen CPGs can induce some hypoallergenic characteristics, as has been shown with the major ragweed allergen Amb a 1, and thereby confer an additional advantage for specific immunotherapy [58].

Modular antigen translocation technology (MAT) can theoretically greatly improve the efficacy of antigen uptake, processing, and presentation, and therefore ensure that an adequate allergen dose can be achieved for a therapeutic effect [59]. The MAT vector encodes a protein-construct comprised of a translocation element that facilitates uptake by antigen presenting cells, a targeting element that can redirect the immune response, and a 6-Histidine N-terminal tail to facilitate purification. The inclusion of appropriate restriction sites allows the introduction of a gene encoding the allergen of choice. The translocation element is a cell penetrating peptide (CPP) that imparts intra-cellular as opposed to extra-cellular characteristics to the construct, thus favoring cellular uptake, while the targeting element is a truncated form of the human invariant chain (Ii) which targets the endosomal compartment of the antigen presenting cell. Efficient antigen processing ensures delivery of an adequate dose to induce a Th1 cytokine profile with enhanced interferon-γ and IL-10 secretion, and diminished IL-4, IL-5 and IL-2 levels. This cytokine profile has been observed in in vitro investigations and is consistent with the responses seen in association with immunotherapy.

Although not intended for specific immunotherapy as such, genetically engineered negative signaling molecules have the potential for the treatment of allergic disease. Cross-linking of FcεRI on the surface of mast cells and basophils with multivalent allergen leads to phosphorylation of tyrosine-based activation motifs (ITAMs) in the cytoplasmic tails of the β and γ receptor subunits and subsequent release of mediators of allergic inflammation. These cells also express the low affinity FcγRIIb receptor, which possesses a tyrosine-based inhibition motif (ITIM) in the cytoplasmic tail. It has been shown that a fusion protein comprised of Fcγ and Fcε sequences was able to co-aggregate the FcεRI and FcγRIIb receptors and inhibit mast cell and basophil activation as a consequence of negative signaling resulting from the tyrosine phosphorylation of the FcγRIIb ITIM [60].This concept was extended and rendered allergen specific by using a chimeric fusion protein comprised of an allergen together with a truncated IgG Fcγ1. The protein was produced by expression of a chimeric gene encoding the γ-hinge-CHγ2-CHγ3 sequence, a 15-amino acid linker and the two chains of Fel d 1. The fusion protein inhibited histamine release from basophils of cat allergic donors and passively sensitized cord blood derived mast cells by more than 75%, and was also shown to be active in vivo in a mouse model [61]. The Fcγ - Fcε fusion constructs are also active in B cells and Langerhans-like dendritic cells which express FcεRII and FcεRI respectively, as well as FcγRIIb. Constructs were effective in inhibiting IgE-class switching and IgE production in B cells, whilst dendritic cells were modulated in a fashion analogous to mast cells and basophils. As yet there is no indication as to what dosage schedules might have to be adopted or how long-acting the treatment effect may be. The suggestion has been made that the technology might be particularly attractive in food allergy where there are currently few therapeutic options.

Conclusions

Recombinant DNA-technology provides a powerful tool for manipulating gene sequences encoding allergens in order to create hypoallergenic variants. Allergen diversity is such that there is no one strategy that can be applied and the development of variants with the desired characteristics remains a highly empirical process. It is important to define a meaningful reduction in IgE-reactivity and essential to use an adequate panel of test methods to screen candidate molecules and confirm their hypoallergenic characteristics. The hypoallergenic variants have the potential to provide a second generation of recombinant allergen vaccines to follow those based on native allergen structures.

References

1. Larche M, Akdis CA, Valenta R (2006) Immunological mechanisms of allergen-specific immunotherapy. Nat Rev Immunol 6:761–71
2. Maasch HJ, Marsh DG (1987) Standardized extracts: Modified allergens – Allergoids. Clin Rev Allergy 5:89–106
3. Akdis CA, Blaser K (2001) Bypassing IgE and targeting T cells for specific immunotherapy of allergy. Trends Immunol 22:175–8
4. Cirkovic TD, Bukilica MN, Gavrovic MD et al (1999) Physicochemical and immunologic characterization of low molecular- weight allergoids of Dactylis glomerata pollen proteins. Allergy 54:128–34
5. Mistrello G, Brenna O, Roncarolo D et al (1996) Monomeric chemically modified allergens: Immunologic and physicochemical characterization. Allergy 51:8–15
6. Rappuoli R, Douce G, Dougan G, et al (1995) Genetic detoxification of bacterial toxins: a new approach to vaccine development. [Review]. Int Arch Allergy Immunol 108:327–33

7. Spangfort MD, Mirza O, Ipsen H, et al (2003) Dominating IgE-binding epitope of Bet v 1, the major allergen of birch pollen, characterized by X-ray crystallography and site-directed mutagenesis. J Immunol 171:3084–90
8. Breiteneder H, Mills EN (2005) Molecular properties of food allergens. J Allergy Clin Immunol 115:14–23
9. Stadler MB, Stadler BM (2003) Allergenicity prediction by protein sequence. FASEB J 17:1141–3
10. Furmonaviciene R, Sewell HF, Shakib F (2000) Comparative molecular modelling identifies a common putative IgE epitope on cysteine protease allergens of diverse sources. Clin Exp Allergy 30:1307–13
11. Arquint O, Helbling A, Crameri R, et al (1999) Reduced in vivo allergenicity of Bet v 1d isoform, a natural component of birch pollen. J Allergy Clin Immunol 104:1239–43
12. Ferreira F, Ebner C, Kramer B, et al (1998) Modulation of IgE reactivity of allergens by site-directed mutagenesis: Potential use of hypoallergenic variants for immunotherapy. FASEB J 12:231–42
13. Holm J, Gajhede M, Ferreras M (2004) Allergy vaccine engineering: Epitope modulation of recombinant Bet v 1 reduces IgE binding but retains protein folding pattern for induction of protective blocking-antibody responses. J Immunol 173:5258–67
14. Rabjohn P, West CM, Connaughton C (2002) Modification of peanut allergen Ara h 3: Effects on IgE binding and T cell stimulation. Int Arch Allergy Immunol 128:15–23
15. Swoboda I, Bugajska-Schretter A, et al (2007) A recombinant hypoallergenic parvalbumin mutant for immunotherapy of IgE-mediated fish allergy. J Immunol 178:6290–6
16. Haselden BM, Kay AB, Larche M (1999) Immunoglobulin E-independent major histocompatibility complex-restricted T cell peptide epitope-induced late asthmatic reactions. J Exp Med 189:1885–94
17. Kay AB, Larche M (2004) Allergen immunotherapy with cat allergen peptides. Springer Semin Immunopathol 25:391–9
18. Verhoef A, Alexander C, Kay AB, et al (2005) T cell epitope immunotherapy induces a CD4+ T cell population with regulatory activity. PLoS Med 2:e78
19. Vrtala S, Hirtenlehner K, Vangelista L (1997) Conversion of the major birch pollen allergen, Bet v 1, into two nonanaphylactic T cell epitope-containing fragments – Candidates for a novel form of specific immunotherapy. J Clin Invest 99:1673–81
20. van Hage-Hamsten M, Kronqvist M, Zetterström O (1999) Skin test evaluation of genetically engineered hypoallergenic derivatives of the major birch pollen allergen, Bet v 1: Results obtained with a mix of two recombinant Bet v 1 fragments and recombinant Bet v 1 trimer in a Swedish population before the birch pollen season. J Allergy Clin Immunol 104:969–77
21. Vrtala S, Focke M, Sperr W, et al (2001) Recombinant hypoallergenic fragments of the major Timothy grass pollen allergen, Phl p 6, for immunotherapy. J Allergy Clin Immunol 107:S257
22. Kinnunen T, Buhot C, Narvanen A (2003) The immunodominant epitope of lipocalin allergen Bos d 2 is suboptimal for human T cells. Eur J Immunol 33:1717–26
23. Kinnunen T, Jutila K, Kwok WW, et al (2007) Potential of an altered peptide ligand of lipocalin allergen Bos d 2 for peptide immunotherapy. J Allergy Clin Immunol 119:965–72
24. Linhart B, Valenta R (2004) Vaccine Engineering Improved by Hybrid Technology. Int Arch Allergy Immunol 134:324–31
25. Hirahara K, Tatsuta T, Takatori T, et al (2001). Preclinical evaluation of an immunotherapeutic peptide comprising 7 T-cell determinants of Cry j 1 and Cry j 2, the major Japanese cedar pollen allergens. J Allergy Clin Immunol 108:94–100
26. Karamloo F, Schmid-Grendelmeier P, Kussebi F (2005) Prevention of allergy by a recombinant multi-allergen vaccine with reduced IgE binding and preserved T cell epitopes. Eur J Immunol 35:3268–76
27. Punnonen J (2000) Molecular breeding of allergy vaccines and antiallergic cytokines. Int Arch Allergy Immunol 121:173–82

28. Ferreira F, Wallner M, Breiteneder H et al (2002) Genetic engineering of allergens: Future therapeutic products. Int Arch Allergy Immunol 128:171–8
29. Gafvelin G, Parmley S, Neimert-Andersson T, et al (2007) Hypoallergens for allergen-specific immunotherapy by directed molecular evolution of mite group 2 allergens. J Biol Chem 282:3778–87
30. Wild C, Wallner M, Hufnagl K, et al (2007) A recombinant allergen chimer as novel mucosal vaccine candidate for prevention of multi-sensitivities. Allergy 62:33–41
31. Vrtala S, Hirtenlehner K, Susani M et al (2001) Genetic engineering of a hypoallergenic trimer of the major birch pollen allergen, Bet v 1. FASEB J 15:2045–7
32. Pauli G, Purohit A, Oster JP, et al (2000) Comparison of genetically engineered hypoallergenic rBet v 1 derivatives with rBet v 1 wild-type by skin prick and intradermal testing: Results obtained in a French population. Clin Exp Allergy 30:1076–84
33. Kahlert H, Weber B, Cromwell O, et al (2003) Evaluation of the allergenicity of hypoallergenic recombinant derivatives of Bet v 1 using basophil activation by CD203c expression measurement. In: Marone G, editor. Clinical Immunology and Allergy in Medicine. Naples, Italy: JGC Editions, 735–40
34. Niederberger V, Horak F, Vrtala S, et al (2004) Vaccination with genetically engineered allergens prevents progression of allergic disease. Proc Natl Acad Sci USA 101(Suppl 2):14677–82
35. Reese G, Ballmer-Weber BK, Wangorsch A, et al (2007) Allergenicity and antigenicity of wild-type and mutant, monomeric, and dimeric carrot major allergen Dau c 1: Destruction of conformation, not oligomerization, is the roadmap to save allergen vaccines. J Allergy Clin Immunol 119:944–51
36. Linhart B, Hartl A, Jahn-Schmid B, et al (2005) A hybrid molecule resembling the epitope spectrum of grass pollen for allergy vaccination. J Allergy Clin Immunol 115:1010–6
37. Ma Y, Gadermaier G, Bohle B et al (2006) Mutational analysis of amino acid positions crucial for IgE-binding epitopes of the major apple (Malus domestica) allergen, Mal d 1. Int Arch Allergy Immunol 139:53–62
38. Son DY, Scheurer S, Hoffmann A, et al (1999) Pollen-related food allergy: Cloning and immunological analysis of isoforms and mutants of Mal d 1, the major apple allergen, and Bet v 1, the major birch pollen allergen. Eur J Nutr 38:201–15
39. Westritschnig K, Focke M, Verdino P, et al (2004) Generation of an allergy vaccine by disruption of the three-dimensional structure of the cross-reactive calcium-binding allergen, Phl p 7. J Immunol 172:5684–92
40. Smith AM, Chapman MD (1996) Reduction in IgE binding to allergen variants generated by site- directed mutagenesis: Contribution of disulfide bonds to the antigenic structure of the major house dust mite allergen Der p 2. Mol Immunol 33:399–405
41. Takai T, Yokota T, Yasue M, et al (1997) Engineering of the major house dust mite allergen Der f2 for allergen-specific immunotherapy. Nat Biotechnol 15:754–8
42. Olsson S, van Hage-Hamsten M, Whitley P (1998) Contribution of disulphide bonds to antigenicity of Lep d 2, the major allergen of the dust mite Lepidoglyphus destructor. Mol Immunol 35:1017–23
43. Bonura A, Amoroso S, Locorotondo G, et al (2001) Hypoallergenic variants of the Parietaria judaica major allergen Par j 1: A member of the non-specific lipid transfer protein plant family. Int Arch Allergy Immunol 126:32–40
44. Drew AC, Eusebius NP, Kenins L, et al (2004) Hypoallergenic variants of the major latex allergen Hev b 6.01 retaining human T lymphocyte reactivity. J Immunol 173:5872–9
45. Korematsu S, Tanaka Y, Hosoi S, et al (2000) C8/119S mutation of major mite allergen Derf-2 leads to degenerate secondary structure and molecular polymerization and induces potent and exclusive Th1 cell differentiation. J Immunol 165:2895–902
46. Kauppinen J, Zeiler T, Rautiainen J, et al (1999) Mutant derivatives of the main respiratory allergen of cow are less allergenic than the intact molecule. Clin Exp Allergy 29:989–96
47. Takai T, Ichikawa S, Yokota T, et al (2000) Unlocking the allergenic structure of the major house dust mite allergen der f 2 by elimination of key intramolecular interactions. FEBS Lett 484:102–7

48. Swoboda I, de Weerd N, Bhalla PL, et al (2002) Mutants of the major ryegrass pollen allergen, Lol p 5, with reduced IgE-binding capacity: Candidates for grass pollen-specific immunotherapy. Eur J Immunol 32:270–80
49. Schramm G, Kahlert H, Suck R, et al (1999) "Allergen engineering": Variants of the timothy grass pollen allergen Phl p 5b with reduced IgE-binding capacity but conserved T cell reactivity. J Immunol 162:2406–14
50. Wald M, Kahlert H, Weber B, et al (2007) Generation of a low Immunoglobulin E-binding mutant of the timothy grass pollen major allergen Phl p 5a. Clin Exp Allergy 37:441–50
51. Marazuela EG, Rodriguez R, Barber D, et al (2007) Hypoallergenic mutants of Ole e 1, the major olive pollen allergen, as candidates for allergy vaccines. Clin Exp Allergy 37:251–60
52. Garcia-Ortega L, Lacadena J, Villalba M, et al (2005) Production and characterization of a noncytotoxic deletion variant of the Aspergillus fumigatus allergen Aspf1 displaying reduced IgE binding. FEBS J 272:2536–44
53. Reisinger J, Horak F, Pauli G, et al (2005) Allergen-specific nasal IgG antibodies induced by vaccination with genetically modified allergens are associated with reduced nasal allergen sensitivity . J Allergy Clin Immunol 116:347–54
54. Gafvelin G, Thunberg S, Kronqvist M, et al (2005) Cytokine and antibody responses in birch-pollen-allergic patients treated with genetically modified derivatives of the major birch pollen allergen Bet v 1. Int Arch Allergy Immunol 138:59–66
55. Weber B, Slamal H, Suck R (2003) Size exclusion chromatography as a tool for quality control of recombinant allergens and hypoallergenic variants. J Biochem Biophys Methods 56:219–32
56. Kettner J, Meyer H, Cromwell O, et al (2007) Specific immunotherapy with recombinant birch pollen allergen rBet v1-FV results of 2 years of treatment (Phase II trial). Allergy 62(Suppl 83):262
57. Kettner J, Meyer H, Narkus A, et al (2007) Specific immunotherapy with recombinant birch pollen allergen rBet v 1-FV is clinically efficacious – results of a Phase III study. Allergy 62(Suppl 83):33
58. Tighe H, Takabayashi K, Schwartz D, et al (2000) Conjugation of immunostimulatory DNA to the short ragweed allergen Amb a 1 enhances its immunogenicity and reduces its allergenicity. J Allergy Clin Immunol 106:124–34
59. Crameri R, Fluckiger S, Daigle I, et al (2007) Design, engineering and in vitro evaluation of MHC class-II targeting allergy vaccines. Allergy 62:197–206
60. Zhu D, Kepley CL, Zhang M, et al (2002) A novel human immunoglobulin Fc gamma Fc epsilon bifunctional fusion protein inhibits Fc epsilon RI-mediated degranulation. Nat Med 8:518–21
61. Zhu D, Kepley CL, Zhang K, et al (2005) A chimeric human–cat fusion protein blocks cat-induced allergy. Nat Med 11:446–9

Reconstructing the Repertoire of Mite Allergens by Recombinant DNA Technology

Seow Theng Ong and Fook Tim Chew

Introduction

Mites are normal inhabitants in our environment and are abundant in house dust as well as barns and grain stores. About 40,000 different mite species have been identified, but more than a million are thought to exist. Nevertheless, only those found significantly among human dwellings are considered important sources of allergens [1]. Among these, two species have been reported almost ubiquitously – *Dermatophagoides pteronyssinus*, and *D. farinae* (from the Family Pyroglyphidae). In tropical homes, the storage mite *Blomia tropicalis* (Family Echymyopodidae) can be prevalent along with the Pyroglyphid mites [2]. In addition, mites in the following families such as Glycyphagidae (*Glycyphagus domesticus* and *Lepidoglyphus destructor*), Acaridae (*Tyrophagus putrescentiae*, *Acarus siro* and *Aleuroglyphus ovatus*), Suidasiidae (*Suidasia pontifica* or *Suidasia medanensis*) and Chortoglyphidae (*Chortoglyphus arcuatus*), as well as a third species from the family Pyroglyphidae (*Euroglyphus maynei*) have been reported to cause allergic responses. Predaceous mites (e.g., *Cheyletus*) and parasitic mites of plants (*Tetranychidae*, spider mites, and *Tarsonemidae*) have also been reported to be present in homes, but how widespread and significant these species are as sources of indoor allergens are yet to be determined.

The role of mites of the genus *Dermatophagoides* as an important source of house dust allergens was established approximately 40 years ago [3]. Since then, multiple epidemiological studies have shown strong casual links between sensitization to its allergens and the development of allergic diseases such as asthma and allergic rhinitis [4]. The examination of house dust mite extracts has indicated that about 4–32 different proteins, with molecular weights ranging from 11 to over 180 kDa,

S.T. Ong and F.T. Chew (✉)
Department of Biological Sciences, National University of Singapore, Allergy and Molecular Immunology Laboratory, Lee Hiok Kwee Functional Genomics Laboratories,
14, Science Drive 4, 117543, Singapore
e-mail: dbscft@nus.edu.sg

R. Pawankar et al. (eds.), *Allergy Frontiers: Future Perspectives*,
DOI 10.1007/978-4-431-99365-0_4, © Springer 2010

can induce and bind IgE antibodies in allergic patients [5–7]. Several studies subsequently revealed that most sera recognize a unique combination of 1–7 bands, although some have broader IgE binding profiles. To date, 22 different groups of allergen have been reported from dust mites [as listed in the World Health Organization – International Union of Immunological Societies (WHO/IUIS) list of allergens, www.allergen.org], in which 19 of them have been identified from the genus *Dermatophagoides*, while two (groups 12 and 19) have only been reported from the storage mite, *B. tropicalis* (see Table 1). Our recent studies, however, showed that more than 40 groups of allergens may be present in the various species of dust mites with allergenic specificities varying from one to the other [8].

Cross-Reactivity: A Common Feature Especially Among Taxonomic Related Mites

The majority of house dust mite allergic patients are co-sensitized to *D. pteronyssinus* and *D. farinae*. High degree of cross-reactivity among the *Dermatophagoides* spp. (*D. pteronyssinus*, *D. farinae*, *D. siboney*, and *D. microceras*) was also reported [9]. A significant relationship between the house dust mites and *E. maynei* has also been found, where all of the suspected allergic patients showed positive skin prick test to both *E. maynei* and the house dust mites.

Several investigators have found little or no cross-reactivity among *Dermatophagoides* spp. and storage mites [10]. Griffin et al. (1989) [11] concluded that there is limited cross-reactivity among *A. siro*, *G. destructor*, and *D. pteronyssinus*, and these mites have common and species-specific allergenic determinants. On the other hand, Lucznska et al. (1990) [12] found that house dust mites seem to cross-react more strongly to *A. siro* and *T. putrescentiae* than to *L. destructor*. In another study, Puerta et al. (1991) [13] reported that the cross-reactivity between *D. farinae* and *B. tropicalis* appears to be greater than that between *D. farinae* and *L. destructor*. A slight cross-reactivity was reported to exist between house dust mites and the mange mites, *Psoroptes cuniculi* and *P. ovis* [14].

Simultaneous sensitization to two or more allergens may originate from cross-reaction or be caused by co-sensitization. Cross-reaction occurs when an antibody originally raised against one allergen binds to a similar allergen from another source; co-sensitization takes place when different IgE antibodies bind to different allergens at the same time. The distinction between cross-reaction and co-sensitization can be determined through in vitro inhibition experiments in which blocking of IgE binding activity occur if the mite proteins are cross-reactive. However, it is important to note that immunoblotting recognized two types of cross-reactivity; one due to proteins and the other due to sugars (glycans on glycoproteins or called cross-reacting carbohydrate determinant).

Table 1 Major groups of dust mite allergens and their biological properties

Group[a]	Biological function	Molecular weight (kD)	IgE binding range (%)	Allergens identified[a]
1	Cysteine protease	25	70–90	Der p 1, Der f 1, Der m 1, Eur m 1, Blo t 1, (Aca s 1, Ale o 1, Sui m 1, and Tyr p 1)[b]
2	Unknown (lipid binding)	14	60–90	Der p 2, Der f 2, Lep d 2, Tyr p 2, Eur m 2, Gly d 2, (Aca s 2, Ale o 2, Blo t 2 and Sui m 2)[b]
3	Trypsin	28, 30	51–90	Der p 3, Der f 3, Eur m 3[b], Blo t 3, (Aca s 3, Ale o 3, Sui m 3, and Tyr p 3)[b]
4	Amylase	57, 60	25–46	Der p 4, Der f 4, Eur m 4, (Aca s 4, Blo t 4, Sui m 4, and Tyr p 4)[b]
5	Unknown	15	9–70	Der p 5, Blo t 5, Lep d 5, (Ale o 5, Der f 5, Gly d 5, Sui m 5, and Tyr p 5)[b]
6	Chymotrypsin	25	30–40	Der p 6, Der p f, (Ale o 6, Blo t 6 and Sui m 6)[b]
7	Unknown	22–31	50–62	Der p 7, Der f 7, Lep d 7, (Aca s 7, Ale o 7, Blo t 7, Sui m 7 and Tyr p 7)[b]
8	Glutathione S-transferase	26	40	Der p 8, (Aca s 8, Ale o 8, Blo t 8, Der f 8, Lep d 8 and Sui m 8)[b]
9	Collagenolytic serine protease	30	>90	Der p 9, (Ale o 9, Blo t 9, Der f 9 and Sui m 9)[b]
10	Tropomyosin	33–37	5–80	Der p 10, Der f 10, Blo t 10, Lep d 10, Tyr p 10, (Aca s 10, Ale o 10, and Sui m 10)[b]
11	Paramyosin	92, 98, 110	80	Der f 11, Der p11, Blo t 11
12	Unknown	14	50	Blo t 12
13	Fatty acid binding protein	14, 15	10–23	Blo t 13, Aca s 13, Lep d 13, Tyr p 13, Der f 13, (Ale o 13, Der p 13, Gly d 13, and Sui m 13)[b]
14	Apolipophorin	177	30[c], 39[d], 70[e]	Der f 14, Eur m 14, Der p 14 and (Blo t 14)[b]
15	98 kDa chitinase	98	?	Der f 15, Der p 15 and (Blo t 15)[b]
16	Gelsolin-like protein/villin	53	35	Der f 16
17	EF-hand calcium binding protein	53	35	Der f 17
18	60kDa chitinase	60	54	Der f 18 and Der p 18
19	antimicrobial peptide	7.2	?	(Blo t 19)[b]
20	Arginine kinase	40	?	(Der p 20, Der f 20, and Ale o 20)[b]
21	Unknown	14	?	Der p 21[b] and Blo t 21
22	Unknown	14	?	(Der p 22, Der f 22, Ale o 22, Aca c 22, and Tyr p 22)[b]

[a]Groups as listed in the WHO/IUIS list of allergens as of March, 2007. http://www.allergen.org/List.htm. Species of dust mites: Aca s (*Acarus siro*), Ale o (*Aleuroglyphus ovatus*), Blo t (*Blomia tropicalis*), Der f (*Dermatophagoides farinae*), Der m (*D. microceras*), Der p (*D. pteronyssinus*), Der s (*D. siboney*), Eur m (*Euroglyphus maynei*), Gly d (*Glycyphagus domesticus*), Lep d (*Lepidoglyphus destructor*), Sui m (*Suidasia medanensis*) and Tyr p (*Tyrophagus putrescentiae*)

[b]Unpublished; but sequence data available in WHO/IUIS list of allergen or GenBank

Data for [c]Mag allergen

[d]recombinant Mag 3 allergen

[e]natural Mag 3 allergen

General Features of Allergens

Allergens are antigens that stimulate the production of, and combine specifically with IgE antibodies. Most allergens reacting with IgE and IgG antibodies are proteins, often with carbohydrate side chains, but in certain circumstances, pure carbohydrates have been considered to be allergens [15]. Nevertheless, allergens are often derived from common and usually harmless substances such as pollens, mold spores, animal dander, dust, foods, insect venoms, and drugs.

There appear to be three restrictions for a molecule to become an allergen: (1) it has to possess a surface to which the antibody can form a complementary surface; (2) it has to have an amino acid sequence in its backbone that is able to bind the MHC II alleles of the responding individual; and (3) the free energy of interaction of the allergen with the antibody should be adequate to ensure binding at low concentrations. However, there is no unifying theory for why some proteins are allergenic and others not. There are also no characteristic features of the allergens other than to be able to reach and stimulate immune cells and mast cells. Any protein, therefore, may be allergenic, especially if it avoids the activation of TH2 suppressive mechanisms [16].

The number of identified allergens is increasing rapidly. In 1995, at least 250–300 allergens of clinical importance have been identified among the weeds, grasses, trees, animal dander, molds, house dust mites, parasites, insect venoms, occupational allergens, drugs, and foods. Today, more than 2,000 allergen (including variants and isoforms) protein or nucleotide sequences have been deposited in the GenBank and other databases. Allergenic proteins could be identified using serum containing high level of IgE antibody in combination with a number of immunochemical assays that separate proteins based on their net charge (isoelectric focusing), size (Western blot analysis), and ability to bind to IgE antibody (competitive inhibition immunoassay).

Mite Allergens as an Important Source of Indoor Allergens

Dust mites are common sources of indoor allergens besides cockroaches, cats, and dogs. Mite allergens are divided into specific groups on the basis of their biochemical composition, sequence homology, and molecular weight. A protein can be included in the Allergen Nomenclature if the prevalence of IgE reactivity is >5% and if it elicits IgE responses in as few as five patients. The nomenclature of the allergens, which is recommended by International Union of Immunologic Societies Subcommittee/World Health Organization (IUIS/WHO), includes the first three letters of the genus, the first letter of the species and an Arabic numeral to indicate the chronological order of purification. For example, Der p 1 is the first isolate from *D. pteronyssinus*. Allergens from different species of the same or different genus which share the common biochemical properties are considered to belong to the same group.

Mite allergens can be detected in many areas of the homes: the carpets, upholstered furniture, and clothing. They are present in the mite bodies, secreta, and excreta, in which the fecal particles contain the greatest proportion of mite allergen. Exposure to ≥2 μg of Der p 1 and/or Der f 1 per gram of dust can be considered as a risk factor for sensitization to mites and bronchial hyperreactivity, exposure to ≥10 μg of group 1 allergens per gram of dust represents a higher level of risk for both sensitization and asthma development in genetically predisposed individuals [17]. Moreover, allergen levels in excess of 10 μg g^{-1} of dust have been identified in many parts of the world.

A total of 22 allergen groups have been described in dust mites. These allergens fall into molecular weights between 10 kDa and 180 kDa, and they have diverse biological functions such as enzymes, enzyme inhibitors, ligand binding proteins, and structural proteins. Our recent studies using a large scale genomic approach however showed that more than 40 groups of mite allergens may be present [8], and this is summarized in Table 2.

A significant number of important mite allergens have been shown to possess enzyme activity. These include the hydrolytic enzymes such as the cysteine protease (group 1 allergen), serine proteases (group 3, 6 and 9 allergens), amylase (group 4 allergen); and nonhydrolytic enzymatic, glutathione S-transferase (group 8 allergen). There have been a lot of speculations that the presence these enzymes among allergens relates to the role of proteolytic enzyme activity for disruption of the cohesion of the bronchial epithelial barriers and the strongest evidence came from several in vitro studies on Der p 1 [18].

However, there is lack of evidence that biological functions of the proteins are closely linked to their ability to induce IgE responses and the enzymatic functions per se are not a prerequisite to induce IgE productions. It is argued that environmental exposure to mite group 2 allergens is 2–10 times lower than that of Der p 1, but it elicits similarly high IgE responses among the mite allergic patients [19]. Furthermore, the function of other important mite allergens such as group 5 and group 7 mite allergens is also entirely unknown. On the other hand, mites group 10 and 11 allergens are cytoskeletal proteins in function and may elicit as high as 80% IgE reactivity.

Furthermore, some of the most efficient allergens from other animals and plants do not have any proteolytic activity. For example, the major grass and tree pollen allergens, Phl p 11 and Bet v 2 are profilins; major peanut allergens Ara h 1, Ara h 2, and Ara h 3 are seed storage proteins; Mag 29, fungal Pen c 19, Cla h 4, and Asp f 12 are heat shock proteins; and cockroach Bla g 4 belongs to the lipocalin family. Several homologs to these have now been identified, cloned, and expressed from dust mites and were also found to bind IgE [8].

Thus, enzymatic activity cannot be considered as a common feature of allergens. In this regard, the potential effects of the enzymatic function of Der p 1 on allergenicity may represent a special case, and the fact that mites secrete several allergenic enzymes may be coincidental [19]. Nevertheless, it is important to remember that among the major functional sets of proteins, enzymes are often more water soluble than structural or membrane based proteins, and that solubility plays a considerable

Table 2 Allergen homologues (apart from those listed in the WHO/IUIS list of allergens) which have been identified from expressed sequence tag catalogs of the dust mite genomes [see reference 8]

Homologous to	Identity
Mag29	Mag29 in *Dermatophagoides farinae*
Alpha-tubulin	Tubulin alpha chain in *Lepidoglyphus destructor*
Alt a 12	Acidic ribosomal protein P1 [*Alternaria alternata*]
Cla h 3/Alt a 10	Aldehyde dehydrogenase [*Cladosporium herbarum, A. alternata*]
Alt a 6/Fus c 1	Acid ribosomal protein P2 [*A. alternata, Fusarium culmorum*]
Act c 1	Cysteine protease [*Actnidia chinesis*]
Cop c 2	Thioredoxin [*Coprinus comatus*]
Mal f 6	Cyclophilin [*Malassezia furfur*]
Gal d 2	Ovalbumin [*Gallus domesticus*]
Heb v 8/Pyr c 4	Profilin [*Hevea brasiliensis, Pyrus communis* etc]
Len c 1	Vicilin [*Lens culinaris*]
Ves m 1	Phospholipase A1 [*Vespula maculifrons*]
Per a 1	Cr-PII [*Periplenata americana*]
Can d a 1	Alcohol dehydrogenase [*Candida albicans*]
Pen c 19/Cla h 4	heat shock protein 70 [*Penicillium citrinum, C. herbarum*]
Asp f 12	heat shock protein 90 [*Aspergillus fumigatus*]
Rho m 1/Alt a 11	Enolase [*Rhodotorula mucilaginosa, A. alternata*]
Ani s 2	Paramyosin [*Anisakis simplex*]
Asp f 6	Superoxide dismutase [*Aspergillus fumigatus*]
Mal d 2	Thaumatin [*Malus domestica*]
Aed a 1	Apyrase precursor [*Aedes aegyptii*]
Api m 6	Unknown [*Apis mellifera*]
Alt a 2	Unknown [*A. alternata*]
Zea m 14, Pru a 3	Nonspecific lipid transfer protein [*Zea mays, Prunus avium*]
Ole e 8	Calcium binding protein [*Olea eurpaea*]
Bla g 2	Aspartic protease [*Blatella germanica*]
Mal f 4	Malate dehydrogenase [*Malassezia furfur*]

role in allergenicity. The biological activity of an allergen, thus, mainly be involved in the process of unspecific induction of the inflammatory response or will augment the immunological shift toward an allergic reaction.

Isoallergens: Many Allergens in Nature Exist in Several Isoforms

Isoallergens may be as different in their sequence and structure as allergens from different species. Consequently, their immunogenicity could differ and they might have to be considered as separate allergens. This is of important when recombinant allergens are to be used in immunotherapy since all isoforms must be represented in the evaluation and treatment of patients.

According to WHO/IUS Allergen Subcommittee (1994), these similar molecules are designated as isoallergens when they share the following common biochemical properties: similar molecular size; identical biological function, if known, for example, enzymatic action; and a recommended guide of ≥67% identity of amino acid sequences. Each isoallergen may also have multiple forms of closely similar sequences resulted from nucleotide mutations. Such mutations are either silent or which can lead to single or multiple amino acid substitutions. These copies are called variants and designated by suffixes of a period followed by four Arabic numerals. The first two numerals 01–99 refer to a particular isoallergen, and the two subsequent numerals 01–99 refer to a particular variant of a particular isoallergen designated by the preceding two numerals.

Isoallergens reported in various sources display different serological properties, some showed equivalent allergenicity (e.g., isoforms of latex allergen Hev b 7) while some reported different antigenicities (e.g., isoforms of ragweed pollen Amb a 1) and different allergenicities (e.g., isoforms of apple allergen Mal d 1). The major birch pollen allergen, Bet v 1, has been shown to exist in at least 11 isoforms. Interestingly, Ferreira and co-workers (1996) [20] reported that three naturally occurring isoforms of Bet v 1 display high T cell antigenicity and low or no IgE binding activity.

Intraspecies sequence variation has been a feature of mite allergens. Sequence polymorphism has been reported for the cDNA encoding group 1, 2, 3, and 5 allergens. Some of the polymorphic residues of group 1 and 2 allergens were in regions of known T cell epitopes. Several recombinant variants of Der p 2 were found to be able to stimulate different degree of T cell proliferative responses and cytokines productions while isoallergens from Lep d 2, however, have been shown to have comparable IgE reactivity in vitro and in vivo. The effect of the polymorphic variants on T cell responses and IgE reactivity may reflect different responsiveness of individuals or could be due to exposure to regional polymorphisms. We have also identified several potential paralogs (duplicate genes) of allergenic components which share very low sequence homology (less than 50% amino acid similarities) but have substantially high IgE binding capacity [8].

Cross-Reactivity: Common Feature Among Proteins Derived from Taxonomically Related Organisms and/or Evolutionary Conserved Proteins (Pan Allergen)

Allergenic cross-reactivity occurs when different proteins have a certain degree of both primary and tertiary structure homology and contain identical or similar specific IgE binding epitopes. Cross-reactivity is a frequent feature among mite allergens, especially in those from taxonomically related species. Generally, it has been known that pyroglyphid mites have low cross-reactivity with nonpyroglyphid mites. Gafvelin and co-workers (2001) [21] reported that extensive cross-reactivity was detected among group 2 allergens from *G. domesticus*, *L. destructor*, and *T. putrescentiae*, but little cross-reactivity was found between these allergens and Der p 2. On the other hand, Smith et al. (2001) [22] demonstrated that the allergenic cross-reactivity among Der p 2, Der f 2, and Eur m 2 is a direct result of the conserved antigenic surface, whereas the lack of cross-reactivity with Lep d 2 and Tyr p 2 could be a result of the multiple amino acid substitutions across the protein surface. Hales et al. (2000) [23] presented that the proliferative response and the level of IL-5 produced after in vitro challenge with group 1 and 7 allergen were equivalent from both *D. pteronyssinus* and *D. farinae* even though the latter mite species is not detected in the environment where the study population live.

Cross-reaction can also caused by evolutionary conserved protein structures. High structural homology between these allergenic proteins present in different, apparently unrelated sources of exposure seems to play an important role in IgE mediated polysensitization. These allergen families, known as pan allergens, represent proteins sharing a high degree of sequence homology. A striking example that accounts for most of the allergenic cross-reactivity among insects and arachnids, with other invertebrates such as mollusks, nematodes, and also foods derived from these invertebrates such as shrimps, other crustaceans, and snails, is the muscle protein tropomyosin [24]. This highly conserved coiled-coil protein exist in both muscle and nonmuscle cells. It has been identified as major allergen in shrimp (Pen a 1, Pen I 1 and Met e 1); crab (Cha f 10; lobster (Pan s 1 and Hom a 1)); oyster (Cra g 1); gastropod (Tur c 1 and Tod p 1); dust mites (Der p 10, Der f 10 and Blo t 10); and cockroaches (Per a 7) [24]. Furthermore, several studies have demonstrated cross-reactivity of IgE to insects and parasites, specifically the nematodes *Anisakis simplex* and *Acaris suis*, which may also be caused by tropomyosin [24]. Thus, cross-reactivity among tropomyosins could largely attribute to shared primary and tertiary structures.

Reese et al. (1999) [24] proposed that exposure and sensitization to a particular food allergen may ultimately lead to sensitization to certain aeroallergens. In view of the data accumulated, they also suggested that the in vitro cross-reactivity among tropomyosins in different invertebrate species not only exists, but also has important clinical implications and may result in the induction of sensitization and allergic reactions to both foods and inhalants in the same patient. Moreover, these studies also help explain some unusual observations of reactivity in the absence of sensitization.

However, similarity per se does not mean that the proteins will cross-react on the IgE level. IgE antibodies to shrimp tropomyosin do not cross react with heterologous mammalian tropomyosins from pork, beef, chicken, or mouse [25]. The reason could be due to immunologic tolerance induced by autologous proteins with a similar fold. Moreover, amino acid substitutions in a protein sequence might markedly affect the outer protein surface and thus reduce antibody reactivity. Therefore, investigation of the nonallergenic counterparts may shed light on the structural features that suppress immune response or conversely contribute to the allergenic activity of the invertebrate tropomyosin.

Molecular Biology for Allergen Research, Diagnosis and Treatment: Expression Systems for Recombinant Allergens Production

A variety of recombinant allergens from plants, mites, mammals, and insects have been expressed in various systems, both prokaryotic and eukaryotic. Many investigators reported a high degree of similarity between the recombinant allergens produced when compared to their natural counterparts in terms of structure, function, and immune reactivity. Table 3 gives an overview of the bioactivity of the recombinant dust mite allergens produced in various expression systems.

E. coli is the oldest and most commonly utilized system for production of recombinant proteins. The bacterial system is easy to handle, cost-effective and the yield can be high. However, over production of foreign proteins in the cytoplasm of *E. coli* often goes together with misfolding and segregation into insoluble aggregates such as inclusion bodies, which can lead to the production of biologically

Table 3 Overview of the productions of recombinant mite allergens: from the aspects of the production yield, bioactivities, and types of expression systems used

Allergen group	Yield	Bioactivity compared to natural	Expression system
1	High	Natural enzymatic and IgE binding	Eukaryotic
2	High	Natural IgE binding	*E. coli*
3	Low[a]	High IgE binding	*E. coli*
4	Moderate	Natural amylase activity; reduced IgE binding	*P. pastoris*
5	High	IgE binding; crystallizable but no natural protein tested	*E. coli* and yeast
6	Low[a]	High IgE binding	*E. coli*
7	High	70–90% of natural IgE binding activity	*E. coli*
8	Unclear	High IgE binding; binds glutathione substrate, but no natural protein tested	*E. coli*
9	Low[a]	High IgE binding	*E. coli*
10	High[a]	Lower IgE binding than natural	*E. coli*
11	Moderate[a]	Lower IgE binding than natural	*E. coli*
12	Unknown	IgE binding in phage immunoassay	Lambda phage
13	Moderate	High IgE binding but no natural protein tested	*E. coli*
14	Peptide fragments	Detectable IgE binding	*E. coli*
15–19	Insufficient Information	Insufficient information	Insufficient Information
20–22	Moderate to high	Moderate to high IgE binding	*E. coli*

[a]Expressed with vector fusion proteins

inactive proteins and require some elaborate low yield renaturation procedure. The limitations described can be critical for recombinant allergen production in particular because many IgE antibody responses are dependent upon the native conformation of the protein.

The advantages of eukaryotic expression systems are that high level expression is common, the proteins are usually folded correctly with disulfide bonds formed, posttranslationally modified including processing signal sequences, adding lipids and carbohydrates, and also purification can often be simplified to a single step procedure, such as affinity chromatography. A variety of eukaryotic expression systems are available, and the most commonly used in allergen studies are the yeast and insect systems. Some of the recombinant allergens expressed in these systems show IgE binding capacity and behave similar biological activities to the native proteins.

To determine the expression system of choice, a few factors have to be taken into consideration based on the time, resources, experience available in the laboratory, the nature of the allergens and the utility of the recombinant allergens produced. Nonetheless, protein expression for each allergen is still a very empirical process. The performance of any one expression method will also vary with the individual target protein and its expression level. Thus, experience in working with expression system is a very important consideration.

Almost all allergens are derived from eukaryotic system sources. Although the eukaryotic expression systems are preferred for retaining the native conformation and/or posttranslational modification of the recombinant protein, eukaryotic systems are normally time consuming and probably requires specialized skills and experiences. For example, Der p 1 produced in yeast, *Saccharomyces cerevisae* showed high IgE binding frequency in contrast to no IgE binding activity when produced in *E. coli*. However, it was insoluble and had to be denatured and renatured [26]. Der p 1 expressed in another yeast, *Pichia pastoris* displayed a hyperglycoslated form which had decreased IgE binding activity and poor induction of histamine release from basophils. It was suggested that the hyperglycosylation hindered the maturation of the protein [27].

On the other hand, there is a large amount of experience with *E. coli* for the prokaryotic systems. Prokaryotic systems do not perform the posttranslational modifications of many eukaryotic proteins and many proteins do not fold properly. In addition, excessive rare codon usage in the target gene could be a cause for low level expression as well as truncation products.

Nevertheless, the prokaryotic expression system is still the first choice for allergen expression in this study, primarily because the main objective is to screen and characterize a panel of allergens identified. The bacterial expression system is able to offer a rapid and cost-effective way since it is relatively easy to use, can be manipulated into variants for optimized production of desired target genes, requires straight forward purification steps and also there are many examples of allergens successfully produced in this system. In the case of the group 2 mite allergen Der p 2, Lep d 2, olive allergen Ole e 3, Ole e 8, and the yeast allergen Mal f 1, no functional and immuno activity differences were observed between protein produced in prokaryotic and eukaryotic expression systems. However, the allergens with predicted post-translational modifications and/or those that show lower immuno activity compare to their natural counterparts should be produced in eukaryotic systems.

Recombinant Allergens Essential for Research and Diagnosis

In the past and even until recently, most studies and all clinical practices still relied heavily on whole mite extracts. The natural extracts, however, are heterogeneous products containing many nonallergenic proteins, carbohydrates, and other macromolecules. The allergens produced from natural sources vary in composition and content. The quality of the extracts is influenced by many factors, including the quality of the starting raw material, extraction procedure, protease content, and storage conditions. These factors strongly influenced the final composition, potency, and stability of allergen preparations and ultimately the outcome of diagnostic tests in vitro and in vivo. These natural materials are also at risk of being contaminated with allergens from other sources and can contain proteolytic enzymes. Such enzymes may be allergenic or nonallergenic, but in either case can cause degradation and loss of potency when administered together with other allergens during immunotherapy.

Many of the problems associated with using natural allergenic products for allergy diagnosis and treatment can be overcome with the use of recombinant allergens. Many important allergens from dust mites, pollen, animal dander, molds and fungi, insect venoms, and foods have now been defined at molecular level through gene cloning (http://www.allergen.org). Advances in molecular technology provide the opportunity for in vitro production of virtually unlimited amounts of a particular allergen of standardized quality and adequate concentration. The cDNA sequence coding for the desired protein is inserted into cultured *E .coli* bacteria, yeast or insect cells, which express the corresponding recombinant protein. These allergens can be purified under defined conditions and with single step procedures such as affinity chromatography. Their purity can be established by SDS-PAGE, HPLC and mass spectrometry.

Recombinant proteins can be easily produced in a large quantity sufficient for various characterizations of their physiochemical, biological, and immunological properties. The IgE binding capacity, T cell responses, and cytokine profiles of many important allergens such as the mite group 1, 2, and 7 allergens, birch pollen Bet v 1 and some peanut allergens have been studied using recombinant proteins. Recombinant allergens are thus powerful reagents to study the mechanism involved in allergic reactions and also to study structure-function relationship. The elucidation of primary structure of allergens opens door to determine the tertiary structures of allergens by NMR techniques, X-ray crystallography or computer-based modeling and also contributes to the understanding of cross-reactivity among apparently unrelated allergenic sources. The allergens of Bet v 1 family and the profilin family have been identified in trees, grasses, and weed pollens and in many fruits and vegetables [28,29]. Extensive cross-reactivity have been reported among these proteins with similar biological functions and some of the protein structures such as Bet v 1, Bet v 2, Pru av 1 and Phl p 2 have also been successfully determined by nuclear magnetic resonance (NMR) and X-ray crystallography.

Beside research applications, recombinant allergens also carry the advantage for being used for diagnostic purposes as they can consistently be produced at high purity and defined concentrations with verifiable protein content. Since 1991, recombinant allergens such as Bet v 1 and Bet v 2 were successfully used for in vitro diagnosis of pollen allergy [30]. Later, the first skin test with recombinant allergen (fungus *Aspergillus fumigatus* Asp f I/a) was described [31]. Several important allergens form various sources are now commercially available for diagnosis purposes, these include mite group 1, 2, 5, and 7 allergens, cat Fel d 1 and albumin, cockroach Bla g 1, 2, 4, and 5 allergens, birch pollen Bet v 1 and Bet v 2, peanut Ara h 1, Ara h 2, and Ara h 3 and, etc., [19]. Hiller et al. in 2002 [32] have applied microarray technology to develop a miniaturized allergy test containing 94 purified allergen molecules that represent the most common allergen sources. This method, which uses very small quantities of the patient's serum, allows the determination and monitoring of the allergic patients' IgE reactivity profiles to large numbers of disease-causing allergens.

The application of molecular biology to the field of allergen characterization has led to the availability of continuously increasing number of recombinant allergen molecules that mimic the immunological properties of their natural counterparts. Furthermore, the allergenic activity of the natural extracts could be completely reproduced with careful formulation and proper selection of the recombinant proteins [19,30] and such approach is especially advantageous to represent the less abundant allergens in the wild extract such as the mite group 3–14 allergens [33].

Molecular Modification of Recombinant Proteins: For Allergen Specific Immunotherapy

Recombinant DNA technology also offers the possibility of developing allergen immunotherapy as well as allergen vaccines seeing that recombinant allergens can consistently be produced at high purity. Once a molecule is cloned, it is possible for the alteration of the primary, secondary, and tertiary structure of the recombinant proteins. Many recent studies have been performed with the objective of producing recombinant modified allergens with reduced allergenicity but conserved T cell antigenicity to access their potential use for improved immunotherapy [34].

The treatment of domestic mite allergic disease combines immunologic and pharmacologic therapy. Several prescription and nonprescription drugs are currently available to relief symptoms associated with allergic reactions such as antihistamines, glucocorticosteroids, β2-adrenoreceptor agonists, and anti-leukotrienes. While drugs provide symptomatic treatment, allergen avoidance and immunotherapy can modify the natural course of the disease. Immunotherapy is indicated for patients with mild to moderate disease who requires seasonal or perennial prophylactic drugs such as allergic rhinitis, asthma, and venom hypersensitivity and have demonstrated evidence of specific IgE antibodies to clinically relevant allergens.

Immunotherapy was first introduced in the early 1900s and has since then been used to treat allergic patients. Immunotherapy is the practice of administering gradually increasing quantities of an allergen vaccine to an allergic subject in order to improve the symptoms associated with the subsequent exposure to the causative allergen. Immunotherapy is currently the only treatment that may affect the natural course of allergic diseases, whether by preventing the development of asthma in patients with allergic diseases or by altering the disease progression. However, the details of its mechanism of action, its efficacy, and its limitation are still not fully understood.

The binding domain of an allergen to IgE antibody or T-cell that induces specific IgE production is known as epitope. Once the primary sequence of an allergen is accessible, various methods can be utilized to map the B and T cell epitopes of the allergen. A good candidate for immunotherapy should possess the characteristics of reduced capacity to bind serum IgE, ensuring a lower risk of IgE mediated side effects, and retention of their T cell epitopes, allowing for a modulation of the immune responses. If the B cell epitopes of a recombinant allergen could be disrupted to produce a protein with lower IgE binding potential, then it could be administered to the patient at a higher dosage. The hypoallergenic proteins would then have a better chance of being processed by a nonprofessional antigen presenting cells (APC). If the processed peptides are presented to circulating T cells by APCs without the proper co-stimulatory molecules, the T cells will become desensitized to that T cell epitope.

Genetic engineering of gene can involve changing specific base pair, that is, mutated genes of allergens, for example, of Bet v 1, Bet v 4, Lol p 5; introduction of new piece of DNA into the existing DNA molecule, that is, chimeric or hybrid genes, for example, of venom Ves v 5 and Pol a 5; disruption of three dimensional structure, that is, conformational variants of Der f 2, Par j 1; and deletions of DNA, that is, truncated gene or gene fragments of Lol p 1, Bet v 1, Phl p 5. Some naturally occurring allergen isoforms (e.g., of Bet v 1) that display high T cell antigenicity and low/no IgE binding activity can also be used as full length hypoallergenic variants for immunotherapy [20].

Promising results have been achieved for the Der f 2 and Bet v 1 mutants. Previous work has suggested that the IgE epitopes of group 2 mite allergen were dependent on conformation rather than contiguous amino acids. Two intramolecular disulfide bonds that were required for Der f 2 structural stability have been disrupted and the mutated protein elicited much lower IgE reactivity from patient sera compare to the wild type protein. The C8–C119 mutant of Der f 2 was shown to give rise to both a markedly reduced SPT and in vitro histamine release but had a completely intact capacity to stimulate T cells [34]. This Der f 2 mutant has also been applied in a murine model and mice sensitized to wild-type rDer f 2 showed decreased bronchoconstriction when intranasally challenged with the C8–C119 mutant, compared with nonmutated rDer f 2 [35].

Similar findings were also observed in studies aiming for the immunotherapeutic potential of mutants from other allergenic sources. Encouraging results have been achieved for Bet v 1 mutants either by splitting the molecule into two fragments or by linking three Bet v 1 molecules together as a trimer where reduced inflammatory and skin test responses were reported [36,37]. Deletion mutants, for example, of Phl p 5, the major timothy grass allergen, have been created outside the dominant T-cell region and shown to have reduced IgE binding capacity but retained T cell reactivity [38]. Site directed mutagenesis has also been performed to disrupt the disulphide bond on the major cow allergen, Bos d 2 and resulted in lower IgE binding without affecting the T cell stimulatory capacity [39].

Conclusion

Recombinant technology has strongly improved our knowledge about the properties of allergens and leading to new perspectives to overcome some difficulties presented by natural extracts in allergy diagnosis, research, and therapy. Recombinant applications have been able to promise several advantages including the consistency in preparations of pharmaceutical quality products, optimizations of the dosage for all components in a preparation and inclusion of only the relevant allergens for therapy, in order to exclude any risk of possible contamination and infectious agents, thus, reducing unwanted side effects. The development of this technology in research and clinical trials will definitely lead to significant advancements in allergy research, diagnosis, and treatment.

References

1. Olsson S, van Hage-Hamsten M (2000) Allergens from house dust and storage mites: similarities and differences, with emphasis on the storage mite *Lepidoglyphus destructor*. Clin Exp Allergy 30:912–929
2. Fernandez-Caldas E, Puerta L, Caraballo L, Lockey RF (2004) Mite Allergens. In: Lockey RF, Bukantz SC, Bousquet J (eds) Allergens and Allergen Immunotherapy 3rd edn. Marcel Dekker, Inc, New York, pp 251–270
3. Voorhorst R, Spieksma FThM, Varekamp H, Leupen MJ, Lyklema AW (1967) The house dust mite (*Dermatophagoides pteronyssinus*) and the allergen it produces: identity with the house dust allergen. J Allergy 39:325–339
4. Platts-Mills TAE, De Weck A (1989) Dust mite allergens and asthma – A world wide problem. Bull World Health Organ 66:769–780
5. Arlian LG, Berstein IL, Geis DP, Vyszenski-Moher DL, Gallagher JS, Martin B (1987) Investigations of culture medium – free HDM. III. Antigens and allergens of body fecal extract of *Dermatophagoides farinae.* J Allergy Clin Immunol 79:457–466
6. Arlian LG, Berstein IL, Geis DP, Vyszenski-Moher DL, Gallagher JS (1987) Investigations of culture medium – free HDM. IV. Cross antigenicity and allergenicity between the HDM, *D. farinae* and *D. pteronyssinus*. J Allergy Clin Immunol 79:467–476

7. Batard T, Hrabina A, Bi XZ, Chabre H, Lemoine P, Couret MN, Faccenda D, Villet B, Harzic P, André F, Goh SY, André C, Chew FT, Moingeon P (2006) Production and characterization of pharmaceutical-grade *Dermatophagoides pteronyssinus* and *Dermatophagoides farinae* house dust mites for allergy vaccines. Int Arch Allergy Immunol 140:295–305
8. Angus AC, Ong ST, Chew FT (2004) Sequence tag catalogs of dust mite expressed genomes: utility in allergen and acarologic studies. Am J Pharmacogenomics 4:357–369
9. Ferrandiz R, Dreborg S (1997) Analysis of individual cross-reacting allergens between *Dermatophagoides siboney* and other mites by immunoblot inhibition. Int Arch Allergy Appl Immunol 113:238–239
10. Chew FT, Yi FC, Chua KY, Fernandez-Caldas E, Arruda LK, Chapman MD, Lee BW (1999) Allergenic differences between the domestic mites *Blomia tropicalis* and *Dermatophagoides pteronyssinus*. Clin Exp Allergy 29:982–989
11. Griffin P, Ford AW, Alterman L, Thompson J, Parkinson C, Blainey AD, Davies RJ, Topping MD (1989) Allergenic and antigenic relationship between three species of storage mite and the house dust mite, *Dermatophagoides pteronyssinus*. J Allergy Clin Immunol 84:108–117
12. Luczynska CM, Griffin P, Davies RJ, Topping MD (1990) Prevelance of specific IgE to storage mites (*A. siro, L.destructor* and *T. longior*) in an urban population and cross-reactivity with the house dust mite (*Dermatophagoides pteronyssinus*). Clin Exp Allergy 20:403–406
13. Puerta L, Fernandez-Caldas E, Caraballo L, Lockey RF (1990) Sensitization to *Blomia tropicalis* and *Lepidoglyphus destructor* in *Dermatophagoides* spp-allergic individuals. J Allergy Clin Immunol 88:943–950
14. Stewart GA, Fisher WF (1986) Cross-reactivity between the house dust mite *Dermatophagoides pteronyssinus* and the mange mites *Psoroptes cuniculi* and *P. ovis*. I. Demonstration of antibodies to the house dust mite allergen D pt 12 in sera from *P. cuniculi* infested rabbits. J Allergy Clin Immunol 78:293–299
15. Aalberse RC, Akkerdaas JH, van Ree R (2001) Cross-reactivity of IgE antibodies to allergens. Allergy 56:478–490
16. Aalberse RC (2000) Structural biology of allergens. J Allergy Clin Immunol 106:228–238
17. Sporik R, Holgate ST, Platts-Mills TAE, Cogswell JJ (1990) Exposure to house dust mite allergen (Der p I) and the development of asthma in childhood: a prospective study. New Engl J Med 323:502–507
18. Wan H, Winton HL, Soeller C, Tovey ER, Gruenert DC, Thompson PJ, Stewart GA, Taylor GW, Garrod DR, Robinson C (1999) Der p 1 facilitates transepithelial allergen delivery by disruption of tight junctions. J Clin Invest 104:123–133
19. Chapman MD, Smith AM, Vailes LD, Arruda LK, Dhanaraj V, Pomes A (2000) Recombinant allergens for diagnosis and therapy of allergic disease. J Allergy Clin Immunol 106:409–418
20. Ferreira F, Hirtenlehner K, Jilek A, Godnik-Cvar J, Breiteneder H, Grimm R, Hoffmann-Sommergruder K, Scheiner O, Kraft D, Breitenbach M, Rheinberger HJ, Ebner C (1996) Dissection of immunoglobulin E and T lymphocyte reactivity of isoforms of the major birch pollen allergen Bet v 1: potential use of hypoallergenic isoforms for immunotherapy. J Exp Med 183:599–609
21. Gafvelin G, Johansson E, Lundin A, Smith AM, Chapman MD, Benjamin DC, Derewenda U, van Hage-Hamsten M (2001) Cross-reactivity of a new group 2 allergen from the dust mite *Glycyphagus domesticus*, Gly d 2 and group 2 alergens from *Dermatophagoides pteronyssinus*, *Lepidoglyphus destructor*, and *Tyrophagus putrescentiae* with recombinant allergens. J Allergy Clin Immunol 107:511–518
22. Smith AS, Benjamin DC, Hozic N, Derewenda U, Smith WA, Thomas WR, Gafvelin G, Hage-Hamsten M, Chapman MD (2001) The molecular basis of antigenic cross-reactivity between the group 2 mite allergens. J Allergy Clin Immunol 107:977–984
23. Hales BJ, Shen HD, Thomas WR (2000) Cross-reactivity of T cell responses to *Dermatophagoides pteronyssinus* and *D. farinae*. Studies with group 1 and 7 allergens. Clin Exp Allergy 30:927–933
24. Reese G, Ayuso R, Lehrer SB (1999) Tropomyosin: an invertebrate pan-allergen. Int Arch Allergy Appl Immunol 119:247–258

25. Ayuso R, Lehrer SB, Tanaka L, Ibañez MD, Pascual C, Burks AW, Sussman GL, Goldberg B, Lopez M, Reese G (1999) IgE antibody response to vertebrate meat proteins including tropomyosin. Ann Allergy Asthma Immunol 83:399–405
26. Chua KY, Kehal PK, Thomas WR, Vaughan PR, Marcreadie IG (1992) High-frequency binding of IgE to the Der p 1 allergen expressed in yeast. J Allergy Clin Immunol 89:95–102
27. Van Oort E, de Heer PG, van Leeuwen WA, Derksen NI, Muller M, Huverneers S, Aalberse RC, van Ree R (2002) Maturation of *Pichia pastoris*-derived recombinant pro-Der p 1 induced by deglycosylation and by the natural cysteine protease Der p 1 from house dust mite. Eur J Biochem 269:671–679
28. Valenta R, Duchene M, Ebner C, Valent P, Sillaber C, Deviller P, Ferreira F, Tejkl M, Edelmann H, Kraft D, Scheiner O (1992) Profilins constitute a novel family of functional plant pan-allergens. J Exp Med 175:377–385
29. Ferreira FD, Hoffmann-Sommergruber K, Breiteneder H, Pettenburger K, Ebner C, Sommergruber W, Steiner R, Bohle B, Sperr WR, Valent P, Kungl AJ, Breitenbach M, Kraft D, Scheiner O (1993) Purification and characterization of recombinant Bet v 1, the major birch pollen allergen. J Biol Chem 268:19574–19580
30. Valenta R, Duchêne M, Vrtala S, Birkner T, Ebner C, Hirschwehr R, Breitenbach M, Rumpold H, Scheiner O, Kraft D (1991) Recombinant allergens for immunoblot diagnosis of tree pollen allergy. J Allergy Clin Immunol 88:889–894
31. Moser M, Crameri R, Menz G, Scheneider T, Dudler T, Virchow C, Gmachl M, Blaser K, Suter M (1992) Cloning and expression of recombinant *Aspergillus fumigatus* allergen I/a (rAsp f I/a) with IgE binding and type I skin test activity. J Immunol 149:454–460
32. Hiller R, Laffer S, Harwanegg C, et al (2002) Microarray allergen molecules: diagnostic gatekeepers allergy treatment. FASEB J 16:414–416
33. Thomas WR, Smith W (1999) Towards defining the full spectrum of important house dust mite allergens. Clin Exp Allergy 29:1583–1587
34. Takai T, Yokota T, Yague M, Nishiyama C, Yuuki T, Mori A, Okudaira H, Okumura Y (1997) Engineering of the major house dust mite allergen Der f 2 for allergen specific immunotherapy. Nat Biotechnol 15:754–758
35. Yasue M, Yokota T, Fukada M, Takai T, Suko M, Okudaria H, Okumura Y (1998) Hyposensitization to allergic reaction in rDEr f 2-sensitized mice by intranasal administration of a mutant of rDER f 2, C8/C119S. Clin Exp Immunol 113:1–9
36. Van Hage-Hamsten M, Kronqvist M, Zetterstrom O, Johansson E, Niederberger V, Vrtala S, Gronlund H, Gronneberg R, Valenta R (1999) Skin test evaluation of genetically engineered hypoallergenic derivatives of the major birch pollen allergen, Bet v 1: results obtained with a mix of two recombinant Bet v 1 fragments and recombinant Bet v 1 trimer in a Swedish population before the birch pollen season. J Allergy Clin Immunol 104:969–977
37. Nopp A, Hallden G, Lundahl J, Johansson E, Vrtala S, Valenta R, Gronneberg R, van Hage-Hamsten M (2000) Comparison of inflammatory responses to genetically engineered hypoallergenic derivates of the major birch pollen allergen Bet v 1 and to recombinant Bet v 1 wild type in skin chamber fluids collected from birch pollen-allergic patients. J Allergy Clin Immunol 106:101–109
38. Schramm G, Kahlet H, Suck R, Weber B, Stuwe HT, Muller WD, Bufe A, Becker WM, Schlaak MW, Jager L, Cromwell O, Fiebig H (1999) "Allergen Engineering": variants of the timothy grass pollen allergen Phl p 5b with reduced IgE binding capacity but conserved T cell reactivity. J Immunol 162:2406–2414
39. Kauppinen J, Zeiler T, Rautiainen J, Rytkonen-Nissinen M, Taivainen A, Mantyjarvi R, Virtanen T (1999) Mutant derivatives of the main respiratory allergen of cow are less allergenic than the intact molecule. Clin Exp Allergy 29:989–996

Immunostimulatory (CpG) DNA-Based Therapies for the Treatment of Allergic Disease

Tomoko Hayashi and Eyal Raz

Abbreviations

AC	Allergic conjunctivitis
AD	Atopic dermatitis
AHR	Airway hyperresponsiveness
APC	Antigen-presenting cell
AR	Allergic rhinitis
BALF	Bronchoalveolar lavage fluid
BCR	B cell receptor
DC	Dendritic cells
DXM	Dexamethasone
IRF	Interferon regulatory factor
LTC4	Leukotriene C4
MAPK	Mitogen-activated protein kinase
MCh	Methacholine
M-trp	1-Methyl-DL-tryptophan
MyD88	Myeloid differentiation primary response gene 88
NF-κB	Nuclear factor-kappa B
PDC	Plasmacytoid dendritic cell
TCR	T cell receptor
TLR	Toll-like receptor
VEGF	Vascular endothelial growth factor

T. Hayashi and E. Raz (✉)
Department of Medicine 0663, University of California San Diego,
9500 Gilman Drive, La Jolla, CA 92093, USA
e-mail: eraz@ucsd.edu

R. Pawankar et al. (eds.), *Allergy Frontiers: Future Perspectives*,
DOI 10.1007/978-4-431-99365-0_5, © Springer 2010

Introduction

Immunological Properties of CpG-ODN

Vertebrates have two types of complementary programs to resist invading pathogens, the innate and adaptive immune systems. The innate immune system recognizes microbial agents via pattern recognition receptors and evokes inflammatory responses that defend the host in an antigen nonspecific manner. In contrast, activation of adaptive immunity is triggered via unique antigen receptors [i.e., T cell receptor (TCR), and B cell receptor (BCR),] that provide antigen-specific responses [1,2]. Toll-like receptors (TLRs) are type-1 transmembrane proteins that are conserved in insects and humans [2]. TLRs are the major sensors of innate immunity and detect a variety of signature microbial compounds shared by multiple microorganisms [3].

Bacterial DNA, as well as their synthetic analogs (i.e., CpG oligonucleotide, CpG-ODN) collectively known as immunostimulatory DNA, are recognized by TLR9, one of 11 TLRs. [3,4]. CpG-ODNs were discovered in complete Freund's adjuvant [5–7]. Expression patterns of TLR9 vary among different species [8]. TLR9 is expressed in limited types of immune cells in humans such as neutrophils, certain colonic or lung epithelial cells, B cells, and plasmacytoid dendritic cells (PDC), whereas in mice it is expressed on macrophages, myeloid dendritic cells, neutrophils, mast cells, and epithelial cells [9–11].

TLR9 is located in the endosome compartment of immune cells. In colonic epithelial cells, TLR9 is expressed on the cell surface and contributes to gut homeostasis via the regulation of tolerance and inflammation [11]. In immune cells, TLR9 signaling induces inflammatory responses that are dependent on the adapter, myeloid differentiation factor 88 (MyD88). TLR9 signaling activates the mitogen-activated protein kinase (MAPK) and nuclear factor-kappa B (NF-κB) pathways as well as certain members of the interferon regulatory factor (IRF) family of transcription factors (IRF3 and IRF7). The NF-κB pathway leads to the expression of inflammatory genes such as TNFα, IL-6, and IL-12, whereas the involvement of IRF-3/7 is essential for type-1 IFN gene induction [8]. These cytokines provoke a strong Th1-like adjuvant effect. CpG-ODN induces a robust and multifaceted innate immune response [12–14] that is characterized by the upregulation of co-stimulatory molecules and the induction of chemokine or chemokine receptor expression by various immune cells [2,15,16]. Recent microarray analysis has identified the induction of 197 genes in murine spleen cells upon administration of CpG-ODN in vivo [17].

The Hygiene Hypothesis and Immunotherapy with CpG-ODN

Over the past three decades, the prevalence and severity of allergic diseases has increased in industrialized countries [18]. One popular, but yet unproven, explanation is the “hygiene hypothesis,” which is based on the assumption that in westernized countries hygiene practices, for example, overuse of antibiotics and aggressive vaccination in early childhood, result in a reduction of microbial burden that would otherwise influence the development of a Th1-biased immunity. This lack of microbial stimulation provokes a Th2-like immunity. Consequently, one would expect these children to be predisposed to allergic disorders [19,20]. However, this simplistic theory is not supported due to the observation of a parallel increase in the prevalence of Th1 disorders such as inflammatory bowel disease and type-1 diabetes seen in these children. Thus, the current formulation of the hygiene hypothesis supports an increase in the prevalence of inflammatory T cell-mediated disease rather than only inflammatory Th2-mediated disease.

The use of TLR ligands such as CpG-ODN can mimic microbial exposure. Increasing amounts of experimental data suggest that administration of CpG-ODN is an effective intervention in animal models of allergic disorders and can even reverse the underlying Th2-biased immune-dysregulation [21,22]. Two distinct strategies for CpG-based therapy have been described, (1) vaccination and (2) immunomodulation (Fig. 1), both of which show promise in a variety of mouse models of allergic diseases [23–26]. Vaccination induces an adaptive immune response that is antigen (allergen) dependent (specific) with long-term duration, whereas immunomodulation results in an innate

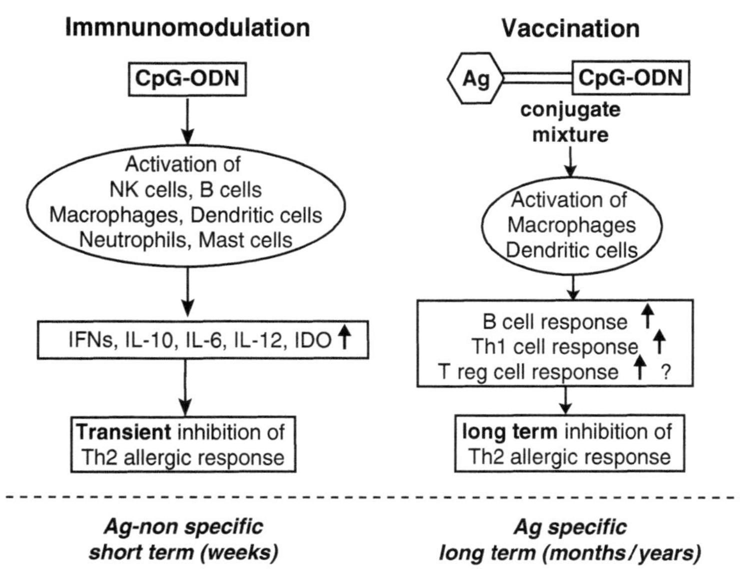

Fig. 1 The principles of CpG-ODN-based immunotherapy; immunomodulation and vaccination. Immunomodulation of allergic inflammation by CpG-ODN is independent of allergens and its effect is transient (up to 6 weeks). CpG-ODN-based vaccination therapy [40] is an allergen-specific therapy, which provides long-term inhibition of allergen-specific hypersensitivities

immune response that is antigen (allergen) independent (nonspecific) with short-term activity.

CpG-ODN Vaccination for Allergic Disease

The principal goal of a vaccination strategy against allergic disease is to elicit a protective and lasting immune response against a specific antigen/allergen. In the past, researchers have modified antigens to make them less allergenic and more immunogenic in order to prevent adverse reactions upon allergen injection, that is, allergen desensitization [27]. Allergen desensitization can be achieved with traditional allergen extracts (i.e., protein-based vaccination). However, this approach is accompanied by critical disadvantages such as the requirement of repeated injections for a long period and the risks of anaphylaxis and related side effects [28,29].

Two strategies were used to develop vaccines against allergens using CpG-ODN as an adjuvant; the injection of a CpG-ODN mixed with allergens, and the injection of allergen-CpG-ODN-conjugates (allergen-immunostimulatory-ODN-conjugate, AIC). Vaccination with allergens mixed or conjugated with CpG-ODN was shown to be effective in suppressing Th2-biased immune profiles and was accompanied by a Th1-biased immune deviation [24,30]. Physical linking of CpG-ODN to allergens dramatically improved the immunogenicity while reducing the allergenicity and the anaphylactogenicity of the related allergen as compared to allergen mixed with CpG-ODN [26,31,32]. The CpG-ODN in the conjugate facilitates antigen/allergen uptake, trafficking to the phagosome where it activates TLR9, and antigen/allergen processing [33]. Professional antigen-presenting cells (APC) thus undergo maturation and efficiently present antigen (allergen) to $CD4^+$ T cells [8]. In mice, the injection of CpG-ODN conjugated to the major short ragweed allergen, Amba1 (the allergen responsible for hay fever), induced IFNγ-producing $CD4^+$ T cells and a higher titer of Amba1-specific IgG2α as compared to Amba1 mixed with CpG-ODN. Furthermore, administration of this AIC to mice sensitized to Amba1 inhibited their preexisting Th2 response, induced a Th1 response (i.e., increased IgG2α and IFNγ production), and decreased IgE and IL-5 production [34]. The AIC was less allergenic than naive protein because the bound ODNs sterically prevented antigen recognition by specific IgE [30,32,34]. Furthermore, AIC preparations resulted in enhanced allergen uptake [35,36] and presentation. Indeed, recent data from a clinical trial with CpG-ODN conjugated to Amba1 (TOLAMBA™) demonstrated significant symptom relief and suppression of the allergic response in patients with allergic rhinitis (AR) [37–40]. This AIC led to a shift from Th2 immunity toward Th1 immunity and appeared to be safe [41]. In addition, this AIC exhibited significantly fewer local reactions upon intradermal skin injection as compared to standardized aqueous ragweed [40,42]. Taken together, AICs demonstrated higher immunogenic and therapeutic efficacy and improved safety as compared to the conventional allergen vaccination (desensitization) approach.

CpG-ODN-Based Immunomodulation

CpG-ODN Suppresses Experimental Asthma

The inflammatory response in allergic asthma is characterized by cellular infiltration of the airways with eosinophils and T lymphocytes [43,44]. A large number of therapies are currently available for the treatment of allergic asthma; corticosteroids for the reversal of allergic inflammation, antihistamines and leukotriene inhibitors for the attenuation of pathology associated with mast cells and eosinophils, and adrenergic receptor agonists for the reversal of bronchospasms [45–47]. However, none of these therapies have been shown to reverse the underlying hypersensitivities to allergens that perpetuate the allergic phenotype.

Immunomodulation by CpG-ODN is allergen-independent and can be delivered systemically [e.g., intraperitoneal (i.p.) injection] or mucosally [i.e., intranasal (i.n.) inoculation] thereby providing rapid protection against experimental asthma upon allergen challenge in sensitized mice [23,25,48]. Administration of CpG-ODN before allergen challenge significantly inhibited both the early and late phases of the asthma reaction, for example, airway hyperresponsiveness (AHR) to inhaled methacholine (MCh) [23,25,48], eosinophilia in bronchoalveolar lavage fluid (BALF), and IgE levels in the serum [49]. CpG-ODN also inhibits IL-4 dependent IgE synthesis by B cells in vitro [50,51]. Administration of CpG-ODN not only inhibited eosinophil infiltration into the airways and lung parenchyma, but also significantly inhibited blood and bone marrow eosinophilia. The inhibition of asthmatic parameters (e.g., AHR) by CpG-ODN was associated with a significant inhibition of Th2 cytokine production (e.g., IL-5) and the induction of allergen-specific IFNγ production. Antibody neutralization studies have shown that the inhibitory effect of CpG-ODN on AHR and Th2 cytokine secretion was mainly mediated by innate cytokines (IFNs and IL-12) secreted by CpG-ODN-activated monocytes/macrophages and NK cells. The reduction of tissue eosinophils by CpG-ODN was immediate and continued for several weeks. In addition, CpG-ODN administration was effective in inhibiting eosinophilic airway inflammation when administered either systemically (i.p.) or mucosally (intranasally) [52–54].

Administration of CpG-ODN after allergen challenge also promotes the resolution of airway inflammation at a level similar to that seen with the glucocorticoid dexamethasone (DXM) [55], a standard therapy for allergic asthma. Mice that had already developed significant levels of eosinophilic airway inflammation did not develop AHR when given either CpG-ODN or DXM [55]. The combined administration of CpG-ODN and DXM was more effective in inhibiting AHR than the administration of either CpG-ODN or DXM alone. Both CpG-ODN and DXM significantly reduced eosinophil infiltration and the levels of Th2 cytokines (i.e., IL-5) in BALF, as well as the number of mucus-producing airway epithelial cells. However, administration of CpG-ODN induced a significant level of IFNγ in BALF whereas DXM did not [55]. Thus, administration of CpG-ODN is as effective as DXM and the administration of both is synergistic in the prevention and reversal of inflammation in experimental asthma.

CpG-ODN Inhibits Airway Remodeling

Allergic asthma is characterized by chronic inflammation followed by airway remodeling. This process results in subepithelial fibrosis, increased smooth muscle mass, and increased in mucous glands [56]. Mice in which chronic experimental asthma was induced developed these features as well as sustained eosinophilic airway inflammation and AHR to MCh. Systemic administration of CpG-ODN significantly inhibited the development of AHR, eosinophilic inflammation, airway mucus production, and most importantly, airway remodeling [57–60]. In addition, CpG-ODN significantly reduced the level of the profibrotic cytokine, transforming growth factor β (TGFβ), in BALF and the lungs [57]. These studies demonstrate that the administration of CpG-ODN prevents not only the Th2-mediated airway inflammation in response to acute allergen challenge but also the consequent airway remodeling associated with chronic allergen exposure.

Administration of CpG-ODN can also reverse established airway remodeling. Its administration to mice with established airway remodeling significantly reduced the degree of airway collagen deposition [61,62]. These findings were accompanied by a reduction in the levels of Th2 attracting chemokines, the number of peribronchial Th2 lymphocytes, and the levels of Th2 cytokines that promote peribronchial fibrosis [57,61].

The inhibitory effect of CpG-ODN in AHR and remodeling was further demonstrated in a primate model of allergic disease [63] using rhesus monkeys, where allergic asthma was induced with house dust mite allergens. The asthmatic monkeys received inhaled CpG-ODN biweekly over a 6 week period. AHR and eosinophil infiltration were reduced twofold in monkeys treated with inhaled CpG-ODN compared to those that were sham-treated. Airways from monkeys treated with CpG-ODN had thinner reticular basement membranes, fewer mucous goblet cells, fewer eosinophils, and fewer mast cells than sham-treated allergic monkeys [63]. These findings indicate that biweekly inhaled CpG-ODN is able to attenuate the magnitude of AHR and airway remodeling seen in a nonhuman primate model of allergic asthma that shares immunopathological mechanisms similar to those in humans.

Airway remodeling in asthma is also associated with increased vascularity and peribronchial angiogenesis. Administration of CpG-ODN before repetitive allergen challenge significantly reduced the levels of peribronchial angiogenesis as well as the levels of bronchoalveolar lavage vascular endothelial growth factor (VEGF) and the number of peribronchial cells expressing VEGF. This effect by CpG-ODN further suppressed the consequences of airway remodeling on lung function [60].

CpG-ODN Inhibits Experimental Allergic Rhinitis

Allergen-sensitized mice that received CpG-ODN had attenuated immediate and late phase responses to intranasal allergen challenge. Specifically, mice given CpG-ODN had less histamine and cysteinyl leukotriene release, and less eosinophilic inflammation in their nasal passages. In addition, splenocytes from mice that received CpG-ODN displayed attenuated allergen-specific IL-4, IL-5, and IL-13 but increased IFNγ secretion [64,65]. Thus, systemic or local delivery of CpG-ODN attenuates both the immediate and the late phase responses in an experimental AR model.

CpG-ODN Inhibits Experimental Allergic Conjunctivitis (AC)

Short ragweed (RW) is the major cause of late summer AC in North America. Magone and colleagues have investigated the ability of CpG-ODN to modulate allergic responses in an RW-induced mouse model of seasonal AC [66]. Systemic or mucosal administration of CpG-ODN before or simultaneously with RW challenge inhibited both the immediate hypersensitivity and late phase responses in the conjunctiva. Furthermore, CpG-ODN administration significantly suppressed the development of RW-specific IgE titers after repeated allergen challenge and improved the clinical symptoms of AC to the same degree observed for DXM.

CpG-ODN Inhibits Atopic Dermatitis

Atopic dermatitis (AD) is a Th2 dominant chronic inflammatory skin disorder associated with elevated levels of serum IgE, infiltration of mast cells and eosinophils, and enhanced expression of Th2 cytokines [67]. An inbred mouse strain, NC/Nga, displays typical AD skin lesions under conventional housing conditions that resembles human AD. Inoue and Aramaki demonstrated that transdermal application of CpG-ODN remarkably reduced the cell infiltration of mast cells/macrophages in the skin of these mice, and converted their immune response from a Th2 phenotype to a Th1 phenotype as demonstrated by cytokine mRNA and serum Ab levels [68]. This intervention also generated regulatory T cells in the skin lesions [68].

Induction of Indoleamine 2,3-Dioxygenase

Initially, the redirection of an allergen-specific Th2 response toward a Th1 response by CpG-ODN was hypothesized to mediate its immunomodulatory activities [23,66]. Recently, it was found that indoleamine 2,3-dioxygenase (IDO), the rate-limiting tryptophan (trp) catabolizing enzyme, is induced in the lungs by CpG-ODN and suppresses Th2 driven allergic asthma [69]. IDO is induced by CpG-ODN as well as some other TLR ligands [70–72]. IDO expression is enhanced by IL-10 but suppressed by IL-4 and IL-13 [73] and is expressed in various cell types including fibroblasts, macrophages, dendritic cells (DC), and epithelial cells [74,75]. IFNγ induced by CpG-ODN amplifies IDO enzymatic activity in the bronchial epithelial cells. The inhibition of IDO activity by a specific inhibitor 1-methyl-DL-tryptophan (M-trp) reversed the immunomodulatory effects of CpG-ODN in experimental asthma as was demonstrated by an increase in AHR, eosinophilic infiltration, and in the levels of IL-5 and IL-13 in the BALF. It was observed that IDO induction by the administration of CpG-ODN reduces the survival of allergen-specific Th2 cells and, consequently, Th2 cytokine production using an adoptive transfer model where Th2 cells are transferred into SCID mice [69]. These data indicate that IDO induced by CpG-ODN mediates its immunomodulatory effects by inducing the death of effector Th2 cells, rather than by inducing a Th1 or regulatory T cell response. Among the TLR ligands tested in this study only CpG-ODN and LPS (a TLR4 ligand) could inhibit experimental asthma. These results correlate with the induction of IDO enzymatic activities by these TLR ligands [69].

Inhibition of the Th2 Phenotype Spread

Epidemiological evidence indicates that the key events contributing to the development of allergic asthma occur in early childhood [76–78]. An accelerated generation of Th2 memory responses against various aeroallergens also occurs during these early years [79–81]. Host genetic and environmental factors are considered critical to the development of asthma [81]. Preexisting Th2/asthmatic responses in early childhood can promote another Th2 response to newly encountered allergens (i.e., Th2 phenotype spread). A recent study documented that administration of CpG-ODN inhibited the production of chemokines involved in the homing of naive $CD4^+$ T and Th2 cells to the bronchial lymph nodes, resulting in the abrogation of the subsequent development of a Th2 phenotype spread, and suggesting that CpG-ODN may be effective in reducing the spread of allergen reactivity (i.e., allergic march) in atopic subjects [79].

Summary and Conclusion

Accumulated experimental data outline the use of CpG-ODN as an effective intervention for the prevention and treatment of allergic disorders. CpG-ODN can be utilized for two distinct interventions, (1) vaccination and (2) immunomodulation (Fig. 1). CpG-ODN-based vaccination provides long-term, allergen specific, therapeutic efficacy as well as improved safety compared to conventional allergen vaccination. Immunomodulation by CpG-ODN provides a short-term, allergen nonspecific therapeutic efficacy. CpG-ODN may intervene in the sequential development of allergic immunopathology (e.g., Th2 phenotype spread, airway remodeling). Because the beneficial effects of CpG-based immunotherapy, that is, vaccination or immunomodulation, are different from each other, we propose that these two therapeutic strategies could be used to complement each other for the treatment of allergic disorders.

Acknowledgments This work is supported by NIH grants AI57709, AI40682, and HL79449.

References

1. Takeda K, Kaisho T, Akira S (2003) Toll-like receptors. *Annual Review Immunology* 21:335–376
2. Ishii KJ, Akira S (2006) Innate immune recognition of, and regulation by, DNA. *Trends in Immunology* 27:525–532
3. Takeda K, Akira S (2005) Toll-like receptors in innate immunity. *International Immunology* 17:1–14
4. Ishii KJ, Uematsu S, Akira S (2006) 'Toll' gates for future immunotherapy. *Current Pharmaceutical Design* 12:4135–4142
5. Tokunaga T, Yamamoto H, Shimada S, et al (1984) Antitumor activity of deoxyribonucleic acid fraction from Mycobacterium bovis BCG. I. Isolation, physicochemical characterization, and antitumor activity. *Journal of the National Cancer Institute* 72:955–962
6. Yamamoto S, Kuramoto E, Shimada S, et al (1988) In vitro augmentation of natural killer cell activity and production of interferon-alpha/beta and -gamma with deoxyribonucleic acid fraction from Mycobacterium bovis BCG. *Japanese Journal of Cancer Research* 79:866–873
7. Tokunaga T, Yano O, Kuramoto E, et al (1992) Synthetic oligonucleotides with particular base sequences from the cDNA encoding proteins of Mycobacterium bovis BCG induce interferons and activate natural killer cells. *Microbiology and Immunology* 36:55–66
8. Kaisho T, Akira S (2006) Toll-like receptor function and signaling. *Journal of Allergy and Clinical Immunology* 117:979–987
9. Hemmi H, Takeuchi O, Kawai T, et al (2000) A toll-like receptor recognizes bacterial DNA. *Nature* 408:740–745
10. Hayashi F, Means TK, Luster AD (2003) Toll-like receptors stimulate human neutrophil function. *Blood* 102:2660–2669
11. Lee J, Mo JH, Katakura K, et al (2006) Maintenance of colonic homeostasis by distinctive apical TLR9 signalling in intestinal epithelial cells. *Nature Cell Biology* 8:1327–1336
12. Krieg AM, Yi AK, Matson S, et al (1995) CpG motifs in bacterial DNA trigger direct B-cell activation. *Nature* 374:546–549
13. Klinman DM, Yi AK, Beaucage SL, et al (1996) CpG motifs present in bacteria DNA rapidly induce lymphocytes to secrete interleukin 6, interleukin 12, and interferon gamma. *Proceedings of the National Academy of Sciences of the United States of America* 93:2879–2883
14. Van Uden J, Raz E (2000) Introduction to immunostimulatory DNA sequences. *Springer Seminars in Immunopathology* 22:1–9
15. Roman M, Martin-Orozco E, Goodman JS, et al (1997) Immunostimulatory DNA sequences function as T helper-1-promoting adjuvants [see comments]. *Nature Medicine* 3:849–854
16. Krieg AM (2002) CpG motifs in bacterial DNA and their immune effects. *Annual Review Immunology* 20:709–760
17. Klaschik S, Gursel I, Klinman DM (2007) CpG-mediated changes in gene expression in murine spleen cells identified by microarray analysis. *Molecular Immunology* 44:1095–1104

18. Howarth PH (1998) Is allergy increasing? – early life influences. *Clinical and Experimental Allergy* 28(Suppl 6):2–7
19. Wills-Karp M, Santeliz J, Karp CL (2001) The germless theory of allergic disease: revisiting the hygiene hypothesis. *Nature Reviews. Immunology* 1:69–75
20. Schaub B, Lauener R, von Mutius E (2006) The many faces of the hygiene hypothesis. *Journal of Allergy and Clinical Immunology* 117:969–977; quiz 978
21. Horner AA, Raz E (2002) Immunostimulatory sequence oligodeoxynucleotide-based vaccination and immunomodulation: two unique but complementary strategies for the treatment of allergic diseases. *Journal of Allergy and Clinical Immunology* 110:706–712
22. Hussain I, Kline JN (2003) CpG oligodeoxynucleotides: a novel therapeutic approach for atopic disorders. *Current Drug Targets Inflammation and Allergy* 2:199–205
23. Broide D, Schwarze J, Tighe H, et al (1998) Immunostimulatory DNA sequences inhibit IL-5, eosinophilic inflammation, and airway hyperresponsiveness in mice. *Journal of Immunology* 161:7054–7062
24. Kline JN, Waldschmidt TJ, Businga TR, et al (1998) Modulation of airway inflammation by CpG oligodeoxynucleotides in a murine model of asthma. *Journal of Immunology* 160:2555–2559
25. Sur S, Wild JS, Choudhury BK, Sur N, Alam R, Klinman DM (1999) Long term prevention of allergic lung inflammation in a mouse model of asthma by CpG oligodeoxynucleotides. *Journal of Immunology* 162:6284–6293
26. Tighe H, Takabayashi K, Schwartz D, Marsden R, Beck L, Corbeil J, Richman DD, Eiden Jr. JJ, Spiegelberg HL, Raz E (2000) Conjugation of protein to immunostimulatory DNA results in a rapid, long-lasting and potent induction of cell-mediated and humoral immunity. *European Journal of Immunology* 30:1939–1947
27. Bousquet J, Lockey R, Malling HJ (1998) Allergen immunotherapy: therapeutic vaccines for allergic diseases. A WHO position paper. *The Journal of Allergy and Clinical Immunology* 102:558–562
28. Nelson HS, Lahr J, Rule R, Bock A, Leung D (1997) Treatment of anaphylactic sensitivity to peanuts by immunotherapy with injections of aqueous peanut extract. *Journal of Allergy and Clinical Immunology* 99:744–751
29. Creticos PS, Reed CE, Norman PS, Khoury J, Adkinson Jr. NF, Buncher CR, Busse WW, Bush RK, Gadde J, Li JT, et al (1996) Ragweed immunotherapy in adult asthma. *The New England Journal of Medicine* 334:501–506
30. Horner AA, Nguyen MD, Ronaghy A, Cinman N, Verbeek S, Raz E (2000) DNA-based vaccination reduces the risk of lethal anaphylactic hypersensitivity in mice. *Journal of Allergy and Clinical Immunology* 106:349–356
31. Horner AA, Datta SK, Takabayashi K, Belyakov IM, Hayashi T, Cinman N, Nguyen MD, Van Uden JH, Berzofsky JH, Richman DD, Raz E (2001) Immunostimulatory DNA-based vaccines elicit multifaceted immune responses against HIV at systemic and mucosal sites. *Journal of Immunology* 167:1584–1591
32. Horner AA, Takabayashi K, Beck L, Sharma B, Zubeldia J, Baird S, Tuck S, Libet L, Spiegelberg HL, Liu FT, Raz E (2002) Optimized conjugation ratios lead to allergen immunostimulatory oligodeoxynucleotide conjugates with retained immunogenicity and minimal anaphylactogenicity. *Journal of Allergy and Clinical Immunology* 110:413–420
33. Datta SK, Redecke V, Prilliman KR, Takabayashi K, Corr M, Tallant T, DiDonato J, Dziarski R, Akira S, Schoenberger SP, Raz E (2003) A subset of toll-like receptor ligands induces cross-presentation by bone marrow-derived dendritic cells. *Journal of Immunology* 170: 4102–4110
34. Tighe H, Takabayashi K, Schwartz D, Van Nest G, Tuck S, Eiden JJ, Kagey-Sobotka A, Creticos PS, Lichtenstein LM, Spiegelberg HL, Raz E (2000) Conjugation of immunostimulatory DNA to the short ragweed allergen amb a 1 enhances its immunogenicity and reduces its allergenicity. *Journal of Allergy and Clinical Immunology* 106:124–134
35. Datta SK, Cho HJ, Takabayashi K, Horner AA, Raz E (2004) Antigen-immunostimulatory oligonucleotide conjugates: mechanisms and applications. *Immunological Reviews* 199:217–226

36. Shirota H, Sano K, Hirasawa N, Terui T, Ohuchi K, Hattori T, Shirato K, Tamura G (2001) Novel roles of CpG oligodeoxynucleotides as a leader for the sampling and presentation of CpG-tagged antigen by dendritic cells. *Journal of Immunology* 167:66–74
37. Creticos PS (2001) The consideration of immunotherapy in the treatment of allergic asthma. *Annals of Allergy, Asthma & Immunology* 87:13–27
38. Tulic MK, Fiset PO, Christodoulopoulos P, Vaillancourt P, Desrosiers M, Lavigne F, Eiden J, Hamid Q (2004) Amb a 1-immunostimulatory oligodeoxynucleotide conjugate immunotherapy decreases the nasal inflammatory response. *Journal of Allergy and Clinical Immunology* 113:235–241
39. Creticos PS, Chen YH, Schroeder JT (2004) New approaches in immunotherapy: allergen vaccination with immunostimulatory DNA. *Immunology and Allergy Clinics of North America* 24:569–581
40. Creticos PS, Schroeder JT, Hamilton RG, Balcer-Whaley SL, Khattignavong AP, Lindblad R, Li H, Coffman R, Seyfert V, Eiden JJ, Broide D (2006) Immunotherapy with a ragweed-toll-like receptor 9 agonist vaccine for allergic rhinitis. *The New England Journal of Medicine* 355:1445–1455
41. Simons FE, Shikishima Y, Van Nest G, Eiden JJ, HayGlass KT (2004) Selective immune redirection in humans with ragweed allergy by injecting Amb a 1 linked to immunostimulatory DNA. *Journal of Allergy and Clinical Immunology* 113:1144–1151
42. Creticos PS, Lichtenstein LM (2003) Progress in the development of new methods of immunotherapy: potential application of immunostimulatory DNA-conjugated to allergens for treatment of allergic respiratory conditions. *Arbeiten aus them Paul-Ehrlich-Institut (Bundesamt fur Sera und Impfstoffe) zu Frankfurt A M*:304–312; discussion 312–303
43. Drazen JM, Arm JP, Austen KF (1996) Sorting out the cytokines of asthma. *Journal of Experimental Medicine* 183:1–5
44. Robinson DS, Hamid Q, Ying S Tsicopoulos A, Barkans J, Bentley AM, Corrigan C, Durham SR, Kay AB (1992) Predominant TH2-like bronchoalveolar T-lymphocyte population in atopic asthma. *The New England Journal of Medicine* 326:298–304
45. Graham LM (2002) Balancing safety and efficacy in the treatment of pediatric asthma. *Journal of Allergy and Clinical Immunology* 109:S560–S566
46. Pullerits T, Praks L, Ristioja V, Lotvall J (2002) Comparison of a nasal glucocorticoid, antileukotriene, and a combination of antileukotriene and antihistamine in the treatment of seasonal allergic rhinitis. *Journal of Allergy and Clinical Immunology* 109:949–955
47. Apter AJ, Szefler SJ (2006) Advances in adult and pediatric asthma. *Journal of Allergy and Clinical Immunology* 117:512–518
48. Serebrisky D, Teper AA, Huang CK, Lee SY, Zhang TF, Schofield BH, Kattan M, Sampson HA, Li XM (2000) CpG oligodeoxynucleotides can reverse Th2-associated allergic airway responses and alter the B7.1/B7.2 expression in a murine model of asthma. *Journal of Immunology* 165:5906–5912
49. Broide DH, Stachnick G, Castaneda D, Nayar J, Miller M, Cho JY, Roman M, Zubeldia J, Hayashi T, Raz E (2001) Systemic administration of immunostimulatory DNA sequences mediates reversible inhibition of Th2 responses in a mouse model of asthma. *Journal of Clinical Immunology* 21:175–182
50. Horner AA, Widhopf GF, Burger JA, Takabayashi K, Cinman N, Ronaghy A, Spiegelberg HL, Raz E (2001) Immunostimulatory DNA inhibits IL-4-dependent IgE synthesis by human B cells. *Journal of Allergy and Clinical Immunology* 108:417–423
51. Lin L, Gerth AJ, Peng SL (2004) CpG DNA redirects class-switching towards "Th1-like" Ig isotype production via TLR9 and MyD88. *European Journal of Immunology* 34: 1483–1487
52. Horner AA, Raz E (2000) Immunostimulatory sequence oligodeoxynucleotide: a novel mucosal adjuvant. *Clinical Immunology* 95:S19–S29
53. Takabayashi K, Libet L, Chisholm D, Zubeldia J, Horner AA (2003) Intranasal immunotherapy is more effective than intradermal immunotherapy for the induction of airway allergen tolerance in Th2-sensitized mice. *Journal of Immunology* 170:3898–3905

54. Kitagaki K, Businga TR, Kline JN (2006) Oral administration of CpG-ODNs suppresses antigen-induced asthma in mice. *Clinical and Experimental Immunology* 143:249–259
55. Ikeda RK, Nayar J, Cho JY, Miller M, Rodriguez M, Raz E, Broide DH (2003) Resolution of airway inflammation following ovalbumin inhalation: comparison of ISS DNA and corticosteroids. *American Journal of Respiratory Cell and Molecular Biology* 28:655–663
56. Elias JA, Zhu Z, Chupp G, Homer RJ (1999) Airway remodeling in asthma. *Journal of Clinical Investigation* 104:1001–1006
57. Cho JY, Miller M, Baek KJ, Han JW, Nayar J, Rodriguez M, Lee SY, McElwain K, McElwain S, Raz E, Broide DH (2004) Immunostimulatory DNA inhibits transforming growth factor-{beta} expression and airway remodeling. *American Journal of Respiratory Cell and Molecular Biology* 30:651–661
58. Jain VV, Businga TR, Kitagaki K, George CL, O'Shaughnessy PT, Kline JN (2003) Mucosal immunotherapy with CpG oligodeoxynucleotides reverses a murine model of chronic asthma induced by repeated antigen exposure. *American Journal of Physiology. Lung cellular and Molecular Physiology* 285:L1137–L1146
59. Banerjee B, Kelly KJ, Fink JN, Henderson Jr. JD, Bansal NK, Kurup VP (2004) Modulation of airway inflammation by immunostimulatory CpG oligodeoxynucleotides in a murine model of allergic aspergillosis. *Infection and Immunity* 72:6087–6094
60. Lee SY, Cho JY, Miller M, McElwain K, McElwain S, Sriramarao P, Raz E, Broide DH (2006) Immunostimulatory DNA inhibits allergen-induced peribronchial angiogenesis in mice. *Journal of Allergy and Clinical Immunology* 117:597–603
61. Youn CJ, Miller M, Baek KJ, Han JW, Nayar J, Lee SY, McElwain K, McElwain S, Raz E, Broide DH (2004) Immunostimulatory DNA reverses established allergen-induced airway remodeling. *Journal of Immunology* 173:7556–7564
62. Broide D (2004) Immunomodulation and reversal of airway remodeling in asthma. *Current Opinion in Allergy and Clinical Immunology* 4:529–532
63. Fanucchi MV, Schelegle ES, Baker GL, Evans MJ, McDonald RJ, Gershwin LJ, Raz E, Hyde DM, Plopper CG, Miller LA (2004) Immunostimulatory oligonucleotides attenuate airways remodelling in allergic monkeys. *American Journal of Respiratory Cell and Molecular Biology* 170:1153
64. Rhee CS, Libet L, Chisholm D, Takabayashi K, Baird S, Bigby TD, Lee CH, Horner AA, Raz E (2004) Allergen-independent immunostimulatory sequence oligodeoxynucleotide therapy attenuates experimental allergic rhinitis. *Immunology* 113:106–113
65. Hussain I, Jain VV, Kitagaki K, Businga TR, O'Shaughnessy P, Kline JN (2002) Modulation of murine allergic rhinosinusitis by CpG oligodeoxynucleotides. *Laryngoscope* 112: 1819–1826
66. Magone MT, Chan CC, Beck L, Whitcup SM, Raz E (2000) Systemic or mucosal administration of immunostimulatory DNA inhibits early and late phases of murine allergic conjunctivitis. *European Journal of Immunology* 30:1841–1850
67. Rudikoff D, Lebwohl M (1998) Atopic dermatitis. *Lancet* 351:1715–1721
68. Inoue J, Aramaki Y (2007) Suppression of skin lesions by transdermal application of CpG-oligodeoxynucleotides in NC/Nga mice, a model of human atopic dermatitis. *Journal of Immunology* 178:584–591
69. Hayashi T, Beck L, Rossetto C, Gong X, Takikawa O, Takabayashi K, Broide DH, Carson DA, Raz E (2004) Inhibition of experimental asthma by indoleamine 2,3-dioxygenase. *Journal of Clinical Investigation* 114:270–279
70. Hissong BD, Byrne GI, Padilla ML, Carlin JM (1995) Upregulation of interferon-induced indoleamine 2,3-dioxygenase in human macrophage cultures by lipopolysaccharide, muramyl tripeptide, and interleukin-1. *Cellular Immunology* 160:264–269
71. Hayashi T, Rao SP, Takabayashi K, Van Uden JH, Kornbluth RS, Baird SM, Taylor MW, Carson DA, Catanzaro A, Raz E (2001) Enhancement of innate immunity against Mycobacterium avium infection by immunostimulatory DNA is mediated by indoleamine 2,3-dioxygenase. *Infection and Immunity* 69:6156–6164

72. Mahanonda R, Sa-Ard-Iam N, Montreekachon P, Pimkhaokham A, Yongvanichit K, Fukuda MM, Pichyangkul S (2007) IL-8 and IDO expression by human gingival fibroblasts via TLRs. *Journal of Immunology* 178:1151–1157
73. Grohmann U, Orabona C, Fallarino F, Vacca C, Calcinaro F, Falorni A, Candeloro P, Belladonna ML, Bianchi R, Fioretti MC, Puccetti P (2002) CTLA-4-Ig regulates tryptophan catabolism in vivo. *Nature Immunology* 3:1097–1101
74. Mellor AL, Munn DH (2001) Extinguishing maternal immune responses during pregnancy: implications for immunosuppression. *Seminars in Immunology* 13:213–218
75. Babcock TA, Carlin JM (2000) Transcriptional activation of indoleamine dioxygenase by interleukin 1 and tumor necrosis factor alpha in interferon-treated epithelial cells. *Cytokine* 12:588–594
76. Taussig LM, Wright AL, Holberg CJ, Halonen M, Morgan WJ, Martinez FD (2003) Tucson Children's Respiratory Study: 1980 to present. *Journal of Allergy and Clinical Immunology* 111:661–675; quiz 676
77. Sears MR, Greene JM, Willan AR, Wiecek EM, Taylor DR, Flannery EM, Cowan JO, Herbison GP, Silva PA, Poulton R (2003) A longitudinal, population-based, cohort study of childhood asthma followed to adulthood. *The New England Journal of Medicine* 349:1414–1422
78. Martinez FD (2003) Toward asthma prevention – does all that really matters happen before we learn to read? *The New England Journal of Medicine* 349:1473–1475
79. Fasce L, Tosca MA, Olcese R, Milanese M, Erba R, Ciprandi G (2004) The natural history of allergy: the development of new sensitizations in asthmatic children. *Immunology Letters* 93:45–50
80. Holt PG, Sly PD, Martinez FD, Weiss ST, Bjorksten B, von Mutius E, Wahn U (2004) Drug development strategies for asthma: in search of a new paradigm. *Nature Immunology* 5:695–698
81. Reed CE (2006) The natural history of asthma. *Journal of Allergy and Clinical Immunology* 118:543–548

Peptide-Based Therapeutic Vaccines for Allergic Diseases: Where Do We Stand?

Hardeep S. Asi and Mark Larché

Introduction: Immunological Homeostasis and Regulatory T cells in Allergy

Immunoglobulin (Ig) E-associated allergic conditions, such as asthma, currently affect more than 25% of individuals in developed nations [1]. These conditions arise when the mechanisms controlling the immune response to innocuous environmental allergens fail, manifesting in hypersensitivity. The equilibrium that is established between T helper (T_H) 2 effector cells on the one hand, and allergen-specific T regulatory cells together with T_H1 effector cells on the other, is central in determining whether hypersensitivity or a healthy immune response develops [2]. Both healthy and allergic individuals possess a range of T cell subsets including T_H1, T_H2 and T regulatory 1 (T_R1) cells, however, the proportions vary (Fig. 1). In healthy individuals, responses to allergen are dominated by T_R1 cells and T_H1 cells, whereas the same response is dominated by allergen-specific T_H2 cells in allergic individuals. Consequently, therapies such as allergen immunotherapy (with natural extracts, recombinant proteins or peptides) that skew the dominant subset in favour of regulatory and T_H1 responses are disease-modifying, and the duration of their action markedly exceeds the treatment period. Furthermore, immunotherapy prevents the development of new sensitizations to different allergens [3] and the progression of allergic rhinitis to asthma [4] which may be attributable to the reconstitution of the T_R1 population.

In addition to the route of exposure and allergen dose, susceptibility to allergic disease is influenced by both genetic and environmental factors [5]. Multiple interactions between genes and also between genes and environmental factors may determine the allergic phenotype. Moreover, the recent increase in the prevalence

H.S. Asi and M. Larché (✉)
Division of Clinical Immunology and Allergy, Department of Medicine, Faculty of Health Sciences, McMaster University, 1200 Main Street West, Hamilton, ON, L8N 3Z5, Canada
e-mail: larche@mcmaster.ca

R. Pawankar et al. (eds.), *Allergy Frontiers: Future Perspectives*,
DOI 10.1007/978-4-431-99365-0_6, © Springer 2010

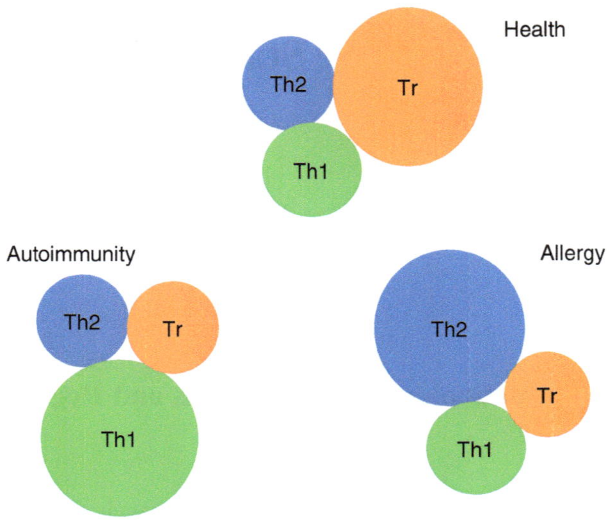

Fig. 1 The delicate balance between T cell subsets. In allergic individuals, the response to common environmental allergens is dominated by allergen-specific T helper 2 (T_H2) cells, which mediate allergy. In healthy individuals, this same response is controlled by T regulatory 1 (T_R1) cells with immunoregulatory capability. Allergen-specific immunotherapy (SIT) modifies the allergic response and skews it towards a regulatory dominated response, thus mimicking the natural response to allergen in healthy individuals.

of allergic conditions in industrialized regions of the world provides further support to the influence of environmental factors in the pathogenesis of allergic diseases. The widespread use of antibiotics, implementation of vaccination programs, and improvement of sanitation in industrialized nations has led to reduced immunological interaction with the infectious organisms with which we have co-evolved [6]. It is hypothesized that this declining exposure results in skewing to T_H2 dominated responses and thus, increased prevalence of hypersensitivity. However, this hypothesis does not explain a simultaneous increase in the prevalence of T_H1-mediated autoimmune disorders [7]. It is most likely that the increase in both T_H1- and T_H2-mediated diseases is a result of immunological dysfunction common to both types of disorder. This is further supported by the observation that simple mutual antagonism between T_H1 and T_H2 responses results in increased disease severity, indicating that T_H1/T_H2 balance is not the core problem [8]. Resolution of allergic disease appears to be associated with increased numbers of regulatory T cells [9]. Furthermore, allergic rhinitis has been associated with defective function of regulatory T cells [10]. Individuals with allergic sensitization to aeroallergens and food allergens have been shown to have a reduced frequency of IL-10 secreting allergen-specific cells with regulatory function [2]. Thus, defective immunoregulation, particularly through compromised regulatory T cell function, may be common to both allergic and autoimmune diseases.

Allergen-Specific Immunotherapy

A significant body of evidence is accumulating which indicates that the dysfunction in immunoregulation in allergic conditions is reversible [11]. Allergic children have demonstrated the ability to "grow out" of their allergies [9], natural exposure to allergens can redirect the allergen-specific immune response and reinstate homeostasis [12], and allergen immunotherapy has been shown to do the same [13] (Fig. 2). Specifically, allergen immunotherapy is of proven efficacy in modifying the outcome of disease and is associated with the induction of regulatory T cell responses [14]. Allergen-specific immunotherapy employs repetitive administration of the sensitizing allergen through subcutaneous injection or the sublingual route. Immunotherapy effectively prevents the onset of further sensitizations to allergen [3] and reduces the chance of developing asthma in patients with allergic rhinitis [4]. Immunotherapy is able to modify diseases through the reduction of seasonal increases in allergen-specific IgE [15]. Furthermore, nasal [16], conjunctival and skin [17] responses to allergen and late-phase responses to allergen in the skin or nasal mucosa are reduced.

Following immunotherapy, T_H2 responses in peripheral blood are reduced [17–19], and T_H1 responses are increased in tissues [17, 20]. Recent studies suggest that these responses occur together with a concomitant increase in the number of cells that produce IL-10, and in some reports transforming growth factor beta (TGF-β) [14, 21, 22]. These immunosuppressive cytokines have been identified in blood and tissue responses to allergen, following therapy [23–25]. This is further supported by the phenomenon that occurs when beekeepers are consistently re-exposed to allergen through recurrent stings. In this case, a mechanism involving IL-10 secreting cells is essential to protect beekeepers from subsequent allergic reactions, such as systemic anaphylaxis [26]. The increase in IL-10 and TGF-β also acts to modify B cell responses by suppressing IgE and inducing isotype switching to IgG4 (through IL-10) and IgA (through TGF-β) (49).

A major limitation of allergen immunotherapy is the incidence of adverse reactions to the treatment as a result of allergic reactions which can include life-threatening anaphylaxis. As a result, the dose of allergen administered is limited and the course of treatment protracted. A number of recent approaches aim to reduce the allergenicity of the treatment without compromising the immunomodulatory effects. One such approach is that of peptide immunotherapy in which short synthetic fragments of the allergen are administered. Peptides representing B cell epitopes of the allergen have not yet been evaluated in clinical studies and will not be considered further in this review. Approaches targeting T cell epitopes have been evaluated in clinical studies of both allergic and autoimmune diseases [27]. Those relevant studies are discussed below.

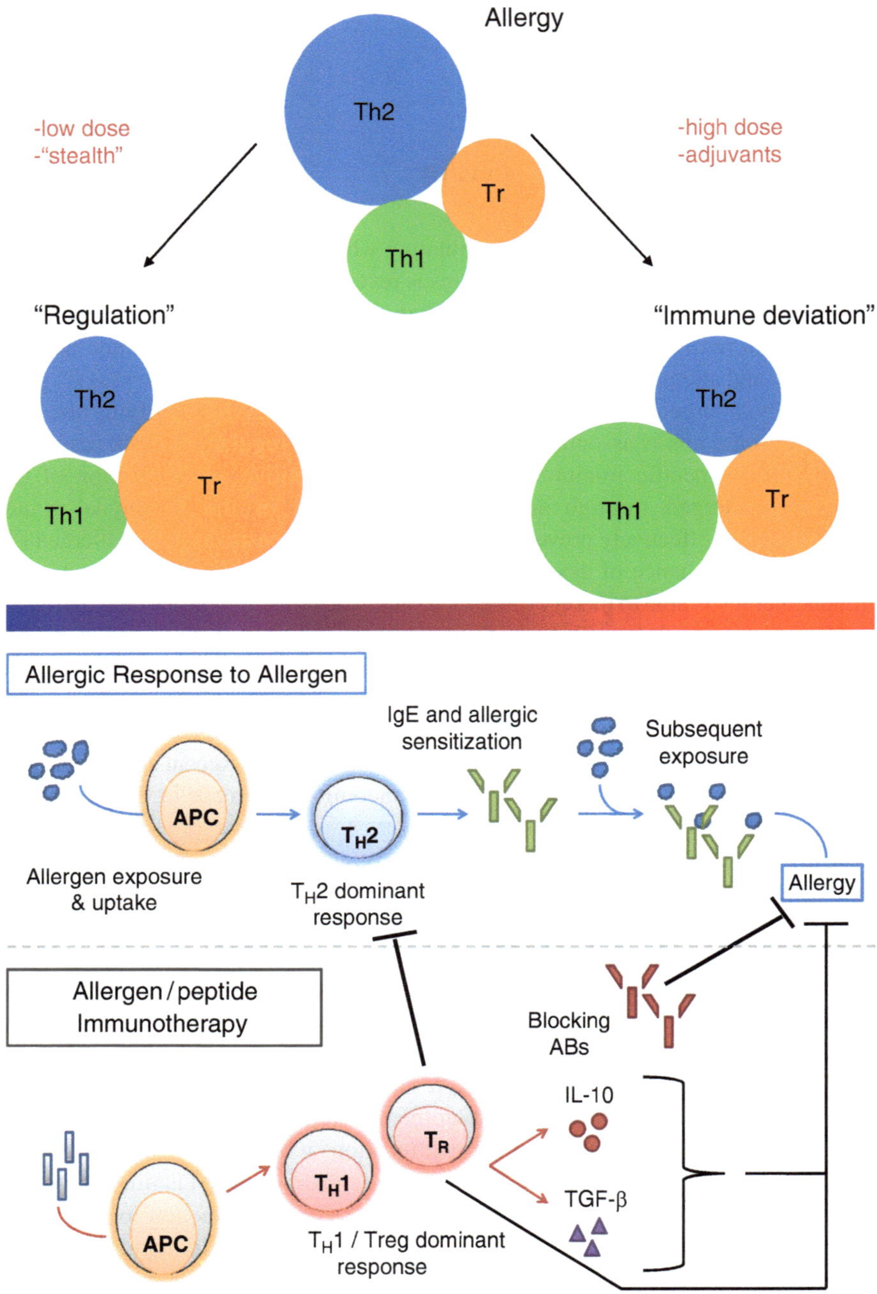

Fig. 2 Representation of the mechanisms of allergen-specific immunotherapy. Antigen presentation by antigen-presenting cells (APCs) to the naïve T cell population results in the differentiation and clonal expansion of T_H2 cells in allergic individuals (not shown). T_H2 cells produce various pro-allergic cytokines, such as interleukin (IL)-4 and IL-5, which cause immunoglobulin class

Peptide Immunotherapy

Peptide immunotherapy in both in vitro and in vivo experiments, has been shown to induce functional, antigen-specific tolerance. In vitro experiments demonstrated that peptides could induce antigen-specific hyporesponsiveness. Cultured T cell clones (in the absence of antigen-presenting cells (APCs) were incubated overnight with high doses of peptide resulting in transient (7 day) non-responsiveness [28]. Subsequently, prophylactic and therapeutic application of peptides in vivo has been evaluated in experimental models of allergy, autoimmunity and transplantation. In the clinic, peptides have been used to treat cat allergy and bee venom allergy.

Cat Allergy

The majority (greater than 90%) of individuals with a clinical history of cat allergy are sensitized (make allergen-specific IgE) to Fel d 1, the major cat allergen. Epitope mapping studies identified numerous T cell epitopes within the molecule [29, 30]. In early clinical studies, two long peptides (IPC-1 and IPC-2) covering a number of T cell epitopes were evaluated in clinical trials. Interestingly, not all T cell epitopes identified in the preceding epitope mapping studies were employed for therapy.

The efficacy of IPC-1/IPC-2 was first evaluated by Norman and his colleagues in a double-blind, placebo-controlled trial [31]. Four weekly subcutaneous injections of placebo or peptides at doses of 7.5, 75 or 750 μg were administered. Modest improvements in symptom and medication scores were observed in the highest dose group, 6 weeks after the treatment. Individual results were heterogeneous with some individuals experiencing marked improvements in symptoms and others not. Treatment was associated with a significant number of adverse events, including chest tightness, nasal congestion, urticaria, flushing and reactions with characteristics of anaphylaxis. These occurred minutes to hours after administration of the peptides. In an associated mechanistic study, a decrease in IL-4 production

Fig. 2 (continued) switching to the epsilon (ε) heavy chain and the production of immunoglobulin (Ig) E from B cells. IL-5 also aids in the activation and recruitment of eosinophils (Eo) from the bone marrow. The release of allergic mediators, in addition to the presence of a T_H2 cytokine milieu, mediates the allergic response. Immunotherapy results in the induction of a T helper 1 (T_H1)/regulatory T cell (T_R) phenotype, causing a skew away from allergen-specific T_H2 responses. Consequently, allergen-specific IgG antibodies form and are able to act as blocking antibodies, preventing the formation of IgE:allergen complexes which degranulate effector cells. IL-10 also possesses a wide range of immunosuppressive capability and is able to downregulate the allergic response. Regulatory T cells are capable of regulating both T_H1 and T_H2 mediated pathogenic responses. *Blue arrows*, response to allergen in allergic individual; *red arrows*, the immunological response to immunotherapy; *black arrows*, the inhibitory effect of regulatory T cells; *negative signs*, represent inhibition (but not proliferation) by peptide-specific T cell lines among subjects in the high group was demonstrated after treatment [32].

Clinical efficacy of the same preparation of peptides was investigated in an inhaled allergen challenge study. The provocative dose (PD_{20}) of allergen resulting in a 20% reduction of forced expiratory volume in one second (FEV_1) was measured before and after a variable cumulative dose of peptides [33]. After therapy, PD_{20} was not significantly different between the treated and placebo groups. However, in the higher dose groups, a significant increase in allergen tolerance between baseline and post-treatment days (statistically significant with the groups but not between treatment and placebo) was observed. IL-4 release was significantly reduced in the high dose group, but there was no change in IFN-γ production.

In a further study, 40 cat-allergic subjects received subcutaneous injections of 250 μg of IPC-1/IPC-2 weekly, for 4 weeks [34]. No change was observed in the primary outcome measurement, in the size of early- and late-phase skin reactivity, following intradermal challenge with whole cat extract. No modulation of allergen-specific cytokine production from peripheral blood mononuclear cells (PBMCs) was observed. Frequent adverse events were reported including symptoms of asthma, rhinitis and pruritus.

In the final published study describing the treatment of 133 cat allergic patients with IPC-1/IPC-2, there was a significant improvement in lung function (FEV_1), but only in individuals with reduced baseline FEV_1 [35]. Subjects received subcutaneous injections of either 75 or 750 μg peptides (total of eight injections). A significant improvement in the subjective ability to tolerate cats was also observed. Subjects selected for this study had moderate to severe disease with high IgE levels. Importantly, approximately 30% of subjects had failed previous whole allergen immunotherapy and more than 40% of the group had asthma. Thus, the patient population for this study could be considered unusually difficult for a phase II study. Adverse events were common and included both immediate IgE-mediated acute reactions and, more frequently, late onset symptoms of asthma which declined with successive doses as observed in other studies.

More recently, a number of clinical studies have been performed with shorter peptides from Fel d 1, administered intradermally to cat allergic asthmatic subjects with mild to moderate disease severity. In the first of these, even a single dose of 5 μg of each of 12 peptides spanning the majority of the Fel d 1 molecule, resulted in significant reductions in the magnitude of the cutaneous late-phase reaction to intradermal allergen challenge. Furthermore reductions in T cell proliferation, Th2 and Th2 cytokines were also reported [36].

Subsequently, in a double-blind, placebo-controlled study, 24 cat allergic asthmatic subjects were subjected to cutaneous allergen challenge, inhaled methacholine PC_{20} and inhaled allergen PD_{20}. Subjects received incremental divided doses totaling 90 μg of each of 12 peptides administered at 3–4 day intervals [37]. Significant reductions in both early and late-phase cutaneous reactions to intradermal challenge with allergen were observed. Subjects treated with peptides felt significantly better able to tolerate exposure to cats after therapy. No significant improvements were observed in subjects who were administered PD_{20} or PC_{20}.

However, the study was not sufficiently powered to detect differences in these secondary outcomes. Analysis of PBMC responses to culture with allergen revealed a decrease in production of IL-4, IL-13 and IFNγ following peptide treatment. This was accompanied by a concomitant increase in production of IL-10 suggesting the induction of an allergen-specific regulatory response.

In a related study [38], a lower dose (41.1 μg) of peptides delivered at 2 week intervals led to a significant improvement in $PC_{20.}$ A significant reduction in the magnitude of the cutaneous late-phase reaction to allergen challenge was also observed. Biopsy of the skin site of allergen challenge revealed increased numbers of CD4+CD25+ T cells following therapy, together with increased numbers of CD4+IFNγ+ T cells and increased expression of TGF-β. Taken together, these observations suggest modulation of allergen-specific immunity at sites of challenge in favour of regulatory and Th1 responses.

Treatment of cat allergic asthmatic subjects with higher doses (approximately 300 μg) of the same peptide preparations have also been performed [39]. Peptides were administered in incremental doses at weekly intervals. Treatment significantly reduced cutaneous late-phase reactions to intradermal allergen challenge as in previous studies. The effect of peptide therapy on late asthmatic responses was evaluated by comparison of bolus inhaled allergen challenge before and after treatment. No effect was observed on the early asthmatic reaction but a significantly reduced late asthmatic reaction was observed within the group who developed a dual asthmatic response to inhaled allergen extract (FEV_1; area under curve 2–8 hours post challenge). Nasal allergen challenge revealed a significant reduction in outcome scores (sneezing, weight of nasal secretions and nasal blockage) but only in those individuals who displayed a single early response to inhaled allergen extract at baseline challenge.

No change in the functional suppressive activity of purified CD4+CD25+ cells was observed following peptide immunotherapy, despite a significant decrease in CD4+ proliferative responses and the production of IL-13 in response to culture of PBMC with allergen, suggesting that CD4+CD25+ "natural" regulatory T cells may not play a significant role in the mechanism of action [40]. However, antigen-specific "adaptive" regulatory T cells were induced. CD4+ cells isolated after peptide therapy were able to suppress allergen-specific proliferative responses of baseline $CD4^{negative}$ cells [41]. These changes were accompanied by an increase in the percentage of CD5+ T cells following therapy. CD5 levels on T cells have previously been shown to regulate the activation threshold of individual T cells, leading to a state of tolerance [42]. PBMC-derived IL-5 production was significantly decreased in this study with a trend towards an increase in IL-10. These data provide evidence that peptide immunotherapy induces a population of CD4+ T cells with regulatory activity.

Insect Venom Allergy

Peptides from the major bee venom allergen phospholipase A_2 (Api m1) have been evaluated in venom allergic individuals. Five subjects received divided incremental doses (cumulative dose 397.1 μg) of a mixture of three peptides at weekly intervals [43]. After treatment, subcutaneous challenge with 10 μg of Api m 1, approximately a third of a sting, was tolerated by all subjects. Three out of five, tolerated a wild bee sting challenge without reaction, the remaining two subjects developed mild systemic allergic reactions. No changes were observed in levels of allergen-specific serum IgE or IgG_4 during therapy but allergen after treatment resulted in a sharp increase in serum concentrations of IgE and IgG_4. Whilst the results of this study is promising, they have to be interpreted with the knowledge that due to the heterogeneous nature of reactions to bee venom, approximately 50% of these subjects might not have been expected to have a reaction on any given challenge.

Four similar peptides were identified in peptide–MHC binding assays [44] and were administered (total dose of 431.1 μg) to 12 subjects in an, open-label, single-blind study controlled with age- and sex-matched untreated controls [45]. Treatment was well tolerated and no adverse events were observed. Whereas allergen-specific T cell proliferative responses and IL-13 and IFNγ responses to allergen were reduced following treatment, the IL-10 response was increased. Late-phase cutaneous reactions to allergen were significantly reduced. Interestingly, despite the fact that the treatment peptides were directed against the T cell epitopes of the allergen, significantly increased levels of allergen-specific IgG and IgG4 were observed transiently following treatment, suggesting that T cell targeted therapies can modulate B cell responses to allergen.

A RUSH (literally "rapid") peptide immunotherapy protocol was evaluated in venom allergic subjects using three polypeptides (long synthetic peptides, LSP) encompassing the entire Api m 1 molecule [46]. No significant change in skin sensitivity to allergen challenge was observed, but a transient increase in T cell proliferation to the peptides was seen. While IFNγ and IL-10 levels increased Th2 cytokines did not. Allergen-specific IgG_4 levels increased throughout the study period. Some local and mild systemic skin reactions were observed.

Conclusion

Allergen immunotherapy is clinically effective and leads to immune deviation from a dominant allergen-specific TH2 response to one dominated by regulatory T cells and/or TH1 cells. However, treatment with whole allergen molecules or extracts is associated with frequent adverse events primarily due to allergenicity. The use of synthetic peptide fragments of the allergen containing the major T cell epitopes is one strategy that is being employed to reduce allergenicity whilst maintaining the ability to modify the immune response. Peptide therapy has been shown to improve a number of surrogate clinical markers such as the cutaneous early and late-phase response to allergen challenge, the late asthmatic response to inhaled allergen or peptides, airway hyperresponsiveness, nasal symptom scores and subjective assessments of symptoms. Mechanistically, peptide immunotherapy appears to modify T cell responses in different ways depending on the tissue; in the blood, IL-10 responses to allergen are increased at the expense of both Th1 and Th2 responses. In the skin at sites of allergen challenge, CD4+CD25+ T cells are increased together with Th1 cells. CD4+ T cells isolated after therapy are able to suppress responses to allergen, supporting the notion that peptide immunotherapy induces allergen-specific regulatory T cells. Peptide therapy has been variably associated with adverse events, which were most likely dependent on the size of the peptides (larger peptides cross linking IgE) and the dose of the peptides (higher doses inducing T cell-dependent bronchoconstriction). Careful consideration of peptide size and dose can effectively eliminate these issues. Further clinical studies are required to fully evaluate the safety and efficacy of this approach.

Conflict Statement

Mark Larché acts as a consultant to, and holds equity in Circassia Ltd., a company developing peptide-based immunotherapy for allergic and autoimmune diseases.

Funding Statement

Mark Larché is currently funded by the Canada Research Chairs Program, AllerGen NCE, Circassia Holdings Ltd., the Canadian Foundation for Innovation and the Canadian Institutes for Health Research (CIHR). The author's research has been funded by Asthma UK, the Medical Research Council (UK).

References

1. Floistrup H, Swartz J, Bergstrom A, Alm JS, Scheynius A, van HM, Waser M, Braun-Fahrlander C, Schram-Bijkerk D, Huber M, Zutavern A, von ME, Ublagger E, Riedler J, Michaels KB, Pershagen G. The Parsifal Study Group. Allergic disease and sensitization in Steiner school children. J Allergy Clin Immunol 2006; 117:59–66
2. Akdis M, Verhagen J, Taylor A, Karamloo F, Karagiannidis C, Crameri R, Thunberg S, Deniz G, Valenta R, Fiebig H, Kegel C, Disch R, Schmidt-Weber CB, Blaser K, Akdis CA. Immune responses in healthy and allergic individuals are characterized by a fine balance between allergen-specific T regulatory 1 and T helper 2 cells. J Exp Med 2004; 199:1567–75
3. Pajno GB, Barberio G, De Luca F, Morabito L, Parmiani S. Prevention of new sensitizations in asthmatic children monosensitized to house dust mite by specific immunotherapy. A six-year follow-up study. Clin Exp Allergy 2001; 31:1392–7
4. Moller C, Dreborg S, Ferdousi HA, Halken S, Host A, Jacobsen L, Koivikko A, Koller DY, Niggemann B, Norberg LA, Urbanek R, Valovirta E, Wahn U. Pollen immunotherapy reduces the development of asthma in children with seasonal rhinoconjunctivitis (the PAT-study). J Allergy Clin Immunol 2002; 109:251–6
5. Cookson W. Genetics and genomics of asthma and allergic diseases. Immunol Rev 2002; 190:195–206

6. von ME. Allergies, infections and the hygiene hypothesis--the epidemiological evidence. Immunobiology 2007; 212:433–9
7. Bach JF. The effect of infections on susceptibility to autoimmune and allergic diseases. N Engl J Med 2002; 347:911–20
8. Hansen G, Berry G, DeKruyff RH, Umetsu DT. Allergen-specific Th1 cells fail to counterbalance Th2 cell-induced airway hyperreactivity but cause severe airway inflammation. J Clin Invest 1999; 103:175–83
9. Karlsson MR, Rugtveit J, Brandtzaeg P. Allergen-responsive CD4+CD25+ regulatory T cells in children who have outgrown cow's milk allergy. J Exp Med 2004; 199:1679–88
10. Ling EM, Smith T, Nguyen XD, Pridgeon C, Dallman M, Arbery J, Carr VA, Robinson DS. Relation of CD4+CD25+ regulatory T-cell suppression of allergen-driven T-cell activation to atopic status and expression of allergic disease. Lancet 2004; 363:608–15
11. Larche M, Akdis CA, Valenta R. Immunological mechanisms of allergen-specific immunotherapy. Nat Rev Immunol 2006; 6:761–71
12. Platts-Mills T, Vaughan J, Squillace S, Woodfolk J, Sporik R. Sensitisation, asthma, and a modified Th2 response in children exposed to cat allergen: a population-based cross-sectional study. Lancet 2001; 357:752–6
13. Durham SR, Walker SM, Varga EM, Jacobson MR, O'Brien F, Noble W, Till SJ, Hamid QA, Nouri-Aria KT. Long-term clinical efficacy of grass-pollen immunotherapy. N Engl J Med 1999; 341:468–75
14. Jutel M, Akdis M, Budak F, Aebischer-Casaulta C, Wrzyszcz M, Blaser K, Akdis CA. IL-10 and TGF-beta cooperate in the regulatory T cell response to mucosal allergens in normal immunity and specific immunotherapy. Eur J Immunol 2003; 33:1205–14
15. Lichtenstein LM, Ishizaka K, Norman PS, Sobotka AK, Hill BM. IgE antibody measurements in ragweed hay fever. Relationship to clinical severity and the results of immunotherapy. J Clin Invest 1973; 52:472–82
16. Durham SR, Ying S, Varney VA, Jacobson MR, Sudderick RM, Mackay IS, Kay AB, Hamid QA. Grass pollen immunotherapy inhibits allergen-induced infiltration of CD4+ T lymphocytes and eosinophils in the nasal mucosa and increases the number of cells expressing messenger RNA for interferon-gamma. J Allergy Clin Immunol 1996; 97:1356–65
17. Varney VA, Hamid QA, Gaga M, Ying S, Jacobson M, Frew AJ, Kay AB, Durham SR. Influence of grass pollen immunotherapy on cellular infiltration and cytokine mRNA expression during allergen-induced late-phase cutaneous responses. J Clin Invest 1993; 92:644–51
18. Secrist H, Chelen CJ, Wen Y, Marshall JD, Umetsu DT. Allergen immunotherapy decreases interleukin 4 production in CD4+ T cells from allergic individuals. J Exp Med 1993; 178:2123–30
19. Ebner C, Siemann U, Bohle B, Willheim M, Wiedermann U, Schenk S, Klotz F, Ebner H, Kraft D, Scheiner O. Immunological changes during specific immunotherapy of grass pollen allergy: reduced lymphoproliferative responses to allergen and shift from TH2 to TH1 in T-cell clones specific for Phl p 1, a major grass pollen allergen. Clin Exp Allergy 1997; 27:1007–15
20. Wachholz PA, Nouri-Aria KT, Wilson DR, Walker SM, Verhoef A, Till SJ, Durham SR. Grass pollen immunotherapy for hayfever is associated with increases in local nasal but not peripheral Th1:Th2 cytokine ratios. Immunology 2002; 105:56–62
21. Akdis CA, Akdis M, Blesken T, Wymann D, Alkan SS, Muller U, Blaser K. Epitope-specific T cell tolerance to phospholipase A2 in bee venom immunotherapy and recovery by IL-2 and IL-15 in vitro. J Clin Invest 1996; 98:1676–83
22. Francis JN, Till SJ, Durham SR. Induction of IL-10+CD4+CD25+ T cells by grass pollen immunotherapy. J Allergy Clin Immunol 2003; 111:1255–61
23. Nasser S, Ying S, Meng Q, Kay AB, Ewan P. Interleukin 10 levels increase in cutaneous biopsies of patients undergoing venom immunotherapy. Eur J Immunol 2001; 31:3704–13
24. Nouri-Aria KT, Wachholz PA, Francis JN, Jacobson MR, Walker SM, Wilcock LK, Staple SQ, Aalberse RC, Till SJ, Durham SR. Grass pollen immunotherapy induces mucosal and peripheral IL-10 responses and blocking IgG activity. J Immunol 2004; 172:3252–9

25. Bellinghausen I, Knop J, Saloga J. The role of interleukin 10 in the regulation of allergic immune responses. Int Arch Allergy Immunol 2001; 126:97–101
26. Akdis CA, Blaser K. IL-10-induced anergy in peripheral T cell and reactivation by microenvironmental cytokines: two key steps in specific immunotherapy. FASEB J 1999; 13:603–9
27. Larche M, Wraith DC. Peptide-based therapeutic vaccines for allergic and autoimmune diseases. Nat Med 2005; 11:S69–S76
28. Lamb JR, Skidmore BJ, Green N, Chiller JM, Feldmann M. Induction of tolerance in influenza virus-immune T lymphocyte clones with synthetic peptides of influenza hemagglutinin. J Exp Med 1983; 157:1434–47
29. Counsell CM, Bond JF, Ohman JL, Greenstein JL, Garman RD. Definition of the human T-cell epitopes of Fel d 1, the major allergen of the domestic cat. J Allergy Clin Immunol 1996; 98:884–94
30. Mark PG, Segal DB, Dallaire ML, Garman RD. Human T and B cell immune responses to Fel d 1 in cat-allergic and non-cat-allergic subjects. Clin Exp Allergy 1996; 26:1316–28
31. Norman PS, Ohman JL, Jr., Long AA, Creticos PS, Gefter MA, Shaked Z, Wood RA, Eggleston PA, Hafner KB, Rao P, Lichtenstein LM, Jones NH, Nicodemus CF. Treatment of cat allergy with T-cell reactive peptides. Am J Respir Crit Care Med 1996; 154:1623–8
32. Marcotte GV, Braun CM, Norman PS, Nicodemus CF, Kagey-Sobotka A, Lichtenstein LM, Essayan DM. Effects of peptide therapy on ex vivo T-cell responses. J Allergy Clin Immunol 1998; 101:506–13
33. Pene J, Desroches A, Paradis L, Lebel B, Farce M, Nicodemus CF, Yssel H, Bousquet J. Immunotherapy with Fel d 1 peptides decreases IL-4 release by peripheral blood T cells of patients allergic to cats. J Allergy Clin Immunol 1998; 102:571–8
34. Simons FE, Imada M, Li Y, Watson WT, HayGlass KT. Fel d 1 peptides: effect on skin tests and cytokine synthesis in cat-allergic human subjects. Int Immunol 1996; 8:1937–45
35. Maguire P, Nicodemus C, Robinson D, Aaronson D, Umetsu DT. The safety and efficacy of ALLERVAX CAT in cat allergic patients. Clin Immunol 1999; 93:222–31
36. Oldfield WL, Kay AB, Larche M. Allergen-derived T cell peptide-induced late asthmatic reactions precede the induction of antigen-specific hyporesponsiveness in atopic allergic asthmatic subjects. J Immunol 2001; 167:1734–9
37. Oldfield WL, Larche M, Kay AB. Effect of T-cell peptides derived from Fel d 1 on allergic reactions and cytokine production in patients sensitive to cats: a randomised controlled trial. Lancet 2002; 360:47–53
38. Alexander C, Ying S, Kay B, Larche M. Fel d 1-derived T cell peptide therapy induces recruitment of CD4+ CD25+; CD4+ interferon-gamma+ T helper type 1 cells to sites of allergen-induced late-phase skin reactions in cat-allergic subjects. Clin Exp Allergy 2005; 35:52–8
39. Alexander C, Tarzi M, Larche M, Kay AB. The effect of Fel d 1-derived T-cell peptides on upper and lower airway outcome measurements in cat-allergic subjects. Allergy 2005; 60:1269–74
40. Smith TR, Alexander C, Kay AB, Larche M, Robinson DS. Cat allergen peptide immunotherapy reduces CD4(+) T cell responses to cat allergen but does not alter suppression by CD4(+) CD25(+) T cells: a double-blind placebo-controlled study. Allergy 2004; 59:1097–101
41. Verhoef A, Alexander C, Kay AB, Larche M. T cell epitope immunotherapy induces a CD4+ T cell population with regulatory activity. PLoS Med 2005; 2:e78
42. Hawiger D, Masilamani RF, Bettelli E, Kuchroo VK, Nussenzweig MC. Immunological unresponsiveness characterized by increased expression of CD5 on peripheral T cells induced by dendritic cells in vivo. Immunity 2004; 20:695–705
43. Muller U, Akdis CA, Fricker M, Akdis M, Blesken T, Bettens F, Blaser K. Successful immunotherapy with T-cell epitope peptides of bee venom phospholipase A2 induces specific T-cell anergy in patients allergic to bee venom. J Allergy Clin Immunol 1998; 101:747–54
44. Texier C, Pouvelle S, Busson M, Herve M, Charron D, Menez A, Maillere B. HLA-DR restricted peptide candidates for bee venom immunotherapy. J Immunol 2000; 164: 3177–84

45. Tarzi M, Klunker S, Texier C, Verhoef A, Stapel SO, Akdis CA, Maillere B, Kay AB, Larche M. Induction of interleukin-10 and suppressor of cytokine signalling-3 gene expression following peptide immunotherapy. Clin Exp Allergy 2006; 36:465–74
46. Fellrath JM, Kettner A, Dufour N, Frigerio C, Schneeberger D, Leimgruber A, Corradin G, Spertini F. Allergen-specific T-cell tolerance induction with allergen-derived long synthetic peptides: results of a phase I trial. J Allergy Clin Immunol 2003; 111:854–61

NKT Ligand Conjugated Immunotherapy

Yasuyuki Ishii

Specific allergen immunotherapy (SIT) is the only existing treatment for the purpose of recovering from antigen-induced allergic disorders. However, the remarkable efficacy of it is not necessarily expected even after long term therapy over a few years. Detailed mechanisms of antigen-specific immune tolerance induced by desensitization also remain unclear. To promote the SIT to the top of the standard therapies for allergic rhinitis and pollinosis, new methods and/or technologies based on the scientific evidences should be added to it. It must be indisputable that the ultimate goal of the SIT is to suppress the on-going IgE antibody formation, and/or to inhibit the secondary IgE antibody responses after the allergen exposure.

It is generally accepted that polarization of the immune response towards type II helper T cells (Th2) is the most important prerequisites for the development of the IgE antibody formation and atopic disorders [1]. Based on this principle, several approaches have been made to reverse the deviation of the T cell response to type I helper T cells (Th1). Among them, ligands for some toll-like receptors (TLRs) are tools available [2]. Chemical conjugate of CpG oligonucleotide (ODN), which induces TLR-9-mediated signal transduction, to antigen, i.e., a device to deliver CpGODN and antigen to the same antigen presenting cells (APCs), was proved to be a potent immunogen for priming Th1-skewed immune response to the antigen [3,4]. Repeated injections of the immunostimulatory sequence (ISS), which encodes CpG motif, conjugated ragweed antigen, Amb a1 to the antigen-primed mice prevented the secondary IgE antibody response to the allergen [5]. Clinical trials of the ISS-Amb a1 conjugate is in progress [6]. Monophosphoryl lipid A (MPL), which is a detoxified derivative of the lipopolysaccharide (LPS) moiety of Salmonella minesota R595 and a ligand for TLR-4, has been utilized as an adjuvant

Y. Ishii
Laboratory for Vaccine Design, RIKEN Research Center for Allergy and Immunology,
1-7-22, Suehiro, Tsurumi, Yokohama, Kanagawa 230-0045, Japan
e-mail: ishiiyas@rcai.riken.jp

R. Pawankar et al. (eds.), *Allergy Frontiers: Future Perspectives*,
DOI 10.1007/978-4-431-99365-0_7, © Springer 2010

for allergen-specific Th1 responses [7]. Allergen-specific Th1-skewing developed by ligands for TLRs with allergens could be powerful tools to suppress both Th2 expansion and IgE antibody formation. However, there are still some concerns relating to adverse effects of the robust Th1 cytokine productions.

Another obvious approach for suppression of the IgE antibody response is to induce immune tolerance and to develop antigen-specific regulatory T cells (Treg). It is well known that intravenous injections of denatured or modified antigen, which lost the major B cell epitope but maintained the T cell epitope of the native antigen, into antigen-primed mice facilitated the differentiation of antigen-specific suppressor (regulatory) T cells, and effectively suppressed the secondary IgE antibody response to the native antigen [8,9]. More recently, it was shown that administration of antigen with heat-killed Listeria monocyotogenes (HKL) as an adjuvant, reversed the already established Th2-dominated response and the IgE antibody formation, and induced a Th1 type immune response to the antigen [10,11]. However, further studies on the cellular mechanisms of the immune deviation revealed that the immunization with HKL and antigen included in incomplete Freund adjuvant induced not only conventional Th1 response but also the differentiation of antigen-specific Treg cells which produce IL-10 and IFN-γ, and that the Treg was responsible for the inhibition of the development of allergen-induced airway hyper-reactivity and for suppression of the IgE antibody response [12]. Possible role of IL-10-producing Treg for suppression of IgE antibody response is supported by the fact that transfer of ovalbumin (OVA)-specific Tr1 clones coincident with OVA immunization inhibited the primary IgE antibody response, whereas transfer of the same number of the antigen-specific Th1 clones failed to do so [13]. Although both Treg and Tr1 might have high potency to suppress Th2 and IgE antibody responses, methods and/or technologies for in vivo development of them have not been fully disclosed yet.

In this chapter, we examine functions of natural killer T cells (NKT) available for Treg development and IgE antibody suppression, and introduce the potential of one prototype for NKT ligand-conjugated immunotherapy.

Identification of NKT Cells

Various subsets of murine NKT cells, which express both T cell receptor (TCR) and NK1.1 marker have been reported [14]. Among NKT cells, Vα14-NKT cells or iNKT cells were identified as a novel lymphocyte lineage and were characterized by using a single invariant Vα14-Jα281 chain in TCR complex [15,16]. $V\alpha14^+$ cells are able to develop in extrathymic lymphoid tissues, including bone marrow and liver, but not spleen, suggesting that Vα14-NKT cells develop through unique selection process distinct from those of conventional T cells. The exclusive expression of the invariant Vα14-Jα281 chain on Vα14-NKT cells and the essential requirement of it were demonstrated in $J\alpha281^{-/-}$ [17], indicating that the expression of invariant Vα14-Jα281 chain is indispensable for the development of Vα14-NKT cells. The precursor of Vα14-NKT cells expresses the granulocyte macrophage colony stimulating factor (GM-CSF) receptor and maturates in the presence of GM-CSF [18]. Vα14-NKT cells have been observed in peripheral lymphoid organs such as bone marrow (20–40%), liver (30–40%), spleen (1–2%), and thymus (0.4%) [16,19]. Vα14-NKT cells belong to the population of $CD4^+$ or $CD4^-CD8^-$ $CD62L^-$ $CD69^+$ $DX5^{dull}$ in the spleen, liver, thymus, and bone marrow cells. The human homologue of Vα14-NKT cells expresses a Vα24-Jα281 chain [20].

Ligands for Vα14-NKT Cells

CD1 molecules present lipids or glycolipids instead of peptides [21]. It has been reported that the number of Vα14-NKT cells are few in several mice with deficiencies in glycolipid metabolism such as Niemann-Pick type C1 protein-deficient mice [22] and prosaposin-deficient mice, which are defective in lipid transfer from membrane to CD1d molecule [23]. As for natural ligands for Vα14-NKT cells, it was firstly suggested that self glycosphingolipids in lysosomal compartment might be involved in the stimulation of Vα14-NKT cells [24]. Moreover, in the mice deficient of β-hexosaminidase b (Hexb) that removes the terminal GalNAc of isoglobo-ceramide iGb4, the generated iGb3 is presented by CD1d molecule and works as an antigen for Vα14-NKT cells [25]. Indeed, Vα14-NKT cells are remarkably deficient in Hexb-deficient mice. It appears that Vα14-NKT cells are positively selected by the self-ligands.

The other ligand for Vα14-NKT cells has been determined as α-galactosylceramide (α-GalCer). The natural product of α-GalCer, agelasphin-9b, (2S,3S,4R)-1-*O*-(alpha-D-galactopyranosyl)-16-methyl-2-[*N*-((*R*)-2-hydroxytetracosanoyl)-amino]-1,3,4 heptadecanetriol, was isolated from the marine sponge Agelas mauritianus as a potent antitumor agent [26]. Several α-GalCer analogs based on the natural α-GalCer were chemically synthesized and assessed by functional analysis, resulting in one α-GalCer, designated as "KRN7000," having a long fatty acyl chain (C_{26}) and sphingosine base (C_{18}) and screened as a ligand for Vα14-NKT cells [27]. Using surface plasmon resonance, mouse CD1 and human CD1d bound not only to the immobilized α-GalCer but also both to the nonantigenic β-GalCer and to phosphatidylethanolamine, indicating that diverse lipids can bind to CD1d [28]. Recent studies have demonstrated that Vα14-NKT cells recognize various glycolipids of microorganisms, such as Sphingomonas bacteria [29] and *Borrelia burgdorferi* [30]. Several α-GalCer analogs have been reported. C-glycoside analog of α-GalCer, α-C-galactosylceramide (α-C-GalCer), acts as natural killer T cell ligand in vivo, and stimulates an enhanced Th1-type response in mice [31,32]. OCH, a sphingosine-truncated analog of α-GalCer, induces IL-4, but not IFN-γ, production of Vα14-NKT cells [33].

IgE Suppression by NKT Cells

Vα14-NKT cells are able to produce both IFN-γ and IL-4 by the stimulation with α-GalCer, e.g., KRN7000 in vitro and in vivo [27]. Since Vα14-NKT cells are primary sources of IL-4 production, Vα14-NKT cells are involved in the enhancement of IgE formation [34]. However, IgE formation of $CD1d^{-/-}$ or $J\alpha281^{-/-}$ mice were quite normal [35–37], suggesting that Vα14-NKT cells are not essential for IgE formation. On the other hand, IFN-γ production of Vα14-NKT cells was indispensable for the suppression of IgE formation after multiple α-GalCer injections [38].

NKT Ligand-Conjugated Immunotherapy

Preparation of α-GalCer-Conjugated Allergen

Since IFN-γ production of Vα14-NKT cells skews Th2 response in allergic diseases to Th1, It is expected that α-GalCer and its analogs might be powerful adjuvant for antigen-specific immunotherapy. In order to test the possible effects of α-GalCer on IgE antibody responses, α-GalCer with or without OVA antigen was intraperitoneally injected into groups of BDF1 (C57BL6 X DBA2) mice 3 days prior to immunization with alum-absorbed DNP-OVA. However, primary anti-DNP IgE, IgG1 and IgG2a antibody responses were not suppressed by pretreatment with α-GalCer regardless of OVA co-injection (personal communication). The previous report also showed that co-injection of the ragweed allergen Amb a 1 with immunostimulatory DNA sequences (ISS)-oligonucleotide (ODN) was much less effective in inducing a Th1 response, whereas Amb a 1-ISS conjugate induced a de novo T(H)1 response and suppressed IgE antibody formation after challenge with Amb a 1 [39]. Attempts were made to generate α-GalCer-conjugated allergen. Since α-GalCer is a strongly hydrophobic reagent unlike ISS-ODN, it was expected that direct conjugation of α-GalCer with hydrophilic allergens would be troublesome. Thus, we prepared liposomes which contained α-GalCer in a lipid monolayer (αGalCer-liposomes) and αGalCer-liposomes encapsulating OVA protein (αGalCer-OVA-liposomes) (Fig. 1).

Potent Activity of α-GalCer-Conjugated Allergen in Primary IgE Antibody Responses

Either αGalCer-liposomes or αGalCer-OVA-liposomes was intraperitoneally injected into groups of BDF1 mice 3 days prior to immunization with alum-absorbed DNP-OVA. Control groups received aqueous α-GalCer or liposomes alone,

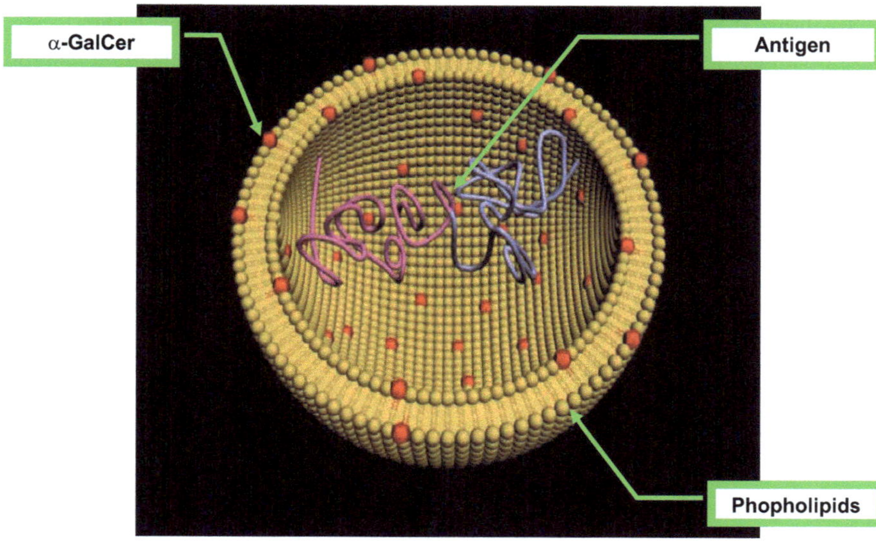

Fig. 1 Structure of αGalCer-liposome containing antigen

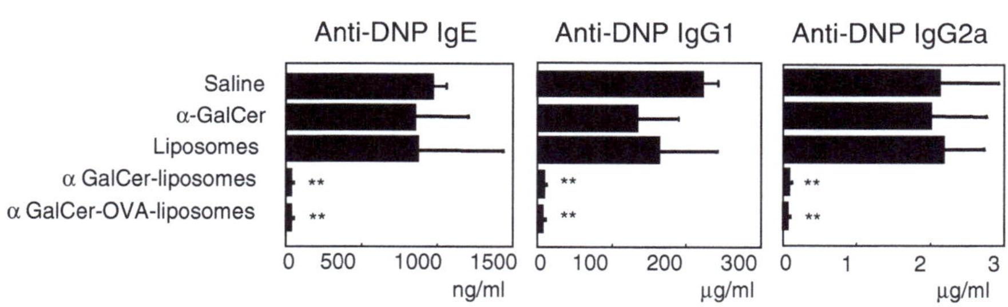

Fig. 2 Suppression of primary antibody responses by administration of αGalCer-liposomes. Groups of BDF1 mice ($n=5$) received samples. Three days later, they were immunized with alum-absorbed DNP-OVA, and the concentration of anti-DNP Abs in their sera was determined by ELISA at day 14. $^{**}p<0.005$ for αGC-liposomes and αGalCer-OVA-liposomes groups versus saline group

prior to immunization. Primary anti-DNP IgE, IgG1 and IgG2a antibody responses were completely suppressed by pre-treatment with αGalCer-liposomes or αGalCer-OVA-liposomes, but not by the pre-treatment with aqueous α-GalCer (Fig. 2). The concentration of total IgE, IgG1 or IgG2a in each group was comparable. These results suggest that αGalCer-liposomes and αGalCer-OVA-liposomes, but not aqueous α-GalCer, might perform novel mechanisms except for the antigen-specific Th1 skewing against primary IgE antibody responses, because OVA antigen in the liposome conjugate was dispensable and IgG2a antibody responses was also completely suppressed.

To clarify if helper T cells were primed by antigen in alum, splenic $CD4^+$ T cells were obtained from each group of the mice 7 days after the immunization, and the cells were cultured for 48 h with irradiated syngenic splenocytes in the presence of DNP-OVA of various concentrations. Determination of the cell proliferation and IL-2 in the culture supernatants showed that the pretreatment with αGalCer-liposomes prevented T cell priming with DNP-OVA, while the pretreatment with aqueous αGalCer rather enhanced the T cell priming with the antigen.

Mechanism of Immune Tolerance Induced by α-GalCer-Conjugated Allergen

IL-10-Producing $CD4^+CD25^+$ T Cells

In the experimental model of anterior chamber-associated immune deviation (ACAID), Sonoda et al [41,42] have shown that NKT cells are required for the development of systemic immune tolerance. They provided definitive evidence that the Vα14-NKT cells involved in the development of immune tolerance, and the NKT cell-derived IL-10 play a critical role in the development of antigen-specific regulatory T cells and immune tolerance. These findings suggested to us the possibility that stimulation of the NKT cells with αGalCer-liposomes at the time of (or prior to) antigen-presentation to naïve T cells, may facilitate the differentiation of Treg, rather than Th, cells that are specific for the antigen. To elucidate the mechanism for the prevention of T cell priming, splenic $CD4^+CD25^+$ T cells of αGC-liposome-treated mice were analyzed 7, 10 and 14 days after the immunization with alum-absorbed DNP-OVA. Analysis for mRNA of splenic $CD4^+CD25^+$ T cells showed that IL-10, but neither IL-4 nor IFN-γ, mRNA expression was augmented on 7 and 14 days after immunization, but the expression level of Foxp3 mRNA of αGC-liposome-treated mice was almost comparable with that of non-treated mice. These results suggest that the elevation of IL-10 expression on $CD4^+CD25^+$ T cells might be involved in the suppression of T cell priming and primary antibody responses.

Antigen-Presenting Cells

In view of the findings in the ACAID system [40,41], we anticipated that presentation of αGalCer to NKT cells by APCs in the vicinity of antigen presentation to OVA-specific naïve T cells, might facilitate the differentiation of OVA-specific Treg cells. Since the formulation of antigen in liposomes enhances antigen uptake by various APCs, such as dendritic cells (DCs), B cells and macrophages, we suspected that the opposite effect of αGalCer-liposomes versus aqueous αGalCer on the antigen-priming of naïve T cells might be due to uptake of αGalCer-liposomes by non-DCs. To test this possibility, either aqueous αGalCer or αGalCer-liposomes was intraperitoneally injected into separate groups of BDF1 mice. DCs, B cells and macrophages were then recovered successively from collagenase-treated splenocytes, respectively. Aliquots of NKT cell fractions were then co-cultured with the purified DCs, B cells or macrophages from the aqueous αGalCer-treated mice or αGalCer-liposome-treated mice, and the concentrations of IFN-γ IL-4 and IL-10 in the culture supernatants were determined. DCs from the αGalCer-liposome-treated mice induced the formations of more cytokines than those from the aqueous αGalCer-treated mice. When B cells from the αGalCer-liposome-treated mice were co-cultured with NKT cell fractions, IL-10 became detectable in the culture supernatant within 24 h, and the concentration of the cytokine markedly increased by 48 h. Since the formation of IL-10 by the co-culture of the B cells with normal spleen cells was prevented by the addition of anti-CD1d antibody, and culture supernatants of the B cells alone did not contain a detectable amount of IL-10, it appears that presentation of CD1d-associated αGalCer on B cells to NKT cells was responsible for the production of IL-10. In contrast, B cells of the mice treated with aqueous αGalCer barely induced the formation of IL-10, when they were co-cultured with NKT cell fractions. The difference between B cells from the αGalCer-liposome-treated mice and those from the aqueous αGalCer-treated mice, with respect to their ability to induce IL-10 formation, is probably due to an enhancement of uptake of α-GalCer in liposome formulation by B cells.

Since the splenic B cells comprised follicular and marginal zone B cells, we determined which subset is involved in the IL-10 formation. BDF1 spleen cells were obtained 24 h after an intraperitoneal injection of αGalCer-liposomes, and $CD11c^{+}$DCs in the splenocytes were depleted. The rest of the splenocytes were then fractionated by histodenz gradient, and B cells in both the high density (HD) and low density (LD) fractions were recovered. The HD-B cells and LD-B cells were then cultured alone or with normal spleen cells, and cytokines in the supernatants were determined, and the concentrations of IFN-γ IL-4 and IL-10 in the culture supernatants were determined. Only LD-B cells induced the formation of IL-10, but neither IL-4 nor IFN-γ was detected in the culture supernatant.

Moreover, LD-B cells were fractionated into $CD21^{high}$ $CD23^{-}$ cell, $CD21^{middle}$ $CD23^{high}$ cell or $CD21^{low}$ $CD23^{-}$ cell fraction by flow cytometry. Each fraction was cultured with NKT cell fractions. IL-10 production was substantially detected in the culture supernatants of CD23-negative cell fractions more than in that of CD23-positive cell fraction. To determine the cell source of IL-10 in this system, LD-B cells were obtained from the spleen of αGalCer-liposome-treated mice by the method described above, and the cells were cultured with NKT cell fractions, from which B cells had been depleted. After 48 h culture, the cells were fractionated into $B220^{-}$ cell and $B220^{+}$ cell fraction. Each cell fraction was analyzed for the presence of IL-10 mRNA by RT-PCR. IL-10 mRNA was detected in $B220^{+}$ cell but not in $B220^{-}$ cell fraction which should contain NKT cells, indicating that presentation of αGalCer on CD23-negative LD-B cells to NKT cells mainly induced the formation of IL-10 by the B cells.

We next determined as to whether the transfer of the LD-B cells pulsed with αGalCer-liposomes might induce the development of the tolerogenic DCs in the spleen of the recipients. LD-B cells were incubated with αGalCer-liposomes, and transferred intravenously into normal mice. After 3 days, the $CD11c^+$ DC-enriched fraction derived from the recipient mice was stained with anti-CD11c and anti-CD45RB mAbs, and analyzed by flow cytometer. Since the $CD11c^{low}B220^+$ $Gr\text{-}1^+$ plasmacytoid DCs should have been depleted from the spleen cells in the process of the enrichment of $CD11c^+$ cells, we wondered if the $CD11c^{low}$ cells might represent $CD45RB^{high}$ tolerogenic DCs. To confirm whether the expansion of $CD11c^{low}CD45RB^{high}$ cells depends on the treatment of αGalCer-liposomes, Vα14NKT-deficient mice received an intraperitoneal injection of αGalCer-liposomes. The proportion of the $CD11c^{low}$ cells did not change by the treatment, indicating that Vα14 NKT cells were indispensable for the expansion of the $CD11c^{low}CD45RB^{high}$ cell population. The results summarized in Table 1 indicate that the trαeatment with αGalCer-liposomes induced a marked increase in $CD11c^{low}CD45RB^{high}$ cells without affecting the number of $CD11c^{high}CD45RB^{low}$ cells, whereas the treatment with aqueous α-GalCer rather induced a significant increase in $CD11c^{high}$ DCs. Characteristics of the $CD11c^{low}CD45RB^{high}$ cells developed by the αGalCer-liposome treatment were determined. The $CD11c^{low}CD45RB^{high}$ cells and $CD11c^{high}$ DCs were recovered by cell sorting from the splenocytes of BDF1 mice 3 days after the injection of αGalCer-liposomes. Analysis of the cell surface molecules of the sorted cells by flow cytometry showed that the expression level of $I\text{-}A^d$, CD40 or CD80 on the $CD11c^{low}CD45RB^{high}$ cells were significantly lower than those on the $CD11c^{high}CD45RB^{low}$ cells, while the expression of CD86 was comparable in the two populations. Upon stimulation with LPS, the $CD11c^{low}CD45RB^{high}$ population produced IL-10 but no IL-12, while the $CD11c^{high}$ DCs secreted IL-12 but no IL-10. These results collectively indicate that $CD11c^{low}CD45RB^{high}$ phenotype population expanded in vivo by the injection of αGalCer-liposomes represents tolerogenic DCs described by Wakkach et al [42], which have a potent to generate antigen-specific Treg cells from naïve $CD4^+$ T cells after the antigen-pulse.

Table 1 αGalCer-liposomes preferentially augment the absolute number of $CD11c^{low}CD45RB^{high}$ cells relative to $CD11c^{high}$ DCs in the spleen of a BDF1 mouse

	Total cells-lineages	$CD11c^{low}CD45RB^{high}$	$CD11c^{high}$
Transfer			
Saline	29.7	1.5(4.9 %)	5.6 (18.8 %)
LD-B	43.1	1.8(4.1 %)	11.4 (26.5 %)
LD-B with αGalCer-liposomes	76.1	10.6 (14.0 %)	9.4(12.4 %)
Injection			
Saline	26.3	1.5(5.5 %)	3.9 (14.9 %)
α-GalCer	51.7	3.6(6.9 %)	8.1 (15.7 %)
Liposomes	44.1	2.9(6.5 %)	6.8 (15.3 %)
αGalCer-liposomes	121.6	30.8(25.3 %)	4.5(3.7 %)

Results represent the number of cells ($\times 10^{-5}$) per mouse spleen

"Total cells-lineages" represent the enriched cells after depletion of CD3, CD19, CD49b, Gr-1, or TER-119-positive cells in splenocytes

"LD-B" represents low-density B cells

Antigen-Specific Suppression by the Treatment with αGarCer-OVA-Liposomes

BDF1 mice were immunized with alum-absorbed DNP-OVA and, after detection of the primary anti-DNP IgE antibody responses at 2 weeks, either αGalCer-liposomes or αGalCer-OVA-liposomes was injected intraperitoneally into the DNP-OVA-primed mice on day 21, 28 and 35. Seven days after the last injection of the liposomes, booster immunization of DNP-OVA was given to all groups, and the secondary anti-DNP-antibody response was assessed 7 days after the booster. Anti-DNP antibody response of all the immunoglobulin isotypes examined, was markedly suppressed by the treatment with αGalCer-OVA-liposomes. The treatment with αGalCer-liposomes slightly suppressed both the IgG1 and IgG2a antibody responses, but failed to affect the IgE antibody response. To determine the carrier-specific nature of the suppression by the treatment with αGalCer-OVA-liposomes, separate groups of BDF1 mice were immunized with alum-absorbed DNP-KLH; one group was treated by three intraperitoneal injections of αGalCer-OVA-liposomes, and another group was treated with αGalCer-liposomes. The results of the secondary antibody responses to DNP-KLH, given 7 days after the liposome treatment, indicated that the treatment with αGalCer-liposomes slightly suppressed the secondary IgG1 and IgG2a antibody responses, but encapsulation of OVA in the liposomes did not enhance the suppressive effect. Neither αGalCer-liposomes nor αGalCer-OVA-liposomes suppressed the secondary IgE antibody response to DNP-KLH (Fig. 3). These results indicate that αGalCer-OVA-liposomes to DNP-OVA-primed mice suppressed their secondary antibody responses to DNP-OVA in antigen (carrier)-specific manner.

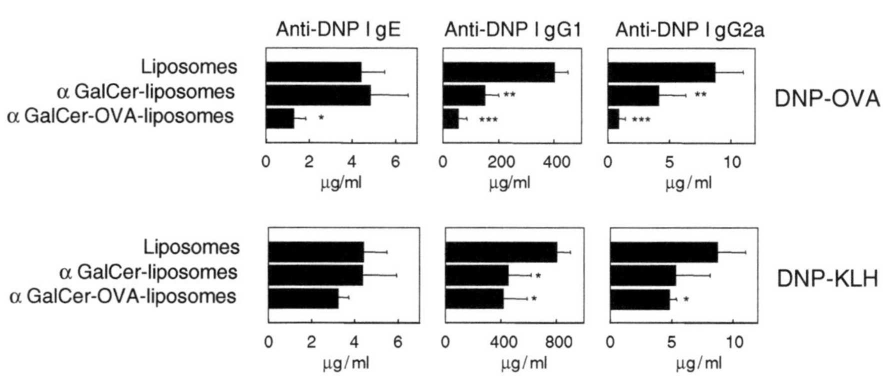

Fig. 3 Carrier-specific suppression of the secondary IgE antibody response by administration of αGalCer-OVA-liposomes. Three groups of BDF1 mice were immunized with alum-absorbed DNP-OVA or DNP-KLH at day 0. They received intraperitoneal injections of "Liposomes," "αGalCer-liposomes" or "αGalCer-OVA-liposomes" on day 21, 28 and 35, and then boosted with either DNP-OVA (0.1 μg) or DNP-KLH (1 μg) on day 42. The concentrations of anti-DNP IgE, IgG1 and IgG2a antibodies in their sera on day 49 were measured by ELISA. $*p<0.05$, $**p<0.005$ and $***p<0.001$ for the αGalCer-liposome or αGalCer-OVA-liposomes group versus liposome group

Conclusions

Recent clinical studies on allergy focused attention on the possible role of Treg cells in prevention of allergic diseases. Ling et al [43] have shown that $CD4^{+}CD25^{-}$ cells from the majority of non-atopic donors caused proliferative response and IL-5 production upon stimulation with allergen-pulsed APC, and that the responses were prevented by the addition of autologous $CD4^{+}CD25^{+}$ cells. In the active allergic pollinosis patients, however, the inhibitory effect of the autologous $CD4^{+}CD25^{+}$ cells was substantially less than that observed in non-atopic individuals. Subsequent studies by Akdis et al [44] identified allergen-specific Th1, Th2 and Tr1 $CD4^{+}$ cells, which produce IFN-γ, IL-4 and IL-10, respectively, upon antigenic stimulation in the peripheral blood of both atopic and healthy individuals, and found that Tr1 cells are a dominant subset in healthy individuals. They proposed the hypothesis that balance between allergen-specific Th2 and Tr1 cells would determine the development of healthy or allergic immune response. These findings support our expectations that αGalCer-liposomes containing an appropriate allergen would be a useful tool for the treatment of allergic patients.

References

1. Stevens TL, Bossie A, Sanders VM, Fernandez-Botran R, Coffman RL, Mosmann TR, et al. Regulation of antibody isotype secretion by subsets of antigen-specific helper T cells. Nature 1988; 334:255–258.
2. Kaisho T, Akira S. Toll-like receptor function and signaling. J Allergy Clin Immunol 2006; 117:979–987.
3. Shirota H, Sano K, Hirasawa N, Terui T, Ohuchi K, Hattori T, et al. B cells capturing antigen conjugated with CpG oligodeoxynucleotides induce Th1 cells by elaborating IL-12. J Immunol 2002; 169:787–794.
4. Cho HJ, Takabayashi K, Cheng PM, Nguyen MD, Corr M, Tuck S, et al. Immunostimulatory DNA-based vaccines induce cytotoxic lymphocyte activity by a T-helper cell-independent mechanism. Nat Biotechnol 2000; 18:509–514.
5. Tighe H, Takabayashi K, Schwartz D, Van Nest G, Tuck S, Eiden JJ, et al. Conjugation of immunostimulatory DNA to the short ragweed allergen amb a 1 enhances its immunogenicity and reduces its allergenicity. J Allergy Clin Immunol 2000; 106:124–134.
6. Marshall JD, Abtahi S, Eiden JJ, Tuck S, Milley R, Haycock F, et al. Immunostimulatory sequence DNA linked to the Amb a 1 allergen promotes T(H)1 cytokine expression while downregulating T(H)2 cytokine expression in PBMCs from human patients with ragweed allergy. J Allergy Clin Immunol 2001; 108:191–197.
7. Wheeler AW Marshall JS, Ulrich JT. A Th1-inducing adjuvant, MPL, enhances antibody profiles in experimental animals suggesting it has the potential to improve the efficacy of allergy vaccines. Int Arch Allergy Immunol 2001; 126:135–139.
8. Takatsu K, Ishizaka K. Reaginic antibody formation in the mouse. VII. Induction of suppressor T cells for IgE and IgG antibody responses. J Immunol 1976; 116:1257–1264.
9. Lee WY, Sehon AH, Akerblom E. Suppression of reaginic antibodies with modified allergens. IV. Induction of suppressor T cells by conjugates of polyethylene glycol (PEG) and monomethoxy PEG with ovalbumin. Int Arch Allergy Appl Immunol 1981; 64:100–114.

10. Yeung VP, Gieni RS, Umetsu DT, DeKruyff RH. Heat-killed Listeria monocytogenes as an adjuvant converts established murine Th2-dominated immune responses into Th1-dominated responses. J Immunol 1998; 161:4146–4152.
11. Hansen G, Yeung VP, Berry G, Umetsu DT, DeKruyff RH. Vaccination with heat-killed Listeria as adjuvant reverses established allergen-induced airway hyperreactivity and inflammation: role of CD8+ T cells and IL-18. J Immunol 2000; 164:223–230.
12. Stock P, Akbari O, Berry G, Freeman GJ, Dekruyff RH, Umetsu DT. Induction of T helper type 1-like regulatory cells that express Foxp3 and protect against airway hyper-reactivity. Nat Immunol 2004; 5:1149–1156.
13. Cottrez F, Hurst SD, Coffman RL, Groux H. T regulatory cells 1 inhibit a Th2-specific response in vivo. J Immunol 2000; 165:4848–4853.
14. Taniguchi M, Harada M, Kojo S, Nakayama T, Wakao H. The regulatory role of Valpha14 NKT cells in innate and acquired immune response. Annu Rev Immunol 2003; 21:483–513.
15. Lantz O, Bendelac, A. An invariant T cell receptor chain is used by a unique subset of major histocompatibility complex class I-specific CD4+ and CD4-CD8- T cells in mice and humans. J Exp Med 1994; 180:1097–1106.
16. Makino Y, Kanno, R., Ito, T, Higashino, K, Taniguchi, M. Predominant expression of invariant $V\alpha14^{+}$ TCR α chain in $NK1.1^{+}$ T cell populations. Int Immunol 1995; 7:1157–1161.
17. Cui J, Shin T, Kawano T, Sato H, Kondo E, Toura I, et al. Requirement for V{alpha}14 NKT Cells in IL-12-Mediated Rejection of Tumors. Science 1997; 278:1623–1626.
18. Sato H, Nakayama T, Tanaka Y, Yamashita M, Shibata Y, Kondo E, et al. Induction of differentiation of pre-NKT cells to mature Valpha 14 NKT cells by granulocyte/macrophage colony-stimulating factor. Proc Natl Acad Sci U S A 1999; 96:7439–7444.
19. Koseki H, Imai K, Nakayama F, Sado T, Moriwaki K, Taniguchi M. Homogenous junctional sequence of the V14+ T-cell antigen receptor {alpha} chain expanded in unprimed mice. Proc Natl Acad Sci U S A 1990; 87:5248–5252. 10.1073/pnas.87.14.5248.
20. Dellabona P, Padovan E, Casorati G, Brockhaus M, Lanzavecchia A. An invariant V alpha 24-J alpha Q/V beta 11 T cell receptor is expressed in all individuals by clonally expanded $CD4^{-}8^{-}$ T cells. J Exp Med 1994; 180:1171–1176.
21. Brigl M, Brenner M. CD1: Antigen presentation and T cell function. Annu Rev Immunol 2004; 22:817–890.
22. Sagiv Y, Hudspeth K, Mattner J, Schrantz N, Stern RK, Zhou D, et al. Cutting edge: impaired glycosphingolipid trafficking and NKT cell development in mice lacking Niemann-Pick type C1 protein. J Immunol 2006; 177:26–30.
23. Zhou D, Cantu C, 3rd, Sagiv Y, Schrantz N, Kulkarni AB, Qi X, et al. Editing of CD1d-bound lipid antigens by endosomal lipid transfer proteins. Science 2004; 303:523–527.
24. Stanic AK, De Silva AD, Park J-J, Sriram V, Ichikawa S, Hirabyashi Y, et al. Defective presentation of the CD1d1-restricted natural Va14Ja18 NKT lymphocyte antigen caused by beta -D-glucosylceramide synthase deficiency. Proc Natl Acad Sci U S A 2003; 100:1849–1854. 10.1073/pnas.0430327100.
25. Zhou D, Mattner J, Cantu Iii C, Schrantz N, Yin N, Gao Y, et al. Lysosomal glycosphingolipid recognition by NKT cells. Science 2004; 306:1786–1789.
26. Morita M, Motoki, K., Akimoto, K., Natori, T., Sakai, T., Sawa, E., Yamaji, K., Koezuka, Y., Kobayashi, E., Fukushima, H. Structure-activity relationship of alpha-galactosylceramide against B16-bearing mice. J Med Chem 1995; 38:2176–2187.
27. Kawano T, Cui J, Koezuka Y, Toura I, Kaneko Y, Motoki K, et al. CD1d-restricted and TCR-mediated activation of V{alpha}14 NKT cells by glycosylceramides. Science 1997; 278:1626–1629.
28. Naidenko OV, Maher JK, Ernst WA, Sakai T, Modlin RL, Kronenberg M. Binding and antigen presentation of ceramide-containing glycolipids by soluble mouse and human CD1d molecules. J Exp Med 1999; 190:1069–1080.
29. Kinjo Y, Wu D, Kim G, Xing G-W, Poles MA, Ho DD, et al. Recognition of bacterial glycosphingolipids by natural killer T cells. Nature 2005; 434:520–525.

30. Kinjo Y, Tupin E, Wu D, Fujio M, Garcia-Navarro R, Benhnia MR-E-I, et al. Natural killer T cells recognize diacylglycerol antigens from pathogenic bacteria. Nat Immunol 2006; 7:978–986.
31. Schmieg J, Yang G, Franck RW, Tsuji M. Superior Protection against Malaria and Melanoma Metastases by a C-glycoside Analogue of the Natural Killer T Cell Ligand {alpha}-Galactosylceramide, J. Exp. Med. 2003; 198:1631–1641.
32. Fujii S-i, Shimizu K, Hemmi H, Fukui M, Bonito AJ, Chen G, et al. Glycolipid {alpha}-C-galactosylceramide is a distinct inducer of dendritic cell function during innate and adaptive immune responses of mice. Proc Natl Acad Sci U S A 2006; 103:11252–11257.
33. Miyamoto K, Miyake S, Yamamura T. A synthetic glycolipid prevents autoimmune encephalomyelitis by inducing TH2 bias of natural killer T cells. Nature 2001; 413:531–534.
34. Bendelac A, Hunziker, R.D., Lantz, O. Increased interleukin 4 and immunoglobulin E production in transgenic mice overexpressing NK1 T cells. J Exp Med 1996; 184:1285–1293.
35. Mendiratta SK, Martin WD, Hong S, Boesteanu A, Joyce S, Van Kaer L. CD1d1 mutant mice are deficient in natural T cells that promptly produce IL-4. Immunity 1997; 6:469–477.
36. Smiley ST, Kaplan MH, Grusby MJ. Immunoglobulin E production in the absence of Interleukin-4-secreting CD1-dependent cells. Science 1997; 275:977–979. 10.1126/science.275.5302.977.
37. Chen Y-H, Chiu NM, Mandal M, Wang N, Wang C-R. Impaired NK1+ T cell development and early IL-4 production in CD1-deficient mice. Immunity 1997; 6:459–467.
38. Cui J, Watanabe N, Kawano T, Yamashita M, Kamata T, Shimizu C, et al. Inhibition of T helper cell type 2 cell differentiation and immunoglobulin E response by ligand-activated Valpha14 natural killer T cells. J. Exp. Med. 1999; 190:783–792.
39. Tighe H, Takabayashi K, Schwartz D, Van Nest G, Tuck S, Eiden JJ, et al. Conjugation of immunostimulatory DNA to the short ragweed allergen Amb a 1 enhances its immunogenicity and reduces its allergenicity. J Allergy Clin Immunol 2000; 106:124–134.
40. Sonoda KH, Exley M, Snapper S, Balk SP, Stein-Streilein J. CD1-reactive natural killer T cells are required for development of systemic tolerance through an immune-privileged site. J Exp Med 1999; 190:1215–1226.
41. Sonoda KH, Faunce DE, Taniguchi M, Exley M, Balk S, Stein-Streilein J. NK T cell-derived IL-10 is essential for the differentiation of antigen-specific T regulatory cells in systemic tolerance. J Immunol 2001; 166:42–50.
42. Wakkach A, Fournier N, Brun V, Breittmayer JP, Cottrez F, Groux H. Characterization of dendritic cells that induce tolerance and T regulatory 1 cell differentiation in vivo. Immunity 2003; 18:605–617.
43. Ling EM, Smith T, Nguyen XD, Pridgeon C, Dallman M, Arbery J, et al. Relation of CD4+CD25+ regulatory T-cell suppression of allergen-driven T-cell activation to atopic status and expression of allergic disease. Lancet 2004; 363:608–615.
44. Akdis M, Verhagen J, Taylor A, Karamloo F, Karagiannidis C, Crameri R, et al. Immune responses in healthy and allergic individuals are characterized by a fine balance between allergen-specific T regulatory 1 and T helper 2 cells. J Exp Med 2004; 199:1567–1575.

Targeting Th2 Cells in Asthmatic Airways

Gaetano Caramori, Kazuhiro Ito, Paolo Casolari, Marco Contoli, Alberto Papi, and Ian M. Adcock

Introduction

Asthma represents a profound worldwide public health problem. The most effective anti-asthmatic drugs currently available include inhaled β_2-agonists and glucocorticoids; these control asthma in about 90–95% of patients. However, the future therapies will need to focus on the 5–10% patients who do not respond well to these treatments and who account for ~50% of the health care costs of asthma [1,2]. Strategies for the primary prevention of asthma remain in the realm of speculation and hypothesis [3]. Drug development for asthma has been directed at improving currently available drugs and finding new compounds that target the Th2-driven airway inflammatory response. Several new compounds have been developed to target specific components of the inflammatory process in asthma [e.g., anti-IgE antibodies (omalizumab), cytokines and/or chemokines antagonists, immunomodulators, antagonists of adhesion molecules], although they have not yet been proven to be particularly effective. In fact, only omalizumab has reached the market; it may be most cost-effective for patients with severe persistent asthma and frequent severe exacerbations requiring hospital care [3–5]. In this chapter, we will review the role of current antiasthma drugs and future new chemical entities that can target Th2 cells in asthmatic airways. Some of these new Th2-oriented strategies may, in the future, not only control symptoms and modify the natural course of asthma, but also potentially prevent or cure the disease.

G. Caramori (✉), P. Casolari, M. Contoli, and A. Papi
Dipartimento di Medicina Clinica e Sperimentale, Centro di Ricerca su Asma e BPCO, Università di Ferrara, Via Savonarola 9, 44100 Ferrara, Italy
e-mail: crm@unife.it

K. Ito and I.M. Adcock
Airway Disease Section, National Heart and Lung Institute, Imperial College of London, London, UK

R. Pawankar et al. (eds.), *Allergy Frontiers: Future Perspectives*,
DOI 10.1007/978-4-431-99365-0_8, © Springer 2010

Effects of Current Antiasthma Drugs on Th2 Cells in Asthmatic Airways

Despite the large number of controlled clinical studies on the effect of many antiasthma drugs (particularly inhaled glucocorticoids) in suppressing airway inflammation in asthmatics, there is a complete absence of controlled clinical studies on the effect of these drugs on the Th2/Tc2 lymphocytes ratio in the airways of asthmatic patients. In particular it is still unknown if inhaled glucocorticoids can decrease the recruitment of Th2 lymphocytes and/or the degree of their differentiation and/or activation.

In vivo animal models of asthma, particularly murine, have been increasingly used to investigate the efficacy of several antiasthma drugs, including their effect on Th2 lymphocytes. However, animal models of asthma have limitations; most are models of acute allergen exposure which are sensitive to anti-interleukin-5 strategies; animals do not spontaneously develop asthma and no model mimics the entire asthma phenotype [6]. For these reasons, the results obtained in animal models of asthma must be confirmed with controlled clinical trials in asthmatic patients.

Effects of Glucocorticoids on Th2 Cells

Inhaled glucocorticoids are the only antiasthma agents that clearly reverse the specific chronic airway inflammation present in asthma. Inhaled glucocorticoids have anti-inflammatory effects in the airway of patients with asthma [3]. In patients treated with inhaled glucocorticoids, there is a marked reduction in the number of mast cells, macrophages, T-lymphocytes, and eosinophils in the sputum, bronchoalveolar lavage (BAL), and bronchial wall [7,8]. Furthermore, glucocorticoids reverse the shedding of epithelial cells, the mucus-cell hyperplasia, and basement-membrane thickening characteristically seen in biopsy specimens from patients with asthma [7,8]. However, some inflammation still persists in the airways of patients with asthma who have poor airway function, despite regular and prolonged treatment with high doses of inhaled or systemic glucocorticoids [8,9]. The inflammatory component of asthmatic airways most responsive to glucocorticoid treatment seems to be eosinophilic inflammation. In patients with persistent asthma, well controlled tapering of inhaled glucocorticoids induces an exacerbation within a few months. This is usually associated with a reversible increase of eosinophilic airway inflammation. Some patients with difficult-to-control asthma may develop exacerbations despite treatment with inhaled glucocorticoids, and these often appear to have an eosinophil-independent inflammatory mechanism [8,9].

Glucocorticoids also have direct inhibitory effects on many of the cells involved in airway inflammation in asthma, including macrophages, T-lymphocytes, eosinophils, mast cells, and airway smooth muscle and epithelial cells. In vitro, glucocorticoids decrease cytokine-mediated survival of eosinophils by stimulating apoptosis.

This process may explain the reduction in the number of eosinophils, particularly low-density eosinophils, in the circulation and lower airways of patients with asthma during glucocorticoid therapy. Inhaled glucocorticoids attenuated the allergen-induced increase in peripheral blood eosinophils and on eosinophil/basophil colony-forming units (Eo/B CFU) [7,8]. They also significantly attenuated the baseline, but not allergen-induced increase, numbers of total CD34(+) cells, CD34(+)IL-3Rα+ cells, and interleukin (IL)-5-responsive Eo/B-CFU in the bone marrow. Glucocorticoids may not inhibit the release of mediators from mast cells, but they do reduce the number of mast cells within the airway [7,8]. CD4+ and CD8+ T lymphocytes in peripheral blood of asthmatic patients are in an activated state and this is downregulated by inhaled glucocorticoids. In fact, treatment with inhaled glucocorticoids reduces the expression of the activation markers CD25 and HLA-DR in both CD4+ and CD8+ T-cell subsets in peripheral blood of patients with asthma. In addition, there is a correlation between the down-regulation of CD4 and CD8 T-lymphocyte activation and the improvement in asthma control. Treatment with inhaled glucocorticoids reduces the number of activated T lymphocytes (CD25+ and HLA-DR+) in the BAL from asthmatic patients [7,8]. However, severe glucocorticoid-dependent and -resistant asthma is associated with persistent airway T-lymphocyte activation [9–11].

In general, glucocorticoids substantially reduce the mast cell/eosinophil/lymphocyte-driven processes, while leaving behind or even augmenting a neutrophil-mediated process. Glucocorticoids enhance neutrophil function through increased leukotriene and superoxide production, as well as inhibition of apoptosis. Glucocorticoids have no effect on sputum neutrophil numbers in patients with severe persistent asthma [9]. Part of the anti-inflammatory activity of glucocorticoids in asthma may also involve reduction in macrophage and resident cell eicosanoid (leukotriene B_4 and thromboxane B_2), and cytokine and chemokine [e.g., IL-1β, IL-4, IL-5, IL-8, GM-CSF, TNF-α, CCL3 (macrophage inflammatory protein-1alpha MIP-1α)], and CCL5 (RANTES) synthesis [7,12]. In addition to their suppressive effects on inflammatory cells, glucocorticoids may also inhibit plasma exudation and mucus secretion in the inflamed airways. However, glucocorticoids have no effect on sputum concentrations of fibrinogen. There is an increase in vascularity in the bronchial mucosa of asthmatics, and high doses of inhaled glucocorticoids may reduce airway wall vascularity in asthmatic patients. Inhaled glucocorticoids also attenuate the increased airway mucosal blood flow present in asthmatic patients [7,8].

Many in vitro studies have indicated that glucocorticoids may participate in guiding the differentiation of T lymphocytes toward the Th2 phenotype [13]. The immunosuppressive effect of glucocorticoids after organ transplantation is mainly due to preferential blockade of Th1 cytokine expression and promotion of a Th2 cytokine-secreting profile. Glucocorticoids, in vitro (a) inhibit IL-12 secretion from monocyte-macrophages and dendritic cells, (b) decrease IL-12 receptor 1- and 2-chain expression, thereby inhibiting IL-12 signalling, (c) inhibit IL-12-induced STAT-4 (transcription factor that drives Th1 differentiation) phosphorylation without affecting STAT-6 (transcription factor that drives Th2 differentiation) phosphorylation , and (d) thereby deviate the immune response predominantly toward the Th2 phenotype [8,12].

In stable asthmatics, systemic glucocorticoid treatment produces a small but significant decrease of 16% in blood CD3+CD4+ and a 12% increase in natural killer (NK)-cell frequency within 3 h. In contrast, the CD3+CD8+ T-cell number and activation marker remain unchanged [14]. In vitro fluticasone inhibits IL-5 and IL-13 and enhances IL-10 synthesis in allergen-stimulated peripheral blood CD4+ T cell cultures in a concentration-dependent manner [15]. Similarly, salmeterol, but not salbutamol, also inhibits IL-5 and IL-13 and enhances IL-10 synthesis in the same cultures [15]. When used in combination, the two drugs demonstrated an additive effect on this pattern of cytokine production [15], perhaps through an effect on Nuclear factor of activated T cells (NFAT) and AP-1 transcription factors [16].

Furthermore, in vitro, glucocorticoids inhibit proliferation and IL-4 and IL-5 secretion by human allergen-specific Th2 lymphocytes [17]. Both beclomethasone and fluticasone inhibit allergen-induced peripheral blood T-cell proliferation and their expression of IL-5 and GM-CSF in asthmatics [18].

Interestingly, the combination of fluticasone and salmeterol significantly inhibits production of IFN-γ, but not that of Th2 cytokines (IL-5 and IL-13) from PBMCs from asthmatic subjects [19]. This is in contrast with the results of an earlier study [20]. When rolipram, a phosphodiesterase 4 (PDE4) inhibitor, is added to the fluticasone-salmeterol combination, this triple combination inhibits IL-13 production by PBMCs from asthmatic patients [19].

In vitro fluticasone alone increases and salmeterol alone does not affect peripheral blood T-cell apoptosis in either normal or asthmatic subjects [21,22]. Their combination significantly increases peripheral blood T-cell apoptosis in comparison with fluticasone alone, and it is also able to reduce the expression of the phosphorylated inhibitory κB alpha (IκBa), thus limiting the nuclear factor κB (NF-κB) activation [22].

Effects of Theophylline on Th2 Cells in Asthmatic Airways

Theophylline has been used in the treatment of asthma for many decades and is still used worldwide. Low-dose theophylline has recently been shown to have significant anti-inflammatory effects in the airways of the asthmatic patients [23,24]. This is supported by a reduced infiltration of eosinophils and CD4+ lymphocytes into the airways of asthmatic patients after allergen challenge subsequent to low doses of theophylline [25,26]. Low doses of theohylline also have reduced the number of CD4+ and CD8+ T lymphocytes and IL-4- and IL-5-containing cells in bronchial biopsies of asthmatic subjects [27,28]. In addition, in an uncontrolled study, in asthmatic patients, regular treatment with low doses of theohylline reduced sputum eosinophils and IL-5 expression, but not sputum CD4+ T lymphocytes and IFN-γ [29]. In patients with severe persistent asthma treated with high doses of inhaled glucocorticoids, withdrawal of theophylline results in increased numbers of activated CD4+ cells and eosinophils in bronchial biopsies [30]. In vitro, low concentrations of theophylline (<25 nM) can inhibit the migration of T lymphocytes to chemotactic factors [31]. Furthermore, theophylline, at high concentrations, has been shown to reduce IL-2 production by T cells and IL-2-dependent T cell proliferation and induces nonspecific suppressor activity in human peripheral blood lymphocytes [32].

In vitro, high concentrations of theophylline suppress CD4+ expression of both Th1 and Th2, excluding IL-5, cytokines probably via inhibition of phosphodiesterases [33,34]. In an animal model of asthma, both low and high doses of aminophylline are effective in preventing late-phase bronchoconstriction, bronchial hyperresponsiveness, and airway inflammation. Furthermore, aminophylline decreases Th2-related cytokine mRNA expression but increases Th1-related cytokines mRNA expression [35].

Effects of Leukotriene-Receptor Antagonists and Synthesis-Inhibitors on Th2 Cells in Asthmatic Airways

Leukotriene-receptor antagonists (pranlukast, zafirlukast, and montelukast) and synthesis-inhibitors (zileuton) reduce the severity of bronchial hyperresponsiveness in asthma. In asthmatic patients, these agents can reduce sputum, bronchial biopsy, and peripheral blood eosinophilia induced by experimental challenge with allergen, aspirin, sulfur dioxide, or leukotriene (LT)E_4 [3,36].

In vitro, the cysteinyl-leukotriene receptor antagonist, pranlukast, can concentration-dependently inhibit the release of Th2 cytokines (IL-3, IL-4, GM-CSF), but not of the Th1 cytokine IL-2, from mite allergen-stimulated PBMCs from asthmatic patients [37]. Also, in an animal model of asthma, treatment with pranlukast reduces IL-5 but has no effect on IFN-γ production [38]. In contrast, high doses of montelukast reduce IL-4, IL-5, and IL-13 levels in the lung and IL-4 and IL-5 expression in BAL [39]. In similar studies, montelukast decreases IL-4 mRNA expression in the lungs while increasing IFN-γ mRNA expression after allergen challenge [40]. Interestingly, the treatment of children with allergic rhinitis with montelukast induces a significant decrease of nasal lavage, IL-4, and IL-13 and a significant increase of IFN-γ levels [41].

Effects of β_2-Agonists on Th2 Cells in Asthmatic Airways

Despite some positive in vivo studies, particularly with formoterol and more recently with salmeterol, the anti-inflammatory effect of short- and long-acting inhaled β_2-agonists has not been convincingly demonstrated in asthmatic airways [3,8]. Although, it was initially proposed that the bronchodilating and symptom-relieving effects of long-acting inhaled β_2-agonists may potentially mask increasing inflammation and delay detection of worsening asthma, there is no evidence that long-acting inhaled β_2-agonists worsen exacerbations of asthma or the chronic airway inflammation in asthma [3].

In vitro studies using resting and activated murine Th1 and Th2 cells have shown that a detectable level of the β_2AR is expressed only on resting and activated Th1 cells, but not the Th2 cells [42,43]. Baseline levels of intracellular cAMP are similar in both subsets, but β_2-agonists induce an increase in cAMP levels in Th1 cells only [43].

Human peripheral blood mononuclear cells when stimulated in vitro with β_2-agonists show decreased levels of IFN-γ and increased levels of IL-4, IL-5, and IL-10, an effect that is thought to be mediated by decreasing IL-12 production thereby suggesting that β_2-agonists promote Th2 cytokine production. β_2-agonists are potent and selective inhibitors of LPS- and CD40-CD40L-stimulated IL-12 production by human macrophages and dendritic cells [44]. In accord with their ability to suppress IL-12 production, when β_2-agonists are added to neonatal cord blood T cells, they selectively inhibit the development of Th1 cells and enhance Th2 cell development [44]. However, in other in vitro studies, β_2-agonists have been shown to inhibit the secretion of IL-4 and IL-5 in T cell lines [45]. Regular treatment of patients with mild asthma with the long-acting β_2-agonist formoterol does not decrease the number of IL-4 immunoreactive cells in their bronchial mucosa [46].

Effects of Cromoglycate and Nedocromil on Th2 Cells in Asthmatic Airways

Cromoglycate (cromolyn) has been shown to inhibit the IgE-mediated mediator release from human mast cells, and to suppress the activation of, and mediator release from, other inflammatory cells (macrophages, eosinophils, monocytes). Prolonged treatment of asthmatic patients with cromoglycate decreases the percentage of blood, sputum, and BAL eosinophils, suggesting a direct anti-inflammatory effect in the human asthmatic airways. Cromoglycate has also been shown to inhibit chloride channels in vitro [8].

Cromoglycate and nedocromil are both very well tolerated and still widely prescribed, in some countries, for the treatment of asthma in children. However, the majority of controlled studies do not show any efficacy of these drugs in the treatment of persistent asthma compared with placebo, although they show some efficacy in exercise-induced bronchoconstriction [8]. In vitro studies also suggest that nedocromil can modulate the differentiation of Th1/Th2 cells [47]; however, there is a complete absence of controlled clinical trials in asthmatic patients using these drugs measuring the Th1/Th2 balance in the lower airways.

Omalizumab

There is a complete absence of controlled clinical trials in asthmatic patients using omalizumab measuring the Th1/Th2 balance in the lower airways.

Effects of Immunosuppressant Drugs on Th2 Cells in Asthmatic Airways

Methotrexate may have a small glucocorticoid sparing effect in adults with asthma who are dependent on oral glucocorticoids. However, the overall reduction in daily steroid use is probably not large enough to reduce steroid-induced adverse effects. This small potential to reduce the impact of steroid side effects is probably also insufficient to offset the adverse effects of methotrexate [2,48]. The absence of an inhibitory effect of methotrexate on a number of inflammatory cells in the blood and mucosa of the asthmatic patients suggests that the steroid-sparing effect of methotrexate is achieved by modulating cell function rather than cell number [8]. Cyclosporin A inhibits the allergen-induced late asthmatic reaction, the allergen-induced increase in IL-5 and GM-CSF in mRNA+ cells in BAL, and the number of eosinophils in blood and bronchial mucosa, but not the early asthmatic reaction [8]. In vitro cyclosporin A inhibits allergen-driven T-cell proliferation, production of IL-2, IL-4, and IL-5 by human CD4+ helper T cells, and IL-5 production in PBMCs from allergen-sensitized atopic asthmatic individuals at physiologic concentrations. In vitro cyclosporin A, at putative therapeutic concentrations, has antiproliferative effects, with equivalent potency, on T-lymphocytes from glucocorticoid-sensitive and -resistant asthmatics, but in vitro T-lymphocyte proliferation assays are not predictive of clinical response to cyclosporin therapy in chronic severe asthma [8,49].

In summary, the glucocorticoid-sparing effect of cyclosporin A is small and of questionable clinical significance. Given the side effects of cyclosporin A, the available evidence does not recommend routine use of this drug in the treatment of oral glucocorticoid-dependent asthma [2,8,50].

New Drugs Which Can Potentially Interfere with Th2 Cells in Asthmatic Airways

Many new drugs are now in development for the treatment of asthma. There has been an intensive search for anti-inflammatory treatments for bronchial asthma that are as effective as glucocorticoids but with fewer side effects. While one approach is to seek glucocorticoids with a greater therapeutic index, the others involve developing different classes of anti-inflammatory drugs [51]. There is also a need for new treatments to deal with the small minority of patients with more severe asthma that is currently not well controlled by high doses of inhaled glucocorticoids and for a safe oral drug that would be effective in all atopic diseases (including asthma, allergic rhinitis, and atopic dermatitis), as they often occur together [51].

Selective inhibition of Th2 lymphocytes function may be effective and well tolerated; there are active research programmes for such drugs in most pharmaceutical companies [52].

Selective Inhibitors of Phosphodiesterase 4

A promising class of novel anti-inflammatory treatments for asthma are the selective inhibitors of PDE4. PDE4 is expressed in macrophages, neutrophils, T cells, and airway smooth muscle cells [8]. These compounds inhibit the hydrolysis of intracellular cAMP, which may result in bronchodilation and suppression of inflammation. There are many compounds in this new class of drugs in the clinical development; however, most of the clinical studies reported have been performed with cilomilast and roflumilast [8]. There are controlled clinical trials suggesting some efficacy of roflumilast in mild to moderate asthma and to prevent exercise-induced asthma in adults [53]. However, the development of cilomilast as an antiasthma drug has apparently been suspended.

There are no significant differences in the expression of PDE4A, PDE4B, and PDE4D in peripheral blood CD4 and CD8 lymphocytes between normal and asthmatic patients [54]. PDE4 subtype expression is lower; however, it shows more intersubject variability in CD8+ cells [54]. Furthermore, in vitro, Th1 lymphocytes show a reduced expression of PDE4C isoform and a lack of PDE4D isoform compared to Th2 lymphocytes [55].

Cyclic adenosine monophosphate (cAMP) is a negative regulator of T-cell activation. However, the effects of cAMP on signaling pathways that regulate cytokine production and cell cycle progression in Th1 and Th2 lymphocytes remain controversial.

In vitro, using allergen-induced human Th1 and Th2 clones, both Th1 and Th2 cytokines production is equally inhibited by selective PDE4 inhibitors [55]. However, the increase in intracellular cAMP is significantly more in Th2 compared with Th1 clones [55]. In vitro, selective PDE4 inhibitors inhibit proliferation and IL-4 and IL-5 secretion by human allergen-specific Th2 lymphocytes and Th1 and Th2 clones [34,56]. Other, in vitro studies suggest that PDE4 inhibitors have complex inhibitory effects on Th1-mediated immunity at the concentration ranges achievable in vivo, whereas Th2-mediated responses are mostly unaffected or even enhanced [57]. The Th2 skewing of the developing immune response is explained by the effects of PDE inhibitors on several factors contributing to T cell priming: the cytokine milieu; the type of costimulatory signal, i.e., up-regulation of CD86 and down-regulation of CD80; and the antigen avidity [57].

In animal studies, PDE4 inhibitors inhibit antigen-mediated T cell proliferation and skew the T cell cytokine profile toward a Th2 phenotype by downregulating the expression or production of Th1 cytokines without affecting Th2 cytokine expression [58,59].

There is a complete absence of controlled clinical trials in asthmatic patients using these drugs measuring the Th1/Th2 balance in the lower airways.

Chemokine Receptor Antagonists Targeting Th2 Cells in Asthmatic Airways

Numerous antibodies, receptor-blocking mutant chemokines, and small molecules are now being evaluated for the treatment of asthma. Chemokines have proven to be amenable drug targets for the development of low molecular weight antagonists by the pharmaceutical industry. CCR3, CCR4, CCR8, and CRTH2 nonpeptide antagonists are involved in the recruitment and/or activation of Th2 cells in the lung and are now being evaluated for the treatment of bronchial asthma; but, so far, no clinical data for these compounds have been reported. However, over the next few years, it is expected that many studies will have been published; at that time, the potential of these exciting new targets will be fully realized [60,61].

CCR3 Antagonists and Asthma

A range of low molecular weight chemicals have been developed to antagonize CCR3, with the aim of selectively inhibiting eosinophil recruitment into tissue sites. However, the results of recent clinical trials with monoclonal antibodies directed against IL-5 question the role of eosinophils in mediating the symptoms of asthma [62]. For this reason, the plans for clinical development of many CCR3 antagonists in asthma have been put on hold [63].

More recently, novel oral CCR3-selective antagonists have been developed, by many pharmaceutical companies including Brystol-Myers Squibb, GSK, and Yamanouchi Pharmaceuticals [64–71], including double CCR3 and H1 receptor antagonists [72]. Some of these compounds are now undergoing clinical trials in asthma.

These compounds are able to prevent the activation and recruitment of eosinophils, but not lymphocytes, in animal models of asthma [66,71,73]. However, in another animal model of asthma, a CCR3 antagonist did not decrease the number of eosinophils in lung tissues but only the antigen-induced clustering of eosinophils along the airway nerves [74]. Immunostaining shows eotaxin in airway nerves and in cultured airway parasympathetic neurons [74]. In vitro both IL-4 and IL-13 increase expression of eotaxin in airway parasympathetic neurons [74]. Thus, signaling via CCR3 mediates eosinophil recruitment to airway nerves and may be a prerequisite for the blockade of inhibitory muscarinic M2 receptors by eosinophil major basic protein [74].

N-nonanoyl-CCL14[10–74] (NNY-CCL14), is an N-terminally truncated and modified peptide derived from the chemokine CCL14 that in vitro inhibits the activity of CCR3 on human eosinophils, because it is able to induce internalization of CCR3 and desensitize CCR3-mediated intracellular calcium release and chemotaxis. In contrast to naturally occurring CCL11, NNY-CCL14 is resistant to degradation by CD26/dipeptidyl peptidase IV (DPP4). This compound is effective in animal models of asthma [75]. N-Nonanoyl-CCL11 (NNY-CCL11) represents another similar compound with dual activity restricted to CCR3 and CCR5. It also has receptor-inactivating capacity and stability against DPP4 degradation [76]. All these new compounds have been developed by Ipf Pharmaceuticals (http://www.ipf-pharmaceuticals.de/index2.html).

Specific targeting of inhibitory receptors on CCR3+ cells may be an alternative approach. For example, cross-linking of inhibitory receptor protein 60 (IR-p60)/CD300a inhibits mast cell and eosinophil activation, and coaggregation of CD300a with CCR3 using a bispecific antibody fragment (LC1) has been shown to be effective in an animal model of asthma [77], but is still untested in human asthma.

TPIASM8 is a new inhaled compound consisting of two modified RNA-targeting oligonucleotides directed against the CCR3 receptor and a common β subunit for the receptors of IL-3, 5, and GM-CSF. TPIASM8 is currently in phase II clinical development for the treatment of asthma (http://www.topigen.com). This novel approach is expected to have advantages over single mediator antagonists.

CCR4 Antagonists and Asthma

The utility of the developing CCR4 antagonists is controversial because CCR4-deficient mice do not show any change in cell recruitment in the lung or induction of airway hyperresponsiveness [78]. However, many CCR4 antagonists are now in preclinical development and have been shown to be effective in reducing the chemotaxis of Th2 cells in vitro and lung eosinophilic inflammation in an animal model of asthma [79–84]. There are no published controlled clinical trials of these compounds in asthma.

CCR8 Antagonists and Asthma

The in vivo role of the CCL1/CCR8 axis in Th2-mediated inflammation is far from clear. CCR8-deficient mice have a marked reduction of airway eosinophil infiltration and allergen-induced airway hyperresponsiveness, but the CCR8 is not essential for the development of airway inflammation in other animal models of asthma [85,86]. Overall, these data, while highlighting a potential major role for CCR8, suggest that multiple chemokines and chemokine receptors may have redundant functions in the pathogenesis of bronchial asthma. CCR8 and CCL1, the CCR8 ligand, antagonists have been recently developed [87–90]. There are no published controlled clinical trials of these compounds in asthma.

CRTH2 Antagonists and Asthma

Ramatroban (Baynas, BAY u3405), an orally active, tromboxan (Tx)A2 antagonist marketed in Japan for the treatment of allergic rhinitis, is also an antagonist for CRTH2, and in vitro inhibits PGD2-induced migration of eosinophils. Ramatroban has been shown to partially attenuate prostaglandin PGD2-induced bronchial hyperresponsiveness in humans, as well as reduce antigen-induced early- and late-phase inflammatory responses in animal models of asthma [91].

A new selective CRTH2 antagonist, named TM30089, is structurally closely related to ramatroban but with less affinity for TP and many other receptors, including the related anaphylatoxin C3a and C5a receptors, selected chemokine receptors, and the cyclooxygenase isoforms 1 and 2, and attenuates airway eosinophilia and mucus cell-hyperplasia in an animal model of asthma [92].

Many novel, selective orally active CRTH2 antagonists have been recently developed [93–99], but there are no published studies on the effect of CRTH2 antagonists in asthmatic patients; the results of the ongoing clinical trials are awaited with interest [97]. A once a day oral molecule ODC9101 is now in phase IIa clinical trials in asthma (http://www.oxagen.co.uk).

CCR5 Agonists and Asthma

Aminooxypentane (AOP)-RANTES/CCL5 is a full agonist of human CCR5 [100], a chemokine receptor expressed selectively on human Th1 lymphocytes. In an animal model of asthma, AOP-RANTES/CCL5 decreases allergen-induced airway inflammation suggesting that targeting CCR5 may also be effective [100].

Sphingosine 1-Phosphate Receptor Agonists

Sphingosine 1-phosphate (S1P) in blood, lymph, and immune tissues stimulates and regulates T cell migration through their S1P(1) (endothelial differentiation gene encoded receptor-1) G protein-coupled receptors (S1P1Rs). S1P1Rs also mediate suppression of T cell proliferation and cytokine production. In fact, S1P decreases CD4 T cell generation of IFN-γ and IL-4 [101].

The novel oral immunomodulator FTY720 is a chemical derivative of myriocin, a metabolite of the ascomycete Isaria sinclairii. The drug has recently been shown to be effective in human kidney transplantation. In contrast to classical immunosuppressants such as cyclosporine A or FK506, FTY720 selectively and reversibly sequesters lymphocytes but not monocytes or granulocytes from blood and spleen into secondary lymphoid organs, thereby preventing their migration toward sites of inflammation and allograft rejection. Moreover, FTY720 does not impair T cell activation, expansion, and memory to systemic viral infections or induce T cell apoptosis at clinically relevant concentrations [102]. FTY720 is a structural analog of sphingosine and following in vivo phosphorylation acts as a agonist at S1P1Rs to block cell motility [102]. This leads to sequestration of lymphocytes in secondary lymphatic tissues and thus, the lymphocytes are kept away from inflammatory lesions. Both Th1 and Th2 cells express a similar pattern of FTY720-targeted S1P1Rs. The inhibitory effect of FTY720, on airway inflammation, airway hyperresponsiveness, and goblet cell hyperplasia in an animal model of asthma, suggest a potential role of this compound in the treatment of asthma [102]. The accompanying lymphopenia could be a serious side effect that would preclude the use of oral FTY720 as an antiasthmatic drug [103]. However, in an animal model of asthma, inhalation of FTY720 prior to or during ongoing allergen challenge suppresses Th2-dependent eosinophilic airway inflammation and bronchial hyperresponsiveness without causing lymphopenia and T cell retention in the lymph nodes [103].

Local treatment with FTY720 inhibits migration of lung dendritic cells to the mediastinal lymph nodes, which in turn inhibits the formation of allergen-specific Th2 cells in lymph nodes. Also, FTY720-treated dendritic cells are less potent in activating naive and effector Th2 cells [103].

Ca^{2+}Release-Activated Ca^{2+} Channels Blockers and Asthma

The pyrazole derivative, YM-58483 (BTP2; http://www.astellas.com), potently inhibits Ca^{2+} release-activated Ca^{2+} (CRAC) channels, IL-2 production in T cells, IL-4 and IL-5 production in stimulated murine Th2 cells, and IL-5 production in stimulated human whole blood cells. YM-58483 inhibited airway eosinophil infiltration, IL-4, and cysteinyl-leukotrienes content and the late-phase asthmatic bronchoconstriction in animal models of asthma [104]. There are no published studies on human asthma using CRAC channel inhibitors.

Transcription Factor Modulators

Asthma is characterized by an increased expression of components of the inflammatory cascade. These inflammatory proteins include cytokines, chemokines, growth factors, enzymes, receptors, and adhesion molecules. The increased expression of these proteins seen in asthma is the result of enhanced gene transcription since many of the genes are not expressed in normal cells but are induced in a cell-specific manner during the inflammatory process. Changes in gene transcription are regulated by transcription factors, which are proteins that bind to DNA and modulate the transcriptional apparatus. Transcription factors may, therefore, play a key role in the pathogenesis of asthma [105,106].

Many transcription factors (for example NF-κB, AP-1, GATA-3, STAT-1 STAT-6, c-MAF, NFATs, SOCS) have been implicated in the differentiation of Th2 lymphocytes and therefore represent therapeutic targets for asthma.

Several new compounds based on interacting with specific transcription factors or their activation pathways are now in development for the treatment of asthma, and some drugs already in clinical use (such as glucocorticoids) work via transcription factors [7]. One concern about this approach is the specificity of such drugs; however, it is clear that transcription factors have selective effects on the expression of certain genes and this may make it possible to be more selective [105,106]. In addition, there are cell-specific transcription factors that may be targeted for inhibition, which can provide selectivity of drug action. One such example is GATA-3, which has been reported to have a restricted cellular distribution. In asthma, it may be possible to target drugs to the airways by inhalation, as is currently utilized for inhaled glucocorticoids to avoid, or minimize, any systemic effects [105,106].

NF-κB and AP-1

Transcription factors, such as NF-κB and activator protein (AP)-1, play an important role in the orchestration of the airway inflammation in asthma. The role of NF-κB and AP-1 should be seen as an amplifying and perpetuating mechanism that will exaggerate the disease-specific inflammatory process. In vitro, AP-1 and NF-κB are also important for the function of Th2 cells [105,106]. There is an evidence for activation of both NF-κB and AP-1 in the bronchial epithelial cells of patients with asthma [105,106].

There are several possible approaches to the inhibition of NF-κB. The most promising approach might be the inhibition of IKKβ by small-molecule inhibitors, which are now in development by several companies [105–108]. Alternative strategies involve the development of small peptide inhibitors of IKKβ/IKKγ association.

Interestingly, in animals, NF-κB decoy oligodeoxynucleotides prevent and treat oxazolone-colitis and thus affect a Th2-mediated inflammatory process [109].

One concern about the long-term inhibition of NF-κB is that effective inhibitors may cause side effects, such as increased susceptibility to infections, as mice that lack NF-κB genes succumb to septicaemia [105–108].

A small-molecule inhibitor, PNRI-299, targeting the oxidoreductase redox effector factor-1, selectively inhibits AP-1 transcription, without affecting NF-κB transcription and significantly reduces airway eosinophil infiltration, mucus hypersecretion, edema, and lung IL-4 levels in a mouse asthma model [110].

In an animal model of asthma, the intratracheally delivered AP-1 decoy oligodeoxynucleotides attenuate eosinophilic airway inflammation, airway hyperresponsiveness, mucous cell hyperplasia, production of allergen-specific immunoglobulins, and synthesis of IL-4, IL-5, and IL-13 in the lung [111].

GATA-3

The transcription factor GATA-3 seems to be of particular importance in the differentiation of human Th2 cells; its expression is increased in the peripheral venous blood T cells from atopic asthmatics [106] and in bronchial biopsies of stable asthmatics compared to controls and increase in BAL cells of asthmatics after allergen challenge [112,113].

Furthermore many studies indicate a critical role for GATA-3 in the development of airway eosinophilia, mucus hypersecretion, and airway hyperresponsiveness in animal models of asthma [114] and suggest that local delivery of GATA-3 antisense oligonucleotides may be a novel approach for the treatment of asthma [115]. This approach has the potential advantage of suppressing the expression of various proinflammatory Th2 cytokines simultaneously rather than suppressing the activity of a single cytokine.

STAT1 Blockers and Asthma

The intracellular signaling intermediates signal transducer, and activator of transcription (STAT)1 mediates many effects of IFN-γ and is implicated in the activation of T-bet, a master regulator of Th1 differentiation. In animal models, Th1 and Th2 cell trafficking is differentially controlled in vivo by STAT1 and STAT6, respectively. STAT6, which regulates Th2 cell trafficking, had no effect on the trafficking of Th1 cells and STAT1 deficiency does not alter Th2 cell trafficking [116].

STAT1 in peripheral tissue regulates the homing of antigen-specific Th1 cells through the induction of a distinct subset of chemokines (CXCL9, CXCL10, CXCL11, and CXCL16) [116]. CXCL10 replacement partially restored Th1 cell trafficking in STAT1-deficient mice in vivo, and deficiency in n, the receptor for CXCL9, CXCL10, and CXCL11, impaired the trafficking of Th1 cells [116].

STAT1 expression and activation are elevated in asthmatic bronchial epithelial cells in some, but not all [117], studies [118]. This has led to the development of decoy oligonucleotides designed to block STAT1 activity. In an animal model of asthma, a single application of this STAT1 decoy oligonucleotides significantly reduces airway hyperresponsiveness, the number of BAL eosinophils and lymphocytes, and the BAL level of IL-5 [119].

This decoy oligonucleotides designated AVT-01 is currently undergoing phase II studies in asthmatic patients (http://www.avontec.de).

STAT-6

STAT6-knockout animals do not express Th2-type chemokines in the lung and as a result do not recruit allergen-specific Th2 cells into the lung following allergen challenge [120]. Furthermore, STAT6-knockout animals fail to develop goblet cell metaplasia in response to IL-13 instillation, and this response can be rescued by epithelial-directed expression of a STAT-6 transgene [121].

Previous data investigating the localization of STAT6 in the human airways have produced divergent results. In two studies, STAT-6 was present only within infiltrating cells of the nose and bronchial mucosa [122,123], while in another two studies STAT-6 was expressed predominantly within the bronchial epithelium of mild asthmatic subjects [124,125]. Therefore, although tempting as a target, a clear rationale for targeting STAT-6 in asthma is not currently available.

In vitro a STAT6-selective antisense significantly reduces eotaxin release from human airway smooth muscle stimulated by IL-13 or IL-4 [126]. Interestingly, in an animal model of asthma, niflumic acid, a relatively specific blocker of calcium-activated chloride channel, inhibits IL-13-induced goblet cell hyperplasia, MUC5AC expression, airway hyperresponsiveness, BAL eosinophilia, and eotaxin increase. Niflumic acid also inhibits STAT6 activation and eotaxin expression in bronchial epithelial cells in vitro [127].

The adipocyte/macrophage fatty acid-binding protein (FABP), aP2, is expressed in bronchial epithelial cells and it is strongly upregulated by both IL-4 and IL-13 in a STAT6-dependent manner. The presence of functional aP2 has been shown very important in an animal model of asthma [128].

c-MAF

The effects of c-MAF appear to be fairly selective, since in vitro studies have demonstrated that this factor is critical for the production of IL-4, but not for IL-5 or IL-13 [129,130]. c-MAF expression in T lymphocytes is regulated by IL-4 levels during Th differentiation. ICOS costimulation potentiates the TCR-mediated initial IL-4 production, possibly through the enhancement of NFATc1 expression [131]. In animals, c-MAF is a Th2 cell-specific transcription factor, which promotes the differentiation of Th2 cells mainly by an IL-4-dependent mechanism [132]. c-MAF-transgenic mice produce higher serum levels of IgE and IgG1, and their Th cells spontaneously developed into Th2 cells in vitro [133]. In contrast, c-MAF-deficient (c-MAF $^{-/-}$) Th cells are unable to differentiate into Th2 cells in the absence of exogenous IL-4. Although c-MAF $^{-/-}$ Th2 cells, differentiated in the presence of exogenous IL-4, produced normal levels of IL-5, IL-10, and IL-13, the production of IL-4 is severely impaired [129]. Furthermore, c-MAF, independent of IL-4, is also essential for normal induction of CD25 (IL-2Rα chain) in developing Th2 cells, which express higher levels than seen in Th1 cells. Blockade of IL-2R signaling selectively inhibits the production of Th2 cytokines, but not IFN-γ or IL-2 [132]. An increased number of c-MAF immunoreactive cells have been observed within the sputum and bronchial biopsies of asthmatic patients compared with control subjects [122,134]. There are no published studies on the effect of selective c-MAF inhibitors in vitro and/or in vivo.

NFATs

NFAT was originally described as a T-cell-specific transcription factor, which is expressed in activated, but not resting, T cells and is required for IL-2 gene transcription. However, we now know that NFAT is not only T cell specific but is also expressed in many other types of cells (e.g., mast cells, monocytes, macrophages, eosinophils, epithelial cells, smooth muscle, and endothelial cells) [135,136].

The NFAT family of transcription factors include the cytoplasmic NFAT transcription factors [NFATc1 (NFATc), NFATc2 (NFATp), NFATc3 (NFAT4, NFATx), NFATc4 (NFAT3), and NFATc5] and nuclear NFAT (NFATn). NFATc proteins are localized in the cytoplasm and activated by stimulation of receptors coupled with calcium mobilization. Receptor stimulation and calcium mobilization result in activation of many intracellular enzymes, including the calcium- and calmodulin-dependent phosphatase calcineurin, a major upstream regulator of NFATc proteins. Stimuli that elicit calcium mobilization result in the rapid dephosphorylation of NFATc proteins and their translocation to the nucleus where they have strong binding affinity to DNA [137,138].

NFATs are ubiquitous regulators of cell differentiation and adaptation [135]; however in stimulated T cells, NFATs are mainly involved in the regulation of proliferation and Th1/Th2 cytokine production [139,140]. For instance, the GM-CSF enhancer contains four composite NFATs/AP-1 DNA binding sites, three of which demonstrate cooperative binding of NFATs and AP-1. The fourth site binds NFATs and AP-1 independently. NFATs show a characteristic ability to interact with AP-1 and NF-κB DNA binding and transactivation. It has been shown that coupled NFAT:AP-1 is more stable and has higher affinity for DNA. Interestingly, preferential activation of NFATc1 correlates with mouse strain susceptibility to allergic responses and IL-4 gene expression [141]. NFATc2 appears to be important for the activation of the Th2 cells [142–147]. In contrast, NFATc3 seems to enhance the expression of the Th1 cytokine genes, IFN-γ, and TNF-α and suppress Th2 cytokine genes such as IL-4 and IL-5 in Th2 cells [148,149].

As substrates for calcineurin, NFATs proteins are major targets of the immunosuppressive drugs such as cyclosporin A (see above) and FK506 because of their ability to inhibit dephosphorylation of NFATs. Bis(trifluoromethyl)pyrazoles (BTPs) are novel inhibitors of both Th1 and Th2 cytokines production [150,151]. Identified initially as inhibitors of IL-2 synthesis, BTPs inhibit IL-2 production with a 10-fold enhancement over cyclosporin A. Additionally, the BTPs show inhibition of IL-4, IL-5, IL-8, and CCL11 production [150,151]. Unlike the IL-2 inhibitors, cyclosporin A and FK506, the BTPs do not directly inhibit the dephosphorylation of NFAT by calcineurin. There are no published studies on NFATc1 inhibitors in asthma.

SOCS Modulation of Th1/Th2 Differentiation

Suppressors of cytokine signaling (SOCS)-1 interacts directly with the Janus kinases (JAK) and inhibits their tyrosine-kinase activity [152]. SOCS1 is an important in vivo inhibitor of type I interferon signaling [153]. A SOCS1 promoter polymorphism (-1478CA>del) is associated with adult asthma [153]. In vitro, these SNPs enhance the transcription of SOCS1 in human lung epithelial cells, but reduces phosphorylation of STAT1 stimulated with IFN-β [153]. SOCS-3 is predominantly expressed in Th2 cells and inhibits Th1 differentiation [154]. SOCS3 also has a role in Th3 differentiation [155,156]. SOCS-3 transgenic mice show increased Th2 responses and an asthma-like phenotype. In contrast, SOCS-3 knockout mice have decreased Th2 development [157]. These data suggest that SOCS-3 may be a new target for the development of antiasthma drugs ([156]. It has been suggested that enhancement of the expression of SOCS-5 in $CD4^+$ T cells might be a useful therapeutic approach to Th2-dominant diseases [158]. In fact, transfer of primed $CD4^+$ T cells constitutively expressing SOCS-5 along with eye drop challenges in a murine allergic conjunctivitis model resulted in attenuated eosinophilic inflammation with enhanced IFN-γ and decreased IL-13 production [159]. However, it should be noted that SOCS-5 appears to be dispensable for the development of Th1 responses in vivo, as demonstrated by use of the SOCS-5 knockout mice [160]. SOCS-5-deficient $CD4^+$ T cells can differentiate into either Th1 or Th2 cells with the same efficiency [160]. These data have been confirmed in an animal model of asthma in which significantly more eosinophils in the airways and higher BAL levels of IL-5 and IL-13 were observed in the SOCS-5 transgenic than the wild-type mice. Airway hyperresponsiveness in the asthma model of SOCS-5 transgenic was also enhanced compared to wild-type mice. Ovalbumin-stimulated $CD4^+$ T cells from the primed SOCS-5 transgenic mice produced significantly more IL-5 and IL-13 than $CD4^+$ T cells from wild-type mice [161]. This finding raises questions about the therapeutic utility of using enhancement of SOCS-5 expression for Th2-mediated diseases, such as asthma.

Peroxisome Proliferator-Activated Receptors

Peroxisome proliferator-activated receptors (PPARs) are transcription factors belonging to the nuclear receptor superfamily. PPARs are activated by an array of polyunsaturated fatty acid derivatives, oxidized fatty acids, and phospholipids and are proposed to be important modulators of allergic inflammatory responses [162]. The three known PPAR subtypes, α, γ, and δ, show different tissue distributions and are associated with selective ligands. PPARs are expressed by eosinophils, T-lymphocytes, and alveolar macrophages, as well as by epithelial, and smooth muscle cells. PPAR-α and -γ are expressed in eosinophils and their activation inhibits in vitro chemotaxis and antibody-dependent cellular cytotoxicity [163]. PPAR-α and -γ are both expressed in monocytes/macrophages. PPAR-γ is expressed in eosinophils and T lymphocytes. In vivo, inflammation induced by leukotriene B_4 (LTB_4), a PPAR-α ligand, is prolonged in PPAR-α-deficient mice, suggesting an anti-inflammatory role for this receptor [164]. In contrast, in mice injected with lipopolysaccharide (LPS), activation of PPAR-α induces a significant increase in plasma tumor necrosis factor- (TNF-α) levels [164].

PPAR-γ ligands significantly inhibit production of IL-5 from T cells activated in vitro [165]. In a murine model of allergic asthma, mice treated orally with ciglitazone, a potent synthetic PPAR-γ ligand, has significantly reduced lung inflammation and mucous production following induction of allergic asthma. T cells from these ciglitazone-treated mice also produce less IFN-γ, IL-4, and IL-2 upon rechallenge in vitro with allergen [165].

Activation of PPAR-γ alters the maturation process of dendritic cells (DCs), the most potent antigen-presenting cells. By targeting DCs, PPAR-γ activation may be involved in the regulation of the pulmonary immune response to allergens [162]. Using a model of sensitization, based on the intratracheal transfer of ovalbumin-pulsed DCs, rosiglitazone, another selective PPAR-γ agonist, reduces the proliferation of antigen-specific T cells in the draining mediastinal lymph nodes but dramatically increases the production of IL-10 by these T cells. After aerosol challenge, the recruitment of BAL eosinophils is strongly reduced compared to control mice. Inhibition of IL-10 activity with anti-IL-10R antibodies partly restored the inflammation [162,166].

PPAR-α and PPAR-γ ligands also decrease antigen-induced airway hyperresponsiveness, lung inflammation and eosinophilia, cytokine production, and GATA-3 expression as well as serum levels of antigen-specific IgE in many different animal models of asthma [163,167–170]. These studies suggest that PPAR-α and PPAR-γ (co)agonists might be a potential anti-inflammatory treatment for asthma [171–173]. Interestingly, in vitro theophylline, procaterol, and dexamethasone induce PPAR-γ expression in human eosinophils [174,175].

MAP Kinase Inhibitors

There are three major mitogen-activated protein (MAP) kinase pathways and there is increasing recognition that these pathways are involved in the pathogenesis of asthma.

p38 MAPK Inhibitors

p38 MAPK kinase is a Ser/Thr kinase involved in many processes thought to be important in lower airways inflammatory responses and tissue remodeling. There is, however, a paucity of reports specifically addressing the role of p38 kinase in asthma [107,176].

There are four members of the p38 MAP kinase family; they differ in their tissue distribution, regulation of kinase activation, and subsequent phosphorylation of downstream substrates. They also differ in terms of their sensitivities toward the p38 MAP kinase inhibitors [107,176]. In general, p38 MAPKs are activated by many stimuli, including cytokines, hormones, and ligands for G protein-coupled receptors; elevated levels of these cytokines are associated with asthma. The synthesis of many inflammatory mediators, such as TNFα, IL-4, IL-5, IL-8, RANTES, and eotaxins, thought to be important in asthma pathogenesis, are regulated through activation of p38 MAPK. p38 MAPK can affect the transcription of these genes but also has major effects on mRNA stability. In addition, p38 MAPK appears to be involved in glucocorticoid resistance in asthma [107,176].

SB 203580, a selective inhibitor of p38 MAP kinase, inhibits the synthesis of many inflammatory cytokines, chemokines, and inflammatory enzymes. Interestingly, in vitro SB203580 appears to have a preferential inhibitory effect on synthesis of Th2 compared to Th1 cytokines, indicating their potential application in the treatment of asthma [177]. Inhaled p38αMAPK antisense oligonucleotide attenuates asthma in an animal model [178]. Several oral and inhaled p38MAPK inhibitors are now in clinical development [179]. Whether this new potential class of anti-inflammatory drugs will be safe in long-term studies in human asthma remains to be established. For the successful use of MAPK inhibitors in clinical trial on patients with asthma, these compounds must be very specific to reduce the side effects of the plethora of physiological MAPK functions. However, options to improve safety include inhaled delivery and use as a steroid-sparing agent.

JNKs

The c-Jun NH_2-terminal kinases (JNKs) phosphorylate and activate members of the AP-1 transcription factor family and other cellular factors implicated in regulating altered gene expression, cellular survival (apoptosis), differentiation and proliferation in response to cytokines, growth factors and oxidative stress, and cancerogenesis. Since many of these are common events associated with the pathogenesis of asthma, the potential of JNK inhibitors as therapeutics has attracted considerable interest. Furthermore, in patients with severe glucocorticoid-resistant asthma, there is an increased expression of the components of the proinflammatory transcription factor AP-1 and enhanced JNK activity [11,180].

The c-jun N-terminal (JNK) group of MAPK consists of three isoforms, encoded by three different genes, of which the JNK1 and 2 isoforms are widely distributed, while JNK3 is mainly located in neuronal tissue. Gene disruption studies in mice demonstrate that JNK is essential for TNFα-stimulated c-Jun phosphorylation and AP-1 activity and is also required for some forms of stress-induced apoptosis. JNKs enhance the transcriptional activity of AP-1 by phosphorylation of the AP-1 component c-Jun on serine residues 63 and 73, thereby increasing AP-1 association with the basal transcriptional complex. JNKs may also enhance the activity of other transcription factors such as ATF-2, Elk-1, and Sap-1a. Many immune and inflammatory genes including cytokines, growth factors, cell surface receptors, cell adhesion molecules, and proteases, such as matrix metalloprotease 1 (MMP-1), are regulated by AP-1 and ATF-2 presumably through the JNK pathway. JNKs do not only affect transcription of cytokine mRNAs but may also enhance the stability of some mRNAs such as that for IL-2 and nitric oxide synthase 2 (NOS2) [107].

JNK activation may also be important in the regulation of the immune response. JNK polarizes the differentiation of CD4+ T cells to a Th1-type immune response by a transcriptional mechanism involving the transcription factor, NFATc1. JNK1 and JNK2 knockout mice have similar phenotypes but some subtle differences exist.For example, JNK2($^{-}$/$_{-}$) CD8+ cells show enhanced proliferation whereas JNK1($^{-}$/$_{-}$) CD8+ cells cannot expand [107].

SP600125 (Signal Pharmaceuticals/Celgene), a JNK inhibitor, inhibited TNFα and IL-2 production in human monocytes and Jurkat cells, respectively and attenuated TNFα- and IL-1β-induced GM-CSF, RANTES, and IL-8 production in primary human airway smooth muscle cells. In addition, in an animal model of chronic asthma, SP-600125 (30 mg/kg sc) reduces BAL accumulation of eosinophils and lymphocytes, cytokine release, serum IgE production, and smooth muscle proliferation after repeated allergen exposure. Similar results were seen with the dual AP-1/NF-κB inhibitor SP100030 [181]. These data indicate that JNK inhibitors may be effective in the treatment of asthma.

A more selective second generation JNK-selective inhibitor [JNK-401(CC-401)] has successfully completed a phase I, double-blind, placebo controlled, ascending single intravenous dose study in healthy human volunteers (http://www.celgene.com). Studies will examine whether JNK-401 will be glucocorticoid-sparing and lacking many of the glucocorticoid side effects in humans.

The JNK pathway is implicated in a number of physiological and pathological functions in a range of human diseases. Due to the extensive cross-talk within this signaling cascade, as well as its cell-type- and response-specific modulation, it is difficult to predict potential adverse events that might arise from pathway inhibition. However, the fact that JNK inhibitors are progressing in clinical trials indicates the utility of targeting this pathway for therapeutic benefit in asthma and will probably be determined in the near future.

Heparin-Like Molecules

Glycosaminoglycans are large, polyanionic molecules expressed throughout the body. The GAG heparin, coreleased with histamine, is synthesized by and stored exclusively in mast cells, whereas the closely related molecule heparan sulfate is expressed, as part of a proteoglycan, on cell surfaces and throughout tissue matrices [182]. An important feature of chemokines is their ability to bind to the glycosaminoglycan side chains of proteoglycans, predominately heparin and heparan sulfate. To date, all chemokines tested bind to immobilized heparin in vitro, as well as cell surface heparan sulfate in vitro and in vivo. These interactions play an important role in modulating the action of chemokines by facilitating the formation of stable chemokine gradients within the vascular endothelium and directing leukocyte migration, by protecting chemokines from proteolysis, by inducing chemokine oligomerisation, and by facilitating transcytosis [183]. There are data suggesting a role for mast cell-derived heparin in enhancing eotaxin-mediated eosinophil recruitment, thereby reinforcing Th2 polarization of inflammatory responses [183]. However, heparan sulfate has been shown in vitro to promote a Th1 response, decreasing the production of IL-4 [184]. Heparin and related molecules have been found to exert anti-inflammatory effects in vitro and in animal models of asthma, and the anti-inflammatory activities of heparin are dissociable from its anticoagulant nature, suggesting that these characteristics could yield novel anti-inflammatory drugs for asthma [185–187]. The inhalation of heparin prevents exercise-induced bronchoconstriction [188–190]. A phase II study in mild asthma using IVX 0142, a novel heparin-derived oligosaccharide, has just been completed (http://clinicaltrials.gov/ct/show/NCT00232999;jsessionid=25FE6BB25329EDD9E1860C6D5851921F?order=1)

Modulators of the Synthesis or Action of Key Proinflammatory Th2 Cell Cytokines

Over one hundred mediators have now been implicated in asthmatic inflammation, including multiple cytokines, chemokines, and growth factors. Blocking a single mediator is therefore unlikely to be very effective in this complex disease, and mediator antagonists have so far not proved to be very effective compared with drugs that have a broad spectrum of anti-inflammatory effects, such as glucocorticoids [191]. However, the potential of blocking Th2 cytokines with proinflammatory action such as of IL-4, IL-5, and IL-13 has still not been completely explored. Also, anti-inflammatory cytokines such as IL-10, IL-12, IL-18, IL-21, IL-23, and IL-27 and interferons may have a therapeutic potential in asthma. TNF-α blockers may also be useful, particularly in severe asthma.

IL-4 Blockers and Asthma

IL-4 analogs, that act as antagonists, which have been developed, fail to induce signal transduction and block IL-4 effects in vitro. These IL-4 antagonists prevent the development of asthma in vivo in animal models [192,193]. However, the development of pascolizumab (SB 240683), a humanized anti-interleukin-4 antibody (Hart 2002), as well as of a blocking variant of human IL-4 (BAY36-1677) has apparently been discontinued.

Soluble IL-4 receptors (sIL-4R) that act as IL-4R antagonists have also been developed [194]; they are effective in an animal model of asthma [195]. A single nebulized dose of sIL-4R prevents the fall in lung function induced by glucocorticoid withdrawal in moderate/severe asthmatics [196]. Subsequent studies have shown that weekly nebulization of sIL-4R improves asthma control over 3 months [197]. However, further studies in patients with milder asthma proved disappointing, and the clinical development of this compound has now been discontinued.

In an animal model of asthma, a IL-4Rα antisense oligonucleotide (IL-4Rα ASO) specifically inhibits IL-4Rα protein expression in lung after inhalation in allergen-challenged mice [198]. Inhalation of IL-4Rα ASO attenuated allergen-induced AHR, suppressed airway eosinophilia and neutrophilia, and inhibited production of airway Th2 cytokines and chemokines in previously allergen-primed and -challenged mice [198]. Histological analysis of lungs from these animals demonstrated reduced goblet cell metaplasia and mucus staining that correlated with inhibition of MUC5AC gene expression in lung tissue. These data support the potential utility of a dual IL-4 and IL-13 oligonucleotide inhibitor in asthma and suggest that local inhibition of IL-4Rα in the lung is sufficient to suppress allergen-induced pulmonary inflammation and AHR in mice [198].

A novel approach is represented by an IL-4 peptide-based vaccine for blocking IL-4 on a persistent basis. Vaccinated mice produce high titers of IgG to IL-4. Serum ovalbumin-specific IgE, eosinophil accumulation in BAL, goblet cell hyperplasia, tissue inflammation, and AHR are markedly suppressed in vaccinated mice in an animal model of asthma [199].

IL-13 Blockers and Asthma

Blocking IL-13, but not IL-4, in animal models of asthma prevents the development of airway hyperresponsiveness after allergen, despite a strong eosinophilic response [121,200,201]. In addition, soluble IL-13Rα2 is effective in blocking the actions of IL-13, including IgE production, pulmonary eosinophilia, and airway hyperresponsiveness in animal models of asthma [202]; the humanized IL-13Rα2 is now entering phase I clinical trials in asthma [203]. Also an anti-IL-13Rα1 antibody is in preclinical development for the treatment of asthma (http://www.zenyth.com).

A human anti-human IL-13 IgG4 monoclonal antibody (CAT-354) that block IL-13 effects in an animal model of asthma [204] is in phase II clinical trials in severe asthma (http://www.cambridgeantibody.com). In addition, Centocor (http://www.centocor.com) has developed an antihuman IL-13 antibody that is effective in animal models of asthma [201,205], and IMA-638 (IgG1, kappa), a humanized antibody to human IL-13 from Wyeth Research, is effective in animal models of asthma [202,206].

As for IL-4 (see above), a novel approach is represented by an IL-13 peptide-based vaccine for blocking IL-13 on a persistent basis. Vaccination significantly inhibits increase in inflammatory cell number and IL-13 and IL-5 levels in BAL. Serum total and ovalbumin-specific IgE are also significantly inhibited. Moreover, allergen-induced goblet cell hyperplasia, lung tissue inflammatory cell infiltration, and AHR are significantly suppressed in vaccinated mice in an animal model of asthma [207].

IL-4 muteins indicate two types of IL-4 variants whose tyrosine at 124 is replaced with aspartate (Y124D) and arginine at 121 is replaced with aspartate (R121D/Y124D). IL-4 muteins act as antagonists for both IL4 and IL-13, because they are able to bind to IL-4R/IL13R, but do not transduce the signal. Bayer initially developed R121D/Y124D (pitrakinra, BY-16-9996, Aerovant), and now the compound is in phase IIa clinical trial for the treatment of asthma under license to Aerovance [203].

Novel "traps" composed of fusions between two distinct receptor components and a portion of the Fc region of the antibody molecule, results in the generation of blockers with markedly increased affinity over that offered by the single component reagents; dual IL-4/IL-13 trap is in the preclinical development for asthma (http://www.regeneron.com).

IL-5

The Th2 cell cytokine, IL-5, plays an important role in eosinophil maturation, differentiation, recruitment, and survival. IL-5 knockout mice appeared to confirm a role in asthma models in which eosinophilia and AHR are markedly suppressed. Humanized anti-IL-5 antibodies have been developed and a single i.v. infusion of one of these (mepolizumab) markedly reduces blood and sputum eosinophilia for several months. Unfortunately, there was no significant effect on the early or late response to allergen challenge, base-line AHR, or FEV_1 [62]. A similar study in moderate/severe persistent asthma showed similar results on eosinophilia but with no improvements in symptoms or lung function [208]. In a subsequent study, eosinophil numbers within the bronchial mucosa were only reduced by ~50% by mepolizumab treatment but again no effect on lung function was noted [209]. These data have raised questions over the importance of eosinophils in asthma. In a controlled clinical trial, administration of mepolizumab, over a period of 6 months, to asthmatic patients, markedly reduces peripheral blood eosinophils without altering the distribution of T-cell subsets and activation status (pattern of Th1 and Th2 cytokine production) of blood lymphocytes [210] mention recent NEJM papers.

In recent studies, RNA interference, using a short hairpin RNA, has been able to block IL-5Rα expression and decrease bone marrow eosinophilopoiesis and blood and BAL eosinophilia in an animal model of asthma showing new potential blockers of IL-5 function [211,212]. These new compounds have still not been tested in human asthma.

IL-6 Antagonists and Asthma

Interleukin-6 and related cytokines, interleukin-11, leukemia inhibitory factor, oncostatin M, ciliary neurotrophic factor, and cardiotrophin-1 are all pleiotropic and exhibit overlapping biological functions. Functional receptor complexes for the IL-6 family of cytokines share the signal transducing component glycoprotein 130 (gp130). Unlike cytokines sharing common β and common γ chains that mainly function in hematopoietic and lymphoid cell systems, the IL-6 family of cytokines function extensively outside these systems as well, owing to the ubiquitous expression of gp130 [213].

The IL-6 receptor complex (IL-6R) consists of either the membrane-bound IL-6 receptor (mIL-6R) or the soluble IL-6 receptor (sIL-6R) complexed with gp130. There are increased levels of sIL-6R in the airways of patients with allergic asthma as compared to those in controls. In addition, local blockade of the sIL-6R in a murine model of asthma led to suppression of Th2 cells in the lung [214]. In contrast, blockade of mIL-6R induced local expansion of Foxp3-positive CD4+CD25+ Tregs with increased immunosuppressive capacities. CD4+CD25+ T cells, but not CD4+CD25- lung T cells, selectively expressed the IL-6Rα chain and showed IL-6-dependent STAT-3 phosphorylation. Finally, in an animal model of asthma, CD4+CD25+ T cells isolated from anti-IL-6R antibody-treated mice exhibited marked immunosuppressive and anti-inflammatory functions [214].

IL-9 Antagonists and Asthma

Numerous in vitro and in vivo studies in both animals and patients with asthma have shown that IL-9 is an important inflammatory mediator in asthma. IL-9 is produced in the lung by a number of different cell types (Th2 lymphocytes, mast cells, eosinophils, and bronchial epithelial cells) and has multiple effects on a wide range of inflammatory and structural cells within the lung, including bronchial epithelial and smooth muscle cells (release of CCL11). IL-9 may be involved in IL-4-triggered IgE production in vitro, mast cells and eosinophils recruitment and activation to the lung, bronchial mucus cell hyperplasia (and MUC4 induction), subepithelial deposition of collagen, and airway hyperresponsiveness [215]. Animal data indicate that IL-9 can promote asthma through IL-13-independent pathways via expansion of mast cells, eosinophils, and B cells and through induction of IL-13 production by hemopoietic cells for mucus production and recruitment of eosinophils by lung epithelial cells [216]. IL-9 mRNA and protein are increased in the bronchial mucosa of atopic asthmatics, where it is expressed predominantly in lymphocytes [217,218]. In addition, BAL IL-9 levels are upregulated in asthmatics following allergen challenge [219].

In animal models of asthma, the overexpression of IL-9 causes BAL eosinophilia, peribronchial accumulation of collagen, and increased BAL levels of CCL5 and CTGF [220]. However, in Th2 cytokine-deficient mice (IL-4, IL-5, IL-9, and IL-13; single to quadruple knockouts), IL-4 alone can activate all Th2 effector functions even in the combined absence of IL-5, IL-9, and IL-13 [221]; the Th2 pulmonary inflammation is unchanged in IL-9-deficient mice, despite a reduced number of lung mast cells and goblet cells [222]. Despite this, in an animal model of asthma, the treatment with an anti-IL-9 antibody reduces airway inflammation and hyperresponsiveness [223,224] suggesting that blockade of IL-9 may be a new therapeutic strategy for bronchial asthma [215]. Interestingly, after allergen exposure, an anti-IL-9 significantly reduces bone marrow eosinophilia in an animal model primarily by decreasing newly produced and mature eosinophils. Anti-IL-9 treatment also reduces blood neutrophil counts, but does not affect BAL neutrophils [225].

IL-10 Modulation and Asthma

New "counterregulatory" models of asthma pathogenesis suggest that dysfunction of IL-10–related regulatory mechanisms might underlie the development of asthma.

IL-10 is produced by several cell types, including monocytes, macrophages, T lymphocytes, dendritic cells, and mast cells. IL-10 is a unique cytokine with a wide spectrum of anti-inflammatory effects. It inhibits the secretion of TNFα and IL-8 from macrophages and tips the balance in favor of antiproteases by increasing the expression of endogenous tissue inhibitors of MMPs (TIMPS). Some of the actions of IL-10 can be explained by an inhibitory effect on NF-κB; however, this does not account for all effects, as IL-10 is very effective at inhibiting IL-5 transcription, which is independent of NF-κB. In mice, many effects of IL-10 appear to be mediated by an inhibitory effect on PDE4, but this does not appear to be the case in human cells [191].

However, in animal models, IL-10, although inhibiting LPS-induced airway inflammation, causes airway mucus metaplasia, inflammation, and fibrosis. These responses are mediated by multiple mechanisms with airway mucus metaplasia being dependent on the IL-13/IL-4Rα/STAT-6 activation pathway, whereas the inflammation and fibrosis are independent of this pathway [226].

IL-10 concentrations are reduced in induced sputum from patients with asthma and with COPD, indicating that this might be a mechanism for increasing lung inflammation in these diseases. In addition, IL-10 production is decreased in peripheral blood mononuclear cells of patients with mild asthma and is further attenuated in severe persistent asthma compared to mild asthma [227,228]. Patients with severe persistent asthma have increased frequency of a haplotype associated with low production of IL-10 by the alveolar macrophages [229]. Furthermore, a defect in glucocorticoid-induced IL-10 production has also been described in blood T lymphocytes from patients with glucocorticoid-resistant asthma [228].

The potent immunosuppressive and anti-inflammatory action of IL-10 has suggested that it may be useful therapeutically in the treatment of asthma. Recombinant human IL-10 has already been licensed for Crohn's disease and psoriasis by daily subcutaneous injection over 4 weeks, and it is reasonably well tolerated causing only a reversible dose-dependent anemia and thrombocytopenia. Another possibility for therapy in the future is the development of other agonists for the IL-10 receptor, or drugs that activate the unique, but so far unidentified, signal transduction pathways activated by this cytokine [191].

Recent data also suggest that vitamin D3 in conjunction with a glucocorticoid may restore the reduced expression of Il-10 seen in T-cells from patients with severe asthma [228].

IL-12 Modulation and Asthma

IL-12 is essential for the development of Th1 immune response, leading to their production of IFN-γ. In addition to priming CD4+ T cells for high IFN-γ production, IL-12 also contributes to their proliferation once they have differentiated into Th1 cells. IL-12 is also capable of inhibiting the Th2-driven allergen-induced airway changes in mice and is therefore considered a new potential drug for the treatment of asthma. In man, IL-12 production is decreased in PBMCs, alveolar macrophages, and bronchial biopsies of patients with mild asthma, and IL-12 synthesis is further attenuated in PBMCs from severe persistent asthma compared to mild asthma [227]. Inhalation of IL-12 has been shown to inhibit allergic inflammation in murine models while decreasing adverse effects seen with systemic administration of this cytokine and adenoviral IL-12 gene transduction may be effective in inducing IL-12 expression in the airways [230]. However, an initial study of inhaled IL-12 in humans with asthma was terminated due to adverse effects, including one death. Furthermore, the use of systemically administered IL-12 in patients with asthma has been limited due to cytokine toxicity and lack of clinical efficacy despite a significant reduction in the number of blood and sputum eosinophils [231]. Another treatment option that has the potential of inducing a Th1 cytokine response is the use of IL-12 linked to polyethylene glycol moieties. This mode of administration is likely to enhance cytokine delivery to the target organ, while decreasing its toxicity. Also intranasal delivery of IL-12 may provide another approach for the treatment of asthma [232].

IL-15

The IL-15 gene is located on chromosome 4q27, approximately distal to the IL2 gene and may be associated with an increased susceptibility to asthma [233,234].

IL-15 shares many biologic activities with IL-2. Both cytokines bind a specific α subunit, and they share the same β and γ common receptor subunits for signal transduction. IL-15, in the presence or absence of TNF-α, reduces spontaneous apoptosis in human eosinophils. The number of cells expressing IL-15 is significantly increased in the bronchial mucosa from patients with Th1-mediated chronic inflammatory diseases of the lung such as sarcoidosis, tuberculosis, and COPD, compared with asthmatic patients and normal subjects [235]. The expression of IL-15 is also increased in the bronchial mucosa of asthmatic patients compared to normal subjects.

In an animal model of asthma, overexpression of IL-15 suppresses Th2-mediated-allergic airway response via induction of CD8+ T cell-mediated Tc1 response [236]. However, in another animal model of asthma, blocking IL-15 prevents the induction of allergen-specific T cells and allergic airway inflammation [237].

NK cells are divided into NK1 and NK2 subsets and the ratio of IL-4 + CD56 + NK2 cells in PBMCs of asthmatic patients is higher than in healthy individuals [238]. STAT6 is also constitutively activated in NK2 clones from asthmatic patients, possibly as a result of IL-15 stimulating their proliferation [238].

There are no clinical studies on the effect of IL-15 pathway modulation in asthmatic patients. Interestingly, a 2-week treatment with the inhaled glucocorticoid fluticasone decreased the numbers of IL-15+ cells in the bronchial mucosa of stable asthmatics [239].

IL-18 Modulation and Asthma

IL-18, originally identified as an IFN-γ-inducing factor, is a unique cytokine that enhances innate immunity and both Th1- and Th2-driven immune responses. IL-18 is able to induce IFN-γ, GM-CSF, TNFα, and IL-1, to activate killing by lymphocytes, and to upregulate the expression of certain chemokine receptors. In contrast, IL-18 induces naive T cells to develop into Th2 cells. IL-18 also induces IL-4 and/or IL-13 production by NK cells, mast cells, and basophils [240].

The same dualism is present in vivo after administration of IL-18 in animal models of asthma. Vaccination with allergen-IL-18 fusion DNA protects against, and reverses established, airway hyperresponsiveness in an animal model of asthma [241]. On the other hand, in other animal models, administration of IL-18 enhances antigen-induced increase in serum IgE and Th2 cytokines and airway eosinophilia in part by increasing antigen-induced TNFα production [242,243]. This suggests that IL-18 may contribute to the development and exacerbation of Th2-mediated airway inflammation in asthma [244,245].

The serum levels of IL-18 are higher in asthmatic patients [246] and increase further during exacerbations (and decrease during the stable phase) compared with normal subjects [247]. Decreased levels of IL-18 in sputum and BAL from asthmatic patients compared to normal controls have also been reported [248,249]. There are no clinical studies on the effect of the administration of human recombinant IL-18 and/or IL-18 antagonists to asthmatic patients.

Class II Family of Cytokine Receptors

Class II family of cytokine receptors (CRF2), now includes 12 proteins: a new human Type I IFN, IFN-κ; molecules related to IL-10 (IL-19, IL-20, IL-22, IL-24, IL-26); and the IFN-λ proteins IFN-λ1 (IL-29), IFN-λ2 (IL-28A), and IFN-λ3

(IL-28B), which have antiviral and cell stimulatory activities reminiscent of type I IFNs, but act through a distinct receptor and are designated as type III IFN by the nomenclature committee of the International Society of Interferon and Cytokine Research [250,251]. In response to ligand binding, the CRF2 proteins form heterodimers, leading to cytokine-specific cellular responses, and these diverse physiological functions are just beginning to be explored. The ligand-binding chains for IL-22, IL-26, and IFN-λ are distinct from that used by IL-10; however, all of these cytokines use a common second chain, IL-10 receptor-2 (IL-10R2; CRF2-4), to assemble their active receptor complexes. Thus, IL-10R2 is a shared component in at least four distinct class II cytokine-receptor complexes. IL-10 binds to IL-10R1; IL-22 binds to IL-22R1; IL-26 binds to IL-20R1; and IFN-λ binds to IFN-λR1 (also known as IL-28R) [253–256]. The binding of these ligands to their respective R1 chains induces a conformational change that enables IL-10R2 to interact with the newly formed ligand-receptor complexes. This in turn activates a signal-transduction cascade that results in rapid activation of several transcription factors, particularly STAT3 [252] and, to a lesser degree, STAT1 [253–256].

IL-19 Modulation and Asthma

IL-19 belongs to the IL-10 family, which includes IL-10, IL-19, IL-20, IL-22, IL-24 [melanoma differentiation-associated gene-7 (MDA-7)], and IL-26 (AK155). The IL-19, IL-20, and IL-24 genes are on chromosome 1q31–32, a region that also contains the IL-10 gene. The two other IL-10-related cytokines, IL-22 and IL-26 genes, are on chromosome 12q15, near the IFN-γ gene [252].

IL-19 and IL-24 bind to the type I IL-20R complex, which is a heterodimer of two previously described orphan class II cytokine receptor subunits: IL-20R1 [IL-20Rα or corticotropin-releasing factor (CRF) 2–8] and IL-20R2 [IL-20Rβ (DIRS1)] [252,257].

In addition, IL-20 and IL-24 but not IL-19, bind to type II IL-20R complex, composed of IL-22R1 and IL-20R2 [252]. In all cases, binding of the ligands results in STAT3 phosphorylation [252].

The IL-19 gene is upregulated in monocytes by LPS and GM-CSF [258] and, in turn, IL-19 induces the production of IL-6, TNF-α, and oxidants in these cells [259]. IL-19 can also induce apoptosis in monocytes [259]. IL-19 also induces the Th2 cytokines IL-4, IL-5, IL-10, and IL-13 production by activated T cells [257,260]. In vitro, A2B adenosine receptors induce IL-19 from bronchial epithelial cells, resulting in TNF-α release [261].

The serum level of IL-19 in patients with stable asthma increases compared with healthy controls [260]. In an animal model of asthma, there is an increased IL-19 expression and transfer of the IL-19 gene into healthy mice upregulated IL-4 and IL-5, but not IL-13; however, IL-19 upregulated IL-13 in “asthmatic” mice [260]. The role of IL-19 blockers in asthma needs to be explored.

IL-21 Modulation and Asthma

The interleukin-2 family of cytokines includes IL-2, IL-4, IL-7, IL-9, IL-13, IL-15, and IL-21. The IL-21 gene is located on human chromosome 4q26–27, near the IL-2 gene. In humans, IL-21 is produced almost exclusively by $CD4^+$ Th1 and Th2 cells. There is very little expression of IL-21 in activated $CD8^+$ cells [262]. The IL-21 receptor complex is a heterodimer containing the IL-21R and the common cytokine receptor γ chain (γc) of the IL-2, IL-4, IL-7, IL-9, and IL-15 receptors [263]. IL-21 binding stimulates activation of JAK1/JAK3 and then preferentially activates STAT-1 and STAT-3 [263]. In addition, IL-21 enhances STAT4 binding to the IFN-γ promoter.

IL-21 modulates the proliferation and differentiation of T cells toward a Th1 phenotype and also stimulates B cells, NK cells, and dendritic cells [262,263]. In addition, IL-21 also stimulates IgG1 production and decreases IgE production [264]. Thus, IL-21 may be a critical cytokine maintaining low IgE levels under physiological and pathological conditions, and importantly, in support of this, IL-21 knockout animals have an increased level of serum IgE and IgE producing B cell expansion [265]. Interestingly, IL-21 knockout and IL-21R knockout animals are healthy and fail to acquire spontaneous inflammatory diseases [264,266].

IL-21 is also a potent stimulator of cell-mediated immunity (effector $CD8^+$ T and NK cells), and it has a potent antitumor activity in many animal models [262,267]; ZymoGenetics (http://www.zymogenetics.com) is developing IL-21 for the treatment of cancer. IL-21 administration in an animal model of asthma reduces titres of antigen-specific IgE and IgG1 antibodies, as well as airway hyperresponsiveness and lung eosinophil recruitment [262]. Thus, IL-21 signaling modulation may be useful for the treatment of asthma [268].

IL-22 Modulation and Asthma

The IL-22 gene (and also the IL-26 gene) is located on human chromosome 12q. The IL-22 heterodimeric receptor is composed of the IL-22R1 (CRF2–9/IL-22R subunit) and the IL-10R2 to generate the IL-22 receptor complex, or IL-20R2 to yield another receptor complex for IL-20 and IL-24 [269]. In addition to its cellular receptor, IL-22 binds to a secreted member of the class II cytokine receptor family, which is called IL-22BP, a soluble receptor which is a naturally occurring IL-22 antagonist.

There are several lines of evidence connecting IL-22 to asthma. Interestingly, in vitro long-term (12 days) exposure of human T cells to IL-19, IL-20, and IL-22 downregulated IFN-gamma but upregulated IL-4 and IL-13 and supported the polarization of naive T cells to Th2-like cells. In contrast, neutralization of endogenous IL-22 activity by IL-22-binding protein decreased IL-4, IL-13, and IFN-gamma synthesis [270].

IL-22 is induced by IL-9, a Th2 cytokine potentially involved in asthma (see above), and by LPS in animal models of asthma [269]. IL-22 induces in vitro and in vivo expression of several acute phase proteins, β-defensins, pancreatitis-associated protein (PAP1), and osteopontin [269]. Some of these proteins are involved in inflammatory and innate immune responses. Inasmuch as IL-22 is implicated in inflammation, the expression of IL-22BP should decrease local inflammation. In this light, it is of interest that IL-22BP expression was detected by in situ hybridization in the mononuclear cells of inflammatory infiltration sites, plasma cells, and a subset of epithelial cells in several tissues including lung [271]. Thus, IL-22 signaling modulation may be useful for the treatment of asthma.

Conclusions

The current asthma therapies are not cures; symptoms return soon after treatment is stopped even after long-term therapy. Although glucocorticoids are highly effective in controling the inflammatory process in asthma, they appear to have little effect on the lower airway remodeling processes that appear to play a role in the pathophysiology of asthma at currently prescribed doses. The development of novel drugs may allow resolution of these changes. In addition, severe glucocorticoid-dependent and -resistant asthma presents a great clinical burden and reducing the side effects of glucocorticoids using novel steroid-sparing agents is needed. Furthermore, the mechanisms involved in the persistence of inflammation are poorly understood and the reasons why some patients have severe life threatening asthma and others have very mild disease are still unknown. Considering the apparently central role of T lymphocytes in the pathogenesis of asthma, drugs targeting disease-inducing Th2 cells are promising therapeutic strategies [272]. However, although animal models of asthma suggest that this is feasible, the translation of these types of studies for the treatment of human asthma remains poor due to the limitations of the models currently used. Since we do not yet understand the underlying causes of asthma, it is unlikely that therapy will lead to a cure.

The myriad of new compounds that are in development directed to modulate Th2 cells recruitment and/or activation will clarify in the near future the relative importance of these cells and their mediators in the complex interactions with the other proinflammatory/anti-inflammatory cells and mediators responsible of the different asthmatic phenotypes. Hopefully, it will soon be possible to identify and manipulate the molecular switches that result in asthmatic inflammation. This may lead to the treatment of susceptible individuals at birth or in the early years and thus prevent the disease from becoming established.

Acknowledgments Supported by Associazione per la Ricerca e la Cura dell'Asma (ARCA, Padua, Italy), The British Lung Foundation, The Clinical Research Committee (Brompton Hospital), Fondo per Ricerca Scientifica di Interesse Locale 2007 (ex60%), GlaxoSmithKline (UK) and Novartis (UK).

References

1. Barnes PJ, Jonsson B, Klim JB (1996) The costs of asthma. Eur Respir J 9:636–642.
2. Gaga M, Zervas E, Grivas S, Castro M, Chanez P (2007) Evaluation and management of severe asthma. Curr Med Chem 14:1049–1059.
3. Global Initiative for Asthma. *Global strategy for Asthma Management and Prevention.* NHLBI/WHO Workshop report. 2002. *NIH Publication* No 02-3659: 1-200. Last update 2006. Freely available online at http://www.ginasthma.com (accessibility verified 15 July 2007).
4. Strunk RC, Bloomberg GR (2006) Omalizumab for asthma. N Engl J Med 354:2689–2695.
5. Avila PC (2007) Does anti-IgE therapy help in asthma? Efficacy and controversies. Annu Rev Med 58:185–203.
6. Kips JC, Anderson GP, Fredberg JJ, Herz U, Inman MD, Jordana M, Kemeny DM, Lotvall J, Pauwels RA, Plopper CG, Schmidt D, Sterk PJ, Van Oosterhout AJ, Vargaftig BB, Chung KF (2003) Murine models of asthma. Eur Respir J 22:374–382.
7. Barnes PJ, Adcock IM (2003) How do corticosteroids work in asthma?Ann Intern Med 139:359–370.
8. Caramori G, Adcock I (2003) Pharmacology of airway inflammation in asthma and COPD. Pulm Pharmacol Ther 16:247–277.
9. Caramori G, Pandit A, Papi A (2005) Is there a difference between chronic airway inflammation in chronic severe asthma and chronic obstructive pulmonary disease? Curr Opin Allergy Clin Immunol 5:77–83.
10. Loke TK, Sousa AR, Corrigan CJ, Lee TH (2002) Glucocorticoid-resistant asthma. Curr Allergy Asthma Rep 2:144–150.
11. Adcock IM, Lane J (2003) Corticosteroid-insensitive asthma: molecular mechanisms. J Endocrinol 178:347–355.
12. Barnes PJ, Chung KF, Page CP (1998) Inflammatory mediators of asthma: an update. Pharmacol Rev 50:515–596.
13. Miyaura H, Itawa M (2002) Direct and indirect inhibition of Th1 development by progesterone and glucocorticoids. J Immunol 168:1087–1094.
14. Karagiannidis C, Ruckert B, Hense G, Willer G, Menz G, Blaser K, Schmidt-Weber CB (2005) Distinct leucocyte redistribution after glucocorticoid treatment among difficult-to-treat asthmatic patients. Scand J Immunol 61:187–196.
15. Peek EJ, Richards DF, Faith A, Lavender P, Lee TH, Corrigan CJ, Hawrylowicz CM (2005) Interleukin-10-secreting "regulatory" T cells induced by glucocorticoids and beta2-agonists. Am J Respir Cell Mol Biol 33:105–111.
16. Jee YK, Gilour J, Kelly A,Bowen H, Richards D, Soh C, Smith P, Hawrylowicz C, Cousins D, Lee T, Lavender P (2005) Repression of interleukin-5 transcription by the glucocorticoid receptor targets GATA3 signaling and involves histone deacetylase recruitment. J Biol Chem 280:23243–23250.
17. Crocker IC, Church MK, Newton S, Townley RG (1998) Glucocorticoids inhibit proliferation and interleukin-4 and interleukin-5 secretion by aeroallergen-specific T-helper type 2 cell lines. Ann Allergy Asthma Immunol 80:509–516.
18. Powell N, Till SJ, Kay AB, Corrigan CJ (2001) The topical glucocorticoids beclomethasone dipropionate and fluticasone propionate inhibit human T-cell allergen-induced production of IL-5, IL-3 and GM-CSF mRNA and protein. Clin Exp Allergy 31:69–76.
19. Goleva E, Dunlap A, Leung DY (2004) Differential control of TH1 versus TH2 cell responses by the combination of low-dose steroids with beta2-adrenergic agonists. J Allergy Clin Immunol 114:183–191.
20. Di Lorenzo G, Pacor ML, Pellitteri ME, Gangemi S, Di Blasi P, Candore G, Colombo A, Lio D, Caruso C (2002) In vitro effects of fluticasone propionate on IL-13 production by mitogen-stimulated lymphocytes. Mediators Inflamm 11:187–190.

21. Melis M, Siena L, Pace E, giomarkaj M, Profita M, Piazzoli A, Todaro M, Stassi G, Bonsignore G, Vignola AM (2002) Fluticasone induces apoptosis in peripheral T-lymphocytes: a comparison between asthmatic and normal subjects. Eur Respir J 19:257–266.
22. Pace E, Gagliardo R, Melis M, La Grutta S, Siena L, Monsignore G, Giomarkaj M, Bousquet J, Vignola AM (2004) Synergistic effects of fluticasone propionate and salmeterol on in vitro T-cell activation and apoptosis in asthma. J Allergy Clin Immunol 114:1216–1223.
23. Barnes PJ (2003) Theophylline: new perspectives for an old drug. Am J Respir Crit Care Med 167:813–818.
24. Barnes PJ (2005) Theophylline in chronic obstructive pulmonary disease: new horizons. Proc Am Thorac Soc 2:334–339; discussion 340–341.
25. Sullivan P, Bekir S, Jaffar Z, Page C, Jeffery P, Costello J (1994) Anti-inflammatory effects of low-dose oral theophylline in atopic asthma. Lancet 343:1006–1008.
26. Jaffar ZH, Sullivan P, Page C, Costello J (1996) Low-dose theophylline modulates T-lymphocyte activation in allergen-challenged asthmatics. Eur Respir J 9:456–462.
27. Djukanovic R, Finnerty JP, Lee C, Wilson S, Madden J, Holgate ST (1995) The effects of theophylline on mucosal inflammation in asthmatic airways: biopsy results. Eur Respir J 8:831–833.
28. Finnerty JP, Lee C, Wilson S, Madden J, Djukanovic R, Holgate ST (1996) Effects of theophylline on inflammatory cells and cytokines in asthmatic subjects: a placebo-controlled parallel group study. Eur Respir J 9:1672–1677.
29. Nie HX, Yang J, Hu SP, Wu XJ (2002) Effects of theophylline on CD4+ T lymphocyte, interleukin-5, and interferon gamma in induced sputum of asthmatic subjects. Acta Pharmacol Sin 23:267–272.
30. Kidney J, Dominguez M, Taylor PM, Rose M, Chung KF, Barnes PJ (1995) Immunomodulation by theophylline in asthma: demonstration by withdrawal of therapy. Am J Respir Crit Care Med 151:1907–1914.
31. Hidi R, Timmermans S, Liu E, Schudt C, Dent G, Holgate ST, Djukanovic R (2000) Phosphodiesterase and cyclic adenosine monophosphate-dependent inhibition of T-lymphocyte chemotaxis. Eur Respir J 15:342–349.
32. Scordamaglia, A, et al. (1988) Theophylline and the immune response: in vitro and in vivo effects. Clin Immunol Immunopathol 48:238–246.
33. Choy DK, Ko F, Li ST, Lp LS, Leung R, Hui D, Lai KN, Lai CK (1999) Effects of theophylline, dexamethasone and salbutamol on cytokine gene expression in human peripheral blood CD4+ T-cells. Eur Respir J 14:1106–1112.
34. Crocker IC, Townley RG, Khan MM (1996) Phosphodiesterase inhibitors suppress proliferation of peripheral blood mononuclear cells and interleukin-4 and -5 secretion by human T-helper type 2 cells. Immunopharmacology 31:223–235.
35. Lin CC, Lin CY, Liaw SF, Chen A (2002) Pulmonary function changes and immunomodulation of Th 2 cytokine expression induced by aminophylline after sensitization and allergen challenge in brown Norway rats. Ann Allergy Asthma Immunol 88:215–222.
36. Holgate ST, Sampson AP (2000) Antileukotriene therapy. Future directions. Am J Respir Crit Care Med 161(suppl):S147–S153.
37. Tohda Y, Nakahara H, Kubo H, Haraguchi R, Fukuoka M, Nakajima S (1999) Effects of ONO-1078 (pranlukast) on cytokine production in peripheral blood mononuclear cells of patients with bronchial asthma. Clin Exp Allergy 29:1532–1536.
38. Matsuse H, Kondo Y,Machida I, Kawano T, Saeki S, Tomari S, Obase Y, Fukushima C, Mizuta Y, Kohno S (2006) Effects of anti-inflammatory therapies on recurrent and low-grade respiratory syncytial virus infections in a murine model of asthma. Ann Allergy Asthma Immunol 97:55–60.
39. Wu AY, Chik SC, Chan AW, Li Z, Tsang KW, Li W (2003) Anti-inflammatory effects of high-dose montelukast in an animal model of acute asthma. Clin Exp Allergy 33:359–366.
40. Nag S, Lamkhioued B, Renzi PM (2002) Interleukin-2-induced increased airway responsiveness and lung Th2 cytokine expression occur after antigen challenge through the leukotriene pathway. Am J Respir Crit Care Med 165:1540–1545.

41. Ciprandi G, Frati F, Marcucci F, Sensi L, Tosca MA, Milanese M, Ricca V (2003) Nasal cytokine modulation by montelukast in allergic children: a pilot study. Allerg Immunol (Paris) 35:295–299.
42. Ramer-Quinn DS, Baker RA, Sanders VM (1997) Activated T helper 1 and T helper 2 cells differentially express the beta-2-adrenergic receptor: a mechanism for selective modulation of T helper 1 cell cytokine production. J Immunol 159:4857–4867.
43. Sanders VM, Baker RA, Ramer-Quinn DS, Kasprowicz DJ, Fuchs BA, Street NE (1997) Differential expression of the beta2-adrenergic receptor by Th1 and Th2 clones: implications for cytokine production and B cell help. J Immunol 158:4200–4210.
44. Panina-Bordignon P, Mazzeo D, Lucia PD, D'Ambrosio D, Lang R, Fabbri L, Self C, Sinigaglia F (1997) Beta2-agonists prevent Th1 development by selective inhibition of interleukin 12. J Clin Invest 100:1513–1519.
45. Holen E, Elsayed S (1998) Effects of beta2 adrenoceptor agonists on T-cell subpopulations. APMIS 106:849–857.
46. Wallin A, Sandstrom T, Cioppa GD, Holgate S, Wilson S (2002) The effects of regular inhaled formoterol and budesonide on preformed Th-2 cytokines in mild asthmatics. Respir Med 96:1021–1025.
47. Farrar JR, Rainey DK, Norris AA (1995) Pharmacologic modulation of Th1 and Th2 cell subsets by nedocromil sodium. Int Arch Allergy Immunol 107:414–415.
48. Davies H, Olson L, Gibson P (2000) Methotrexate as a steroid sparing agent for asthma in adults. Cochrane Database Syst Rev 2:CD000391.
49. Kay AB (2006) The role of T lymphocytes in asthma. Chem Immunol Allergy 91:59–75.
50. Evans DJ, Cullinan P, Geddes DM (2001) Cyclosporin as an oral corticosteroid sparing agent in stable asthma. Cochrane Database Syst Rev 2:CD002993.
51. Barnes PJ (2006) New therapies for asthma. Trends Mol Med 12:515–20.
52. Caramori G, Ito K, Adcock IM (2004) Targeting Th2 cells in asthmatic patients. Curr Drug Targets Inflamm Allergy 3:243–255.
53. Bateman ED, Izquierdo L, Harnest U, Hofbauer P, Magyar P, Schmid-Wirlitsch C, Leichtl S, Bredenboker D (2006) Efficacy and safety of roflumilast in the treatment of asthma.Ann Allergy Asthma Immunol 96:679–686.
54. Landells LJ, Szilagy CM, Jones NA, Banner KH, Allen JM, Doherty A, O'Connor BJ, Spina D, Page CP (2001) Identification and quantification of phosphodiesterase 4 subtypes in CD4 and CD8 lymphocytes from healthy and asthmatic subjects. Br J Pharmacol 133:722–729.
55. Essayan DM, Kagey-Sobotka A, Lichtenstein LM, Huang SK (1997) Differential regulation of human antigen-specific Th1 and Th2 lymphocyte responses by isozyme selective cyclic nucleotide phosphodiesterase inhibitors. J Pharmacol Exp Ther 282:505–512.
56. Essayan DM, Kagey-Sobotka A, Lichtenstein LM, Huang SK (1997) Regulation of interleukin-13 by type 4 cyclic nucleotide phosphodiesterase (PDE) inhibitors in allergen-specific human T lymphocyte clones. Biochem Pharmacol 53:1055–1060.
57. Bielekova B, Lincoln A, McFarland H, Martin R (2000) Therapeutic potential of phosphodiesterase-4 and -3 inhibitors in Th1-mediated autoimmune diseases. J Immunol 164:1117–1124.
58. Marcoz P, Prigent AF, Lagarde M, Nemoz G (1993) Modulation of rat thymocyte proliferative response through the inhibition of different cyclic nucleotide phosphodiesterase isoforms by means of selective inhibitors and cGMP-elevating agents. Mol Pharmacol 44:1027–1035.
59. Sommer N, Martin R, McFarland HF, Quigley L, Cannella B, Raine CS, Scott DE, Loschmann PA, Racke MK (1997) Therapeutic potential of phosphodiesterase type 4 inhibition in chronic autoimmune demyelinating disease. J Neuroimmunol 79:54–61.
60. Adcock IM, Caramori G (2004) Chemokines and asthma. Curr Drug Targets Inflamm Allergy 3:257–261.
61. Charo IF, Ransohoff RM (2006) The many roles of chemokines and chemokine receptors in inflammation. N Engl J Med 354:610–621.
62. Leckie MJ, ten Brinke A, Khan J, Diamant Z, O'Connor BJ, Walls CM, Mathur AK, Cowley HC, Chung KF, Djukanovic R, Hansel TT, Holgate ST, Sterk PJ, Barnes PJ (2000) Effects of an interleukin-5 blocking monoclonal antibody on eosinophils, airway hyper-responsiveness, and the late asthmatic response. Lancet 356:2144–2148.

63. Erin EM, Williams TJ, Barnes PJ, Hansel TT (2002) Eotaxin receptor (CCR3) antagonism in asthma and allergic disease. Curr Drug Targets Inflamm Allergy 1:201–214.
64. Batt DG, Houghton GC, Roderick J, Santella JB 3rd, Wacker DA, Welch PK, Orlovsky YI, Wadman EA, Trzaskos JM, Davies P, Decicco CP, Carter PH (2005) N-Arylalkylpiperidine urea derivatives as CC chemokine receptor-3 (CCR3) antagonists. Bioorg Med Chem Lett 15:787–791.
65. De Lucca GV, Kim UT, Johnson C, Vargo BJ, Welch PK, Covington M, Davies P, Solomon KA, Newton RC, Trainor GL, Decicco CP, Ko SS (2002) Discovery and structure-activity relationship of N-(ureidoalkyl)-benzyl-piperidines as potent small molecule CC chemokine receptor-3 (CCR3) antagonists. J Med Chem 45:3794–3804.
66. De Lucca GV, Kim UT, Vargo BJ, Duncia JV, Santella JB 3rd, Gardner DS, Zheng C, Liauw A, Wang Z, Emmett G, Wacker DA, Welch PK, Covington M, Stowell NC, Wadman EA, Das AM, Davies P, Yeleswaram S, Graden DM, Solomon KA, Newton RC, Trainor GL, Decicco CP, Ko SS (2005) Discovery of CC chemokine receptor-3 (CCR3) antagonists with picomolar potency. J Med Chem 48:2194–2211.
67. De Lucca GV (2006) Recent developments in CCR3 antagonists. Curr Opin Drug Discov Devel 9:516–524.
68. Nakamura T, Ohbayashi M, Toda M, Hall DA, Horgan CM, Ono SJT (2005) A specific CCR3 chemokine receptor antagonist inhibits both early and late phase allergic inflammation in the conjunctiva. Immunol Res 33:213–221.
69. Pruitt JR, Batt DG, Wacker DA, et al. (2007) CC chemokine receptor-3 (CCR3) antagonists: Improving the selectivity of DPC168 by reducing central ring lipophilicity. Bioorg Med Chem Lett 17:2992–2997.
70. Suzuki K, Morokata T, Morihira K, Sato I, Takizawa S, Kaneko M, Takahashi K, Shimizu Y (2006) In vitro and in vivo characterization of a novel CCR3 antagonist, YM-344031. Biochem Biophys Res Commun 339:1217–1223.
71. Wegmann M, Goggel R, Sel S, Sel S, Erb KJ, Kalkbrenner F, Renz H, Garn H (2007) Effects of a low-molecular-weight CCR-3 antagonist on chronic experimental asthma. Am J Respir Cell Mol Biol 36:61–67.
72. Suzuki K, Morokata T, Morihira K, Sato I, Takizawa S, Kaneko M, Takahashi K, Shimizu Y (2007) A dual antagonist for chemokine CCR3 receptor and histamine H(1) receptor. Eur J Pharmacol 563:224–232.
73. Das AM, Vaddi KG, Solomon KA, Krauthauser C, Jiang X, McIntyre KW, Yang XX, Wadman E, Welch P, Covington M, Graden D, Yeleswaram K, Trzaskos JM, Newton RC, Mandlekar S, Ko SS, Carter PH, Davies P (2006) Selective inhibition of eosinophil influx into the lung by small molecule CC chemokine receptor 3 antagonists in mouse models of allergic inflammation. J Pharmacol Exp Ther 318:411–417.
74. Fryer AD, Stein LH, Nie Z, Curtis DE, Evans CM, Hodgson ST, Jose PJ, Belmonte KE, Fitch E, Jacoby DB (2006) Neuronal eotaxin and the effects of CCR3 antagonist on airway hyperreactivity and M2 receptor dysfunction. J Clin Invest 116:228–236.
75. Forssmann U, Hartung I, Balder R, Fuchs B, Escher SE, Spodsberg N, Dulkys Y, Walden M, Heitland A, Braun A, Forssmann WG, Elsner J (2004) n-Nonanoyl-CC chemokine ligand 14, a potent CC chemokine ligand 14 analogue that prevents the recruitment of eosinophils in allergic airway inflammation. J Immunol 173:3456–3466.
76. Manns J, Rieder S, Escher S, Eilers B, Forssmann WG, Elsner J, Forssmann U (2007) The allergy-associated chemokine receptors CCR3 and CCR5 can be inactivated by the modified chemokine NNY-CCL11. Allergy 62:17–24.
77. Munitz A, Bachelet I, Levi-Schaffer F (2006) Reversal of airway inflammation and remodeling in asthma by a bispecific antibody fragment linking CCR3 to CD300a. J Allergy Clin Immunol 118:1082–1089.
78. Conroy DM, Jopling LA, Lloyd CM, Hodge MR, Andrew DP, Williams TJ, Pease JE, Sabroe I (2003) CCR4 blockade does not inhibit allergic airways inflammation. J Leukoc Biol 74:558–563.

79. Allen S, Newhouse B, Anderson AS, Fa'uber B, Allen A, Chantry D, Eberhardt C, Odino J, Burgess LE (2004) Discovery and SAR of trisubstituted thiazolidinones as CCR4 antagonists. Bioorg Med Chem Lett 14:1619–1624.
80. Newhouse B, Allen S, Fa'uber B, Anderson AS, Eary CT, Hansen JD, Schiro J, Gaudino JJ, Laird E, Chantry D, Eberhardt C, Burgess LE (2004) Racemic and chiral lactams as potent, selective and functionally active CCR4 antagonists. Bioorg Med Chem Lett 14:5537–5542.
81. Purandare AV, Gao A, Wan H,Somerville JE, Burke C, Seachord C, Vaccaro W, Wityak J, Poss MA (2005) Identification of chemokine receptor CCR4 antagonist. Bioorg Med Chem Lett 15:2669–2672.
82. Purandare AV, Wan H, Gao A, Somerville JE, Burke C, Vaccaro W, Yang X, McIntyre KW, Poss MA (2006) Optimization of CCR4 antagonists: side-chain exploration. Bioorg Med Chem Lett 16:204–207.
83. Purandare AV, Somerville JE (2006) Antagonists of CCR4 as immunomodulatory agents. Curr Top Med Chem 6:1335–1344.
84. Purandare AV, Wan H, Somerville JE, Burke C, Vaccaro W, Yang X, McIntyre KW, Poss MA (2007) Core exploration in optimization of chemokine receptor CCR4 antagonists. Bioorg Med Chem Lett 17:679–682.
85. Chung CD, Kuo F, Kumer J, Motani AS, Lawrence CE, Henderson WR Jr, Venkataraman C (2003) CCR8 is not essential for the development of inflammation in a mouse model of allergic airway disease. J Immunol 170:581–587.
86. Goya I, Villares R, Zaballos A, Gutierrez J, Kremer L, Gonzalo JA, Varona R, Carramolino L, Serrano A, Pallares P, Criado LM, Kolbeck R, Torres M, Coyle AJ, Gutierrez-Ramos JC, Martinez-A C, Marquez G (2003) Absence of CCR8 does not impair the response to ovalbumin-induced allergic airway disease. J Immunol 170:2138–2146.
87. Fox JM, Najarro P, Smith GL, Struyf S, Proost P, Pease JE (2006) Structure/function relationships of CCR8 agonists and antagonists. Amino-terminal extension of CCL1 by a single amino acid generates a partial agonist. J Biol Chem 281:36652–36661.
88. Ghosh S, Elder A, Guo J, Mani U, Patane M, Carson K, Ye Q, Bennett R, Chi S, Jenkins T, Guan B, Kolbeck R, Smith S, Zhang C, LaRosa G, Jaffee B, Yang H, Eddy P, Lu C, Uttamsingh V, Horlick R, Harriman G, Flynn D (2006) Design, synthesis, and progress toward optimization of potent small molecule antagonists of CC chemokine receptor 8 (CCR8). J Med Chem 49:2669–2672.
89. Marro ML, Daniels DA, Andrews DP, Chapman TD, Gearing KL (2006) In vitro selection of RNA aptamers that block CCL1 chemokine function. Biochem Biophys Res Commun 349:270–276.
90. Norman P (2007) CCR8 antagonists. Exp Opin Ther Patents 17:465–469.
91. Sugimoto H, Shichijo M, Iino T, Manabe Y, Watanabe A, Shimazaki M, Gantner F, Bacon KB (2003) An orally bioavailable small molecule antagonist of CRTH2, ramatroban (BAY u3405), inhibits prostaglandin D2-induced eosinophil migration in vitro. J Pharmacol Exp Ther 305:347–352.
92. Uller L, Mathiesen JM, Alenmyr L, Korsgren M, Ulven T, Hogberg T, Andersson G, Persson CG, Kostenis E (2007) Antagonism of the prostaglandin D2 receptor CRTH2 attenuates asthma pathology in mouse eosinophilic airway inflammation. Respir Res 8:16.
93. Armer RE, Ashton MR, Boyd EA, Brennan CJ, Brookfield FA, Gazi L, Gyles SL, Hay PA, Hunter MG, Middlemiss D, Whittaker M, Xue L, Pettipher R (2005) Indole-3-acetic acid antagonists of the prostaglandin D2 receptor CRTH2. J Med Chem 48:6174–6177.
94. Birkinshaw TN, Teague SJ, Beech C, Bonnert RV, Hill S, Patel A, Reakes S, Sanganee H, Dougall IG, Phillips TT, Salter S, Schmidt J, Arrowsmith EC, Carrillo JJ, Bell FM, Paine SW, Weaver R (2006) Discovery of potent CRTh2 (DP2) receptor antagonists. Bioorg Med Chem Lett 16:4287–4290.
95. Ly TW, Bacon KB (2005) Small-molecule CRTH2 antagonists for the treatment of allergic inflammation: an overview. Expert Opin Investig Drugs 14:769–773.

96. Mathiesen, JM, Ulven T, Martini L, Gerlach LO, Heinemann A, Kostenis E (2005) Identification of indole derivatives exclusively interfering with a G protein-independent signaling pathway of the prostaglandin D2 receptor CRTH2. Mol Pharmacol 68:393–402.
97. Pettipher R, Hansel TT, Armer R (2007) Antagonism of the prostaglandin D2 receptors DP1 and CRTH2 as an approach to treat allergic diseases. Nat Rev Drug Discov 6:313–325.
98. Ulven T, Receveur JM, Grimstrup M, Rist O, Frimurer TM, Gerlach LO, Mathiesen JM, Kostenis E, Uller L, Hogberg T (2006) Novel selective orally active CRTH2 antagonists for allergic inflammation developed from in silico derived hits. J Med Chem 49:6638–6641.
99. Ulven T, Kostenis E (2006) Targeting the prostaglandin D2 receptors DP and CRTH2 for treatment of inflammation. Curr Top Med Chem 6:1427–1444.
100. Chvatchko Y, Proudfoot AE, Buser R, Juillard P, Alouani S, Kosco-Vilbois M, Coyle AJ, Nibbs RJ, Graham G, Offord RE, Wells TN (2003) Inhibition of airway inflammation by amino-terminally modified RANTES/CC chemokine ligand 5 analogues Is not mediated through CCR3. J Immunol 171:5498–5506.
101. Dorsam G, Graeler MH, Seroogy C, Kong Y, Voice JK, Goetzl EJ (2003) Transduction of multiple effects of sphingosine 1-phosphate (S1P) on T cell functions by the S1P1 G protein-coupled receptor. J Immunol 171:3500–3507.
102. Sawicka E, Zuany-Amorim C, Manlius C, Trifilieff A, Brinkmann V, Kemeny DM, Walker C (2003) Inhibition of Th1- and th2-mediated airway inflammation by the sphingosine 1-phosphate receptor agonist FTY720. J Immunol 171:6206–6214.
103. Idzko M, Hammad H, van Nimwegen M, Kool M, Muller T, Soullie T, Willart MA, Hijdra D, Hoogsteden HC, Lambrecht BN (2006) Local application of FTY720 to the lung abrogates experimental asthma by altering dendritic cell function. J Clin Invest 116:2935–2944.
104. Yoshino T, Ishikawa J, Ohga K, Morokata T, Takezawa R, Morio H, Okada Y, Honda K, Yamada T (2007) YM-58483, a selective CRAC channel inhibitor, prevents antigen-induced airway eosinophilia and late phase asthmatic responses via Th2 cytokine inhibition in animal models. Eur J Pharmacol 560:225–233.
105. Barnes PJ (2006) Transcription factors in airway diseases. Lab Invest 86:867–872.
106. Caramori G, Ito K, Adcock IM (2004) Transcription factors in asthma and COPD. IDrugs 7:764–770.
107. Adcock IM, Chung KF, Caramori G, Ito K (2006) Kinase inhibitors and airway inflammation. Eur J Pharmacol 533:118–132.
108. Caramori G, Adcock IM, Ito K (2004) Anti-inflammatory inhibitors of IkappaB kinase in asthma and COPD. Curr Opin Investig Drugs 5:1141–1147.
109. Fichtner-Feigl S, Fuss IJ, Preiss JC, Strober W, Kitani A (2005) Treatment of murine Th1- and Th2-mediated inflammatory bowel disease with NF-kappa B decoy oligonucleotides. J Clin Invest 115:3057–3071.
110. Nguyen C, Teo JL, Matsuda A, Eguchi M, Chi EY, Henderson WR Jr, Kahn M (2003) Chemogenomic identification of Ref-1/AP-1 as a therapeutic target for asthma. Proc Natl Acad Sci U S A 100:1169–1173.
111. Desmet C, Gosset P, Henry E, Garze V, Faisca P, Vos N, Jaspar F, Melotte D, Lambrecht B, Desmecht D, Pajak B, Moser M, Lekeux P, Bureau F (2005) Treatment of experimental asthma by decoy-mediated local inhibition of activator protein-1. Am J Respir Crit Care Med 172:671–678.
112. Erpenbeck VJ, Hohlfeld JM, Discher M, Krentel H, Hagenberg A, Braun A, Krug N (2003) Increased messenger RNA expression of c-maf and GATA-3 after segmental allergen challenge in allergic asthmatics. Chest 123(suppl 3):370S-371S.
113. Erpenbeck VJ, Hagenberg A, Krentel H, Discher M, Braun A, Hohlfeld JM, Krug N (2006) Regulation of GATA-3, c-maf and T-bet mRNA expression in bronchoalveolar lavage cells and bronchial biopsies after segmental allergen challenge. Int Arch Allergy Immunol 139:306–316.
114. Kiwamoto T, Ishii Y, Morishima Y, Yoh K, Maeda A, Ishizaki K, Iizuka T, Hegab AE, Matsuno Y, Homma S, Nomura A, Sakamoto T, Takahashi S, Sekizawa K (2006) Transcription factors T-bet and GATA-3 regulate development of airway remodeling. Am J Respir Crit Care Med 174:142–151.

115. Finotto S, De Sanctis GT, Lehr HA, Herz U, Buerke M, Schipp M, Bartsch B, Atreya R, Schmitt E, Galle PR, Renz H, Neurath MF (2001) Treatment of allergic airway inflammation and hyperresponsiveness by antisense-induced local blockade of GATA-3 expression. J Exp Med 193:1247–1260.
116. Mikhak Z, Fleming CM, Medoff BD, Thomas SY, Tager AM, Campanella GS, Luster AD (2006) STAT1 in peripheral tissue differentially regulates homing of antigen-specific Th1 and Th2 cells. J Immunol 176:4959–4967.
117. Lim S, Caramori G, Tomita K, Jazrawi E, Oates T, Chung KF, Barnes PJ, Adcock IM (2004) Differential expression of IL-10 receptor by epithelial cells and alveolar macrophages. Allergy 59:505–514.
118. Sampath D, Castro M, Look DC, Holtzman MJ (1999) Constitutive activation of an epithelial signal transducer and activator of transcription (STAT) pathway in asthma. J Clin Invest 103:1353–1361.
119. Quarcoo D, Weixler S, Groneberg D, Joachim R, Ahrens B, Wagner AH, Hecker M, Hamelmann E (2004) Inhibition of signal transducer and activator of transcription 1 attenuates allergen-induced airway inflammation and hyperreactivity. J Allergy Clin Immunol 114:288–295.
120. Mathew A, MacLean JA, DeHaan E, Tager AM, Green FH, Luster AD (2001) Signal transducer and activator of transcription 6 controls chemokine production and T helper cell type 2 cell trafficking in allergic pulmonary inflammation. J Exp Med 193.
121. Wills-Karp M (2004) Interleukin-13 in asthma pathogenesis. Immunol Rev 202:175–190.
122. Christodoulopoulos P, Cameron L, Nakamura Y, Lemiere C, Muro S, Dugas M, Boulet LP, Laviolette M, Olivenstein R, Hamid Q (2001) Th2 cytokine-associated transcription factors in atopic and nonatopic asthma: evidence for differential signal transducer and activator of transcription 6 expression. J Allergy Clin Immunol 107:586–591.
123. Ghaffar O, Christodoulopoulos P, Lamkhioued B, Wright E, Ihaku D, Nakamura Y, Frenkiel S, Hamid Q (2000) In vivo expression of signal transducer and activator of transcription factor 6 (STAT6) in nasal mucosa from atopic allergic rhinitis: effect of topical corticosteroids. Clin Exp Allergy 30:86–93.
124. Mullings RE, Wilson SJ, Puddicombe SM, Lordan JL, Bucchieri F, Djukanovic R, Howarth PH, Harper S, Holgate ST, Davies DE (2001) Signal transducer and activator of transcription 6 (STAT-6) expression and function in asthmatic bronchial epithelium. J Allergy Clin Immunol 108:832–838.
125. Caramori G, Lim S, Tomita K, Ito K, Oates T, Chung K, Barnes PJ, Adcock IM (2000) STAT6 expression in T-cells subsets, alveolar macrophages and bronchial biopsies from normal and asthmatic subjects. Eur Respir J 16(suppl 31):162s, abstract.
126. Peng Q, Matsuda T, Hirst SJ (2004) Signaling pathways regulating interleukin-13-stimulated chemokine release from airway smooth muscle. Am J Respir Crit Care Med 169:596–603.
127. Nakano T, Inoue H, Fukuyama S, Matsumoto K, Matsumura M, Tsuda M, Matsumoto T, Aizawa H, Nakanishi Y (2006) Niflumic acid suppresses interleukin-13-induced asthma phenotypes. Am J Respir Crit Care Med 173:1216–1221.
128. Shum BO, Mackay CR, Gorgun CZ, Frost MJ, Kumar RK, Hotamisligil GS, Rolph MS (2006) The adipocyte fatty acid-binding protein aP2 is required in allergic airway inflammation. J Clin Invest 116:2183–2192.
129. Kim JI, Ho IC, Grusby MJ, Glimcher LH (1999) The transcription factor c-Maf controls the production of IL-4 but not other Th2 cytokine. Immunity 10:745–751.
130. Kishikawa H, Sun J, Choi A, Miaw SC, Ho IC (2001) The cell type-specific expression of the murine IL-13 gene is regulated by GATA-3. J Immunol 167:4414–4420.
131. Nurieva RI, Duong J, Kishikawa H, Dianzani U, Rojo JM, Ho I, Flavell RA, Dong C (2003) Transcriptional regulation of th2 differentiation by inducible costimulator. Immunity 18:801–811.
132. Hwang ES, White IA, Ho IC (2002) An IL-4-independent and CD25-mediated function of c-maf in promoting the production of Th2 cytokines. Proc Natl Acad Sci U S A 99:13026–13030.

133. Ho IC, Lo D, Glimcher LH (1998) c-maf promotes T helper cell type 2 (Th2) and attenuates Th1 differentiation by both interleukin 4-dependent and -independent mechanisms. J Exp Med 188:1859–1866.
134. Taha R, Hamid Q, Cameron L, Olivenstein R (2003) T helper type 2 cytokine receptors and associated transcription factors GATA-3, c-MAF, and signal transducer and activator of transcription factor-6 in induced sputum of atopic asthmatic patients. Chest 123: 2074–2082.
135. Horsley V, Pavlath GK (2002) NFAT: ubiquitous regulator of cell differentiation and adaptation. J Cell Biol 156:771–774.
136. Seminario MC, Guo J, Bochner BS, Beck LA, Georas SN (2001) Human eosinophils constitutively express nuclear factor of activated T cells p and c. J Allergy Clin Immunol 107:143–152.
137. Crabtree GR, Olson EN (2002) NFAT signaling: choreographing the social lives of cells. Cell 109(suppl):S67–S79.
138. Hogan PG, Chen L, Nardone J, Rao A (2003) Transcriptional regulation by calcium, calcineurin, and NFAT. Genes Dev 17:2205–2232.
139. Mori A, Kaminuma O, Mikami T, Inoue S, Okumura Y, Akiyama K, Okudaira H (1999) Transcriptional control of the IL-5 gene by human helper T cells: IL-5 synthesis is regulated independently from IL-2 or IL-4 synthesis. J Allergy Clin Immunol 103(suppl):S429–S436.
140. Ogawa K, Kaminuma O, Okudaira H, Kikkawa H, Ikezawa K, Sakurai N, Mori A (2002) Transcriptional regulation of the IL-5 gene in peripheral T cells of asthmatic patients. Clin Exp Immunol 130:475–483.
141. Keen JC, Sholl L, Wills-Karp M, Georas SN (2001) Preferential activation of nuclear factor of activated T cells c correlates with mouse strain susceptibility to allergic responses and interleukin-4 gene expression. Am J Respir Cell Mol Biol 24:58–65.
142. Diehl S, Chow CW, Weiss L, Palmetshofer A, Twardzik T, Rounds L, Serfling E, Davis RJ, Anguita J, Rincon M (2002) Induction of NFATc2 expression by interleukin 6 promotes T helper type 2 differentiation. J Exp Med 196:39–49.
143. Hodge MR, Ranger AM, Charles de la Brousse F, Hoey T, Grusby MJ, Glimcher LH (1996) Hyperproliferation and dysregulation of IL-4 expression in NF-Atp-deficient mice. Immunity 4:397–405.
144. Rengarajan J, Mowen KA, McBride KD, Smith ED, Singh H, Glimcher LH (2002) Interferon regulatory factor 4 (IRF4) interacts with NFATc2 to modulate interleukin 4 gene expression. J Exp Med 195:1003–1012.
145. Rengarajan J, Tang B, Glimcher LH (2002) NFATc2 and NFATc3 regulate T(H)2 differentiation and modulate TCR-responsiveness of naive T(H) cells. Nat Immunol 3:48–54.
146. van Rietschoten JG, Smits HH, van de Wetering D, Westland R, Verweij CL, den Hartog MT, Wierenga EA (2001) Silencer activity of NFATc2 in the interleukin-12 receptor beta 2 proximal promoter in human T helper cells. J Biol Chem 276:34509–34516.
147. Xanthoudakis S, Viola JP, Shaw KT, Luo C, Wallace JD, Bozza PT, Luk DC, Curran T, Rao A (1996) An enhanced immune response in mice lacking the transcription factor NFAT1. Science 272:892–895.
148. Chen J, Amasaki Y, Kamogawa Y, Nagoya M, Arai N, Arai K, Miyatake S (2003) Role of NFATx (NFAT4/NFATc3) in expression of immunoregulatory genes in murine peripheral CD4+ T cells. J Immunol 170:3109–3117.
149. Ranger AM, Oukka M, Rengarajan J, Glimcher LH (1998) Inhibitory function of two NFAT family members in lymphoid homeostasis and Th2 development. Immunity 9:627–635.
150. Chen Y, Smith ML, Chiou GX, Ballaron S, Sheets MP, Gubbins E, Warrior U, Wilkins J, Surowy C, Nakane M, Carter GW, Trevillyan JM, Mollison K, Djuric SW (2002) TH1 and TH2 cytokine inhibition by 3,5-bis(trifluoromethyl)pyrazoles, a novel class of immunomodulators. Cell Immunol 220:134–142.
151. Djuric SW, BaMaung NY, Basha A, Liu H, Luly JR, Madar DJ, Sciotti RJ, Tu NP, Wagenaar FL, Wiedeman PE, Zhou X, Ballaron S, Bauch J, Chen YW, Chiou XG, Fey T, Gauvin D, Gubbins E, Hsieh GC, Marsh KC, Mollison KW, Pong M, Shaughnessy TK, Sheets MP,

Smith M, Trevillyan JM, Warrior U, Wegner CD, Carter GW (2000) 3,5-Bis(trifluoromethyl) pyrazoles: a novel class of NFAT transcription factor regulator. J Med Chem 43:2975–2981.
152. Kubo M, Hanada T, Yoshimura A (2003) Suppressors of cytokine signaling and immunity. Nat Immunol 4:1169–1176.
153. Harada M, Nakashima K, Hirota T, Shimizu M, Doi S, Fujita K, Shirakawa T, Enomoto T, Yoshikawa M, Moriyama H, Matsumoto K, Saito H, Suzuki Y, Nakamura Y, Tamari M (2007) Functional polymorphism in the suppressor of cytokine signaling 1 gene associated with adult asthma. Am J Respir Cell Mol Biol 36:491–496.
154. Kubo M, Inoue H (2006) Suppressor of cytokine signaling 3 (SOCS3) in Th2 cells evokes Th2 cytokines, IgE, and eosinophilia. Curr Allergy Asthma Rep 6:32–39.
155. Inoue H, Kubo M (2004) SOCS proteins in T helper cell differentiation: implications for allergic disorders? Expert Rev Mol Med 6:1–11.
156. Inoue H, Fukuyama S, Matsumoto K, Kubo M, Yoshimura A (2007) Role of endogenous inhibitors of cytokine signaling in allergic asthma. Curr Med Chem 14:181–189.
157. Seki Y, Inoue H, Nagata N, Hayashi K, Fukuyama S, Matsumoto K, Komine O, Hamano S, Himeno K, Inagaki-Ohara K, Cacalano N, O'Garra A, Oshida T, Saito H, Johnston JA, Yoshimura A, Kubo M.(2003) SOCS-3 regulates onset and maintenance of T(H)2-mediated allergic responses. Nat Med 9:1047–54.
158. Seki Y, Hayashi K, Matsumoto A, Seki N, Tsukada J, Ransom J, Naka T, Kishimoto T, Yoshimura A, Kubo M (2002) Expression of the suppressor of cytokine signaling-5 (SOCS5) negatively regulates IL-4-dependent STAT6 activation and Th2 differentiation. Proc Natl Acad Sci USA 99:13003–13008.
159. Ozaki A, Seki Y, Fukushima A, Kubo M (2005) The control of allergic conjunctivitis by suppressor of cytokine signaling (SOCS) 3 and SOCS-5 in a murine model. J Immunol 175:5489–5497.
160. Brender C, Columbus R, Metcalf D, Handman E, Starr R, Huntington N, Tarlinton D, Odum N, Nicholson SE, Nicola NA, Hilton DJ, Alexander WS (2004) SOCS-5 is expressed in primary B and T lymphoid cells but is dispensable for lymphocyte production and function. Mol Cell Biol 24:6094–103.
161. Ohshima M, Yokoyama A, Ohnishi H, Hamada H, Kohno N, Higaki J, Naka T (2007) Overexpression of suppressor of cytokine signalling-5 augments eosinophilic airway inflammation in mice. Clin Exp Allergy 37:735–742.
162. Hammad H, De Heer HJ, Soullie T, Angeli V, Trottein F, Hoogsteden HC, Lambrecht BN (2004) Activation of peroxisome proliferator-activated receptor-gamma in dendritic cells inhibits the development of eosinophilic airway inflammation in a mouse model of asthma. Am J Pathol 164:263–271.
163. Woerly G, Honda K, Loyens M, Papin JP, Auwerx J, Staels B, Capron M, Dombrowicz D (2003) Peroxisome proliferator-activated receptors alpha and gamma down-regulate allergic inflammation and eosinophil activation. J Exp Med 198:411–421.
164. Trifilieff A, Bench A, Hanley M, Bayley D, Campbell E, Whittaker P (2003) PPAR-alpha and -gamma but not -delta agonists inhibit airway inflammation in a murine model of asthma: in vitro evidence for an NF-kappaB-independent effect. Br J Pharmacol 139:163–171.
165. Mueller C, Weaver V, Vanden Heuvel JP, August A, Cantorna MT (2003) Peroxisome proliferator-activated receptor gamma ligands attenuate immunological symptoms of experimental allergic asthma. Arch Biochem Biophys 418:186–196.
166. Kim SR, Lee KS, Park HS, Park SJ, Min KH, Jin SM, Lee YC (2005) Involvement of IL-10 in peroxisome proliferator-activated receptor gamma-mediated anti-inflammatory response in asthma. Mol Pharmacol 68:1568–1575.
167. Honda K, Marquillies P, Capron M, Dombrowicz D (2004) Peroxisome proliferator-activated receptor gamma is expressed in airways and inhibits features of airway remodeling in a mouse asthma model. J Allergy Clin Immunol 113:882–888.
168. Lee KS, Park SJ, Hwang PH, Yi HK, Song CH, Chai OH, Kim JS, Lee MK, Lee YC (2005) PPAR-gamma modulates allergic inflammation through up-regulation of PTEN. FASEB J 19:1033–1035.

169. Lee KS, Park SJ, Kim SR, Min KH, Jin SM, Lee HK, Lee YC (2006) Modulation of airway remodeling and airway inflammation by peroxisome proliferator-activated receptor gamma in a murine model of toluene diisocyanate-induced asthma. J Immunol 177:5248–5257.
170. Lee KS, Kim SR, Park SJ, Park HS, Min KH, Jin SM, Lee MK, Kim UH, Lee YC (2006) Peroxisome proliferator activated receptor-gamma modulates reactive oxygen species generation and activation of nuclear factor-kappaB and hypoxia-inducible factor 1alpha in allergic airway disease of mice. J Allergy Clin Immunol 118:120–127.
171. Spears M, McSharry C, Thomson NC (2006) Peroxisome proliferator-activated receptor-gamma agonists as potential anti-inflammatory agents in asthma and chronic obstructive pulmonary disease. Clin Exp Allergy 36:1494–1504.
172. Belvisi MG, Hele DJ, Birrell MA (2006) Peroxisome proliferator-activated receptor gamma agonists as therapy for chronic airway inflammation. Eur J Pharmacol 533:101–109.
173. Khanna S, Sobria ME, Bharatam PV (2005) Additivity of molecular fields: CoMFA study on dual activators of PPARalpha and PPARgamma. J Med Chem 48:3015–3025.
174. Ueki S, Usami A, Oyamada H, Saito N, Chiba T, Mahemuti G, Ito W, Kato H, Kayaba H, Chihara J (2006) Procaterol upregulates peroxisome proliferator-activated receptor-gamma expression in human eosinophils. Int Arch Allergy Immunol 140(suppl 1):S35–S41.
175. Usami A, Ueki S, Ito W, Kobayashi Y, Chiba T, Mahemuti G, Oyamada H, Kamada Y, Fujita M, Kato H, Saito N, Kayaba H, Chihara J (2006) Theophylline and dexamethasone induce peroxisome proliferator-activated receptor-gamma expression in human eosinophils. Pharmacology 77:33–37.
176. Adcock IM, Caramori G (2004) Kinase targets and inhibitors for the treatment of airway inflammatory diseases: the next Generation of drugs for severe asthma and COPD? Biodrugs 18:167–180.
177. Schafer PH, Wadsworth SA, Wang L, Siekierka SJ (1999) p38 alpha mitogen-activated protein kinase is activated by CD28-mediated signaling and is required for IL-4 production by human CD4+CD45RO+ T cells and Th2 effector cells. J Immunol 162:7110–7119.
178. Duan W, Chan JH, McKay K, Crosby JR, Choo HH, Leung BP, Karras JG, Wong WS (2005) Inhaled p38alpha mitogen-activated protein kinase antisense oligonucleotide attenuates asthma in mice. Am J Respir Crit Care Med 171:571–578.
179. Duan W, Wong WS (2006) Targeting mitogen-activated protein kinases for asthma. Curr Drug Targets 7:691–698.
180. Lane SJ, Adcock IM, Richards D, Hawrylowicz C, Barnes PJ, Lee TH (1998) Corticosteroid-resistant bronchial asthma is associated with increased c-fos expression in monocytes and T lymphocytes. J Clin Invest 102:2156–2164.
181. Huang TJ, Adcock IM, Chung KF (2001) A novel transcription factor inhibitor, SP100030, inhibits cytokine gene expression, but not airway eosinophilia or hyperresponsiveness in sensitized and allergen-exposed rat. Br J Pharmacol 134:1029–1036.
182. Rose MJ, Page C (2004) Glycosaminoglycans and the regulation of allergic inflammation. Curr Drug Targets Inflamm Allergy 3:221–225.
183. Ellyard JI, Simson L, Johnston K, Freeman C, Parish CR (2007) Eotaxin selectively binds heparin: An interaction that protects eotaxin from proteolysis and potentiates chemotactic activity in vivo. J Biol Chem 282(20):15238–15247.
184. Rashid RM, Lee JM,Fareed J, Young MR (2007) In vitro heparan sulfate modulates the immune responses of normal and tumor-bearing mice. Immunol Invest 36:183–201.
185. Lever R, Page C (2001) Glycosaminoglycans, airways inflammation and bronchial hyperresponsiveness. Pulm Pharmacol Ther 14:249–254.
186. Diamant Z, Page CP (2000) Heparin and related molecules as a new treatment for asthma. Pulm Pharmacol Ther 13:1–4.
187. Page C (2000) The role of proteoglycans in the regulation of airways inflammation and airways remodelling. J Allergy Clin Immunol 105(suppl):S518–S521.
188. Ahmed T, Garrigo J, Danta I (1993) Preventing bronchoconstriction in exercise-induced asthma with inhaled heparin. N Engl J Med 329:90–95.

189. Ahmed T, Gonzales BJ, Danta I (1999) Prevention of exercise-induced bronchoconstriction by inhaled low-molecular-weight heparin. Am J Respir Crit Care Med 160:576–581.
190. Garrigo J, Danta I, Ahmed T (1996) Time course of the protective effect of inhaled heparin on exercise-induced asthma. Am J Respir Crit Care Med 153:1702–1707.
191. Barnes PJ (2003) Cytokine-directed therapies for the treatment of chronic airway diseases. Cytokine Growth Factor Rev 14:511–522.
192. Grunewald SM, Werthmann A, Schnarr B, Klein CE, Brocker EB, Mohrs M, Brombacher F, Sebald W, Duschl A (1998) An antagonistic IL-4 mutant prevents type I allergy in the mouse: inhibition of the IL-4/IL-13 receptor system completely abrogates humoral immune response to allergen and development of allergic symptoms in vivo. J Immunol 160:4004–4009.
193. Lindell D, Gundel R, Fitch N, Harris P (1999) The IL-4 receptor antagonist (Bay 16–9996) reverses airway hyperresponsiveness in a primate model of asthma. Am J Respir Crit Care Med 159(suppl): abstract A230.
194. Steinke JW, Borish L (2001) Th2 cytokines and asthma. Interleukin-4: its role in the pathogenesis of asthma, and targeting it for asthma treatment with interleukin-4 receptor antagonists. Respir Res 2:66–70.
195. Henderson WR, Jr, Chi EY, Maliszewski CR (2000) Soluble IL-4 receptor inhibits airway inflammation following allergen challenge in a mouse model of asthma. J Immunol 164:1086–1095.
196. Borish LC, Nelson HS, Lanz MJ, Claussen L, Whitmore JB, Agosti JM, Garrison L (1999) Interleukin-4 receptor in moderate atopic asthma. A phase I/II randomized, placebo-controlled trial. Am J Respir Crit Care Med 160:1816–1823.
197. LC, Nelson HS, Corren J, Bensch G, Busse WW, Whitmore JB, Agosti JM (2001) IL-4R Asthma Study Group. Efficacy of soluble IL-4 receptor for the treatment of adults with asthma. J Allergy Clin Immunol 107:963–970.
198. Karras JG, Crosby JR, Guha M, Tung D, Miller DA, Gaarde WA, Geary RS, Monia BP, Gregory SA (2007) Anti-inflammatory activity of inhaled IL-4 receptor-alpha antisense oligonucleotide in mice. Am J Respir Cell Mol Biol 36:276–285.
199. Ma Y, Hayglass KT, Becker AB, Halayko AJ, Basu S, Simons FER, Peng Z (2007) Novel cytokine peptide-based vaccines: an interleukin-4 vaccine suppresses airway allergic responses in mice. Allergy 62:675–682.
200. Grunig G, Warnock M, Wakil AE, Venkayya R, Brombacher F, Rennick DM, Sheppard D, Mohrs M, Donaldson DD, Locksley RM, Corry DB (1998) Requirement for IL-13 independently of IL-4 in experimental asthma. Science 282:2261–2263.
201. Yang G, Volk A, Petley T, Emmell E, Giles-Komar J, Shang X, Li J, Das AM, Shealy D, Griswold DE, Li L (2004) Anti-IL-13 monoclonal antibody inhibits airway hyperresponsiveness, inflammation and airway remodeling. Cytokine 28:224–232.
202. Kasaian MT, Donaldson DD, Tchistiakova L, Marquette K, Tan XY, Ahmed A, Jacobson BA, Widom A, Cook TA, Xu X, Barry AB, Goldman SJ, Abraham WM (2007) Efficacy of IL-13 neutralization in a sheep model of experimental asthma. Am J Respir Cell Mol Biol 36:368–376.
203. Izuhara K, Arima K, Kanaji S, Ohta S, Kanaji T (2006) IL-13: a promising therapeutic target for bronchial asthma. Curr Med Chem 13:2291–2298.
204. Blanchard C, Mishra A, Saito-Akei H, Monk P, Anderson I, Rothenberg ME (2005) Inhibition of human interleukin-13-induced respiratory and oesophageal inflammation by anti-human-interleukin-13 antibody (CAT-354). Clin Exp Allergy 35:1096–1103.
205. Yang G, Li L, Volk A, Emmell E, Petley T, Giles-Komar J, Rafferty P, Lakshminarayanan M, Griswold DE, Bugelski PJ, Das AM (2005) Therapeutic dosing with anti-interleukin-13 monoclonal antibody inhibits asthma progression in mice. J Pharmacol Exp Ther 313:8–15.
206. Bree A, Schlerman FJ, Wadanoli M, Tchistiakova L, Marquette K, Tan XY, Jacobson BA, Widom A, Cook TA, Wood N, Vunnum S, Krykbaev R, Xu X, Donladson DD, Goldman SJ, Sypek J, Kasain MT (2007) IL-13 blockade reduces lung inflammation after Ascaris suum challenge in cynomolgus monkeys. J Allergy Clin Immunol 119:1251–1257.

207. Ma Y, Hayglass KT, Becker AB, Fan Y, Yang X, Basu S, Srinivasan G, Simons FE, Halayko AJ, Peng Z (2007) Novel recombinant IL-13 peptide-based vaccine reduces airway allergic inflammatory responses in mice. Am J Respir Crit Care Med 176(5):439–445.
208. Kips JC, O'Connor BJ, Langley SJ, Woodcock A, Kerstjens HA, Postma DS, Danzig M, Cuss F, Pauwels RA (2003) Effect of SCH55700, a humanized anti-human interleukin-5 antibody, in severe persistent asthma: a pilot study. Am J Respir Crit Care Med 2003;167:1655–1659. [Comment in: Am J Respir Crit Care Med 167:1586–1587].
209. Flood-Page PT, Menzies-Gow AN, Kay AB, Robinson DS (2003) Eosinophil's role remains uncertain as anti-interleukin-5 only partially depletes numbers in asthmatic airway. Am J Respir Crit Care Med 2003;167:199–204. [Comment in: Am J Respir Crit Care Med 167:102–103].
210. Buttner C, Lun A, Splettstoesser T, Kunkel G, Renz H (2003) Monoclonal anti-interleukin-5 treatment suppresses eosinophil but not T-cell functions. Eur Respir J 21:799–803.
211. Mao H, Wen FO, Liu CT, Liang ZA, Wang ZL, Yin KS (2006) Effect of interleukin-5 receptor-alpha short hairpin RNA-expressing vector on bone marrow eosinophilopoiesis in asthmatic mice. Adv Ther 23:938–956.
212. Mao H, Wen FO, Li SY, Liang ZA, Liu CT, Yin KS, Wang ZL (2007) A preliminary study towards downregulation of murine bone marrow eosinophilopoiesis mediated by small molecule inhibition of interleukin-5 receptor alpha gene in vitro. Respiration 74:320–328.
213. Taga T, Kishimoto T (1997) Gp130 and the interleukin-6 family of cytokines. Annu Rev Immunol 15:797–819.
214. Doganci A, Eigenbrod T, Krug N, De Sanctis GT, Hausding M, Erpenbeck VJ, Haddad el-B, Lehr HA, Schmitt E, Bopp T, Kallen KJ, Herz U, Schmitt S, Luft C, Hecht O, Hohlfeld JM, Ito H, Nishimoto N, Yoshikazi K, Kishimoto T, Rose-John S, Renz H, Neurath MF, Galle PR, Finotto S (2005) The IL-6R alpha chain controls lung CD4+CD25+ Treg development and function during allergic airway inflammation in vivo. J Clin Invest 115:313–325. [Erratum in: J Clin Invest 115:1388. Lehr, Hans A; added].
215. McNamara PS, Smyth RL (2005) Interleukin-9 as a possible therapeutic target in both asthma and chronic obstructive airways disease. Drug News Perspect 18:615–621.
216. Steenwinckel V, Louahed J, Orabona C, Huax F, Warnier G, McKenzie A, Lison D, Levitt R, Renauld JC (2007) IL-13 mediates in vivo IL-9 activities on lung epithelial cells but not on hematopoietic cells. J Immunol 178:3244–3251.
217. Shimbara A, Christodoulopoulos P, Soussi-Gounni A, Olivenstein R, Nakamura Y, Levitt RC, Nicolaides NC, Holroyd KJ, Tsicopoulos A, Lafitte JJ, Wallaert B, Hamid QA (2000) IL-9 and its receptor in allergic and nonallergic lung disease: increased expression in asthma. J Allergy Clin Immunol 105:108–15.
218. Ying S, Meng Q, Kay AB, Robinson DS (2002) Elevated expression of interleukin-9 mRNA in the bronchial mucosa of atopic asthmatics and allergen-induced cutaneous late-phase reaction: relationships to eosinophils, mast cells and T lymphocytes. Clin Exp Allergy 32:866–871.
219. Erpenbeck VJ, Hohlfeld JM, Volkmann B, Hagenberg A, Geldmacher H, Braun A, Krug N (2003) Segmental allergen challenge in patients with atopic asthma leads to increased IL-9 expression in bronchoalveolar lavage fluid lymphocytes. J Allergy Clin Immunol 111:1319–27.
220. van den Brule S, Heymans J, Havaux X, Renauld JC, Lison D, Huax F, Denis O (2007) Pro-fibrotic effect of IL-9 overexpression in a model of airway remodeling. Am J Respir Cell Mol Biol 37(2):202–209.
221. Fallon PG, Jolin HE, Smith P, Emson CL, Townsend MJ, Fallon R, Smith P, McKenzie AN (2002) IL-4 induces characteristic Th2 responses even in the combined absence of IL-5, IL-9, and IL-13. Immunity 17:7–17.
222. Townsend JM, Fallon GP, Matthews JD, Smith P, Jolin EH, McKenzie NA (2000) IL-9-deficient mice establish fundamental roles for IL-9 in pulmonary mastocytosis and goblet cell hyperplasia but not T cell development. Immunity 13:573–578.
223. Cheng G, Arima M, Honda K, Hirata H, Eda F, Yoshida N, Fukushima F, Ishii Y, Fukuda T (2002) Anti-interleukin-9 antibody treatment inhibits airway inflammation and hyperreactivity in mouse asthma model. Am J Respir Crit Care Med 166:409–416.

224. Kung TT, Luo B, Crawley Y, Garlisi CG, Devito K,Minnicozzi M, Egan RW, Kreutner W, Chapman RW (2001) Effect of anti-mIL-9 antibody on the development of pulmonary inflammation and airway hyperresponsiveness in allergic mice. Am J Respir Cell Mol Biol 25:600–605.
225. Sitkauskiene B, Radinger M, Bossios A, Johansson AK, Sakalauskas R, Lotvall J (2005) Airway allergen exposure stimulates bone marrow eosinophilia partly via IL-9. Respir Res 6:33.
226. Lee CG, Homer RJ, Cohn L, Link H, Jung S, Craft JE, Graham BS, Johnson TR, Elias JA (2002) Transgenic overexpression of interleukin (IL)-10 in the lung causes mucus metaplasia, tissue inflammation, and airway remodeling via IL-13-dependent and -independent pathways. J Biol Chem 277:35466–35474.
227. Tomita K, Lim S, Hanazawa T, Usmani O, Stirling R, Chung KF, Barnes PJ, Adcock IM (2002) Attenuated production of intracellular IL-10 and IL-12 in monocytes from patients with severe asthma. Clin Immunol 102:258–266.
228. Xystrakis E, Kusumakar S, Boswell S, Peek E, Urry Z, Richards DF, Adikibi T, Pridgeon C, Dallman M, Loke TK, Robinson DS, Barrat FJ, O'Garra A, Lavender P, Lee TH, Corrigan C, Hawrylowicz CM (2006) Reversing the defective induction of IL-10-secreting regulatory T cells in glucocorticoid-resistant asthma patients. J Clin Invest 116:146–155.
229. Lim S, Crawley E, Woo P, Barnes PJ (1998) Haplotype associated with low interleukin-10 production in patients with severe asthma. Lancet 352:113.
230. Ogawa H, Nishimura N, Nishioka Y, Azuma M, Yanagawa H, Sone S (2003) Adenoviral interleukin-12 gene transduction into human bronchial epithelial cells: up-regulation of pro-inflammatory cytokines and its prevention by corticosteroids. Clin Exp Allergy 33:921–929.
231. Bryan SA, O'Connor BJ, Matti S, Leckie MJ, Kanabar V, Khan J, Warrington SJ, Renzetti L, Ranes A, Bock JA (2000) Effects of recombinant human interleukin-12 on eosinophils, airway hyperresponsiveness, and the late asthmatic response. Lancet 356:2149–2153.
232. Matsuse H, Kong X, Hu J, Wolf SF, Lockey RF, Mohapatra SS (2003) Intranasal IL-12 produces discreet pulmonary and systemic effects on allergic inflammation and airway reactivity. Int Immunopharmacol 3:457–468.
233. Christensen U, Haagerup A, Binderup HG, Vestbo J, Kruse TA, Borgium AD (2006) Family based association analysis of the IL2 and IL15 genes in allergic disorders. Eur J Hum Genet 14:227–235.
234. Kurz T, Strauch K, Dietrich H, Braun S, Hierl S, Jerkic SP, Wienker TF, Deichmann KA, Heinzmann A (2004) Multilocus haplotype analyses reveal association between 5 novel IL-15 polymorphisms and asthma. J Allergy Clin Immunol 113:896–901.
235. Muro S, Taha R, Tsicopoulos A, Olivenstein R, Tonnel AB, Christodoulopoulos P, Wallaert B, Hamid Q (2001) Expression of IL-15 in inflammatory pulmonary diseases. J Allergy Clin Immunol 108:970–975.
236. Ishimitsu R, Nishimura H, Yajima T, Watase T, Kawauchi H, Yoshikai Y (2001) Overexpression of IL-15 in vivo enhances Tc1 response, which inhibits allergic inflammation in a murine model of asthma. J Immunol 166:1991–2001.
237. Ruckert R, Brandt K, Braun A, Hoymann HG, Herz U, Budagian V, Durkop H, Renz H, Bulfone-Paus S (2005) Blocking IL-15 prevents the induction of allergen-specific T cells and allergic inflammation in vivo. J Immunol 174:5507–5515.
238. Wei H, Zhang J, Xiao W, Feng J, Sun R, Tian Z (2005) Involvement of human natural killer cells in asthma pathogenesis: natural killer 2 cells in type 2 cytokine predominance. J Allergy Clin Immunol 115:841–847.
239. O'Sullivan S, Cormican L, Burke CM, Poulter LW (2004) Fluticasone induces T cell apoptosis in the bronchial wall of mild to moderate asthmatics. Thorax 59:657–661.
240. Bombardieri M, McInnes IB, Pitzalis C (2007) Interleukin-18 as a potential therapeutic target in chronic autoimmune/inflammatory conditions. Expert Opin Biol Ther 7:31–40.
241. Maecker HT, Hansen G, Walter DM, DeKruyff RH, Levy S, Umetsu DT (2001) Vaccination with allergen-IL-18 fusion DNA protects against, and reverses established, airway hyperreactivity in a murine asthma model. J Immunol 166:959–965.

242. Tsutsui H, Yoshimoto T, Hayashi N, Mizutani H, Nakanishi K (2004) Induction of allergic inflammation by interleukin-18 in experimental animal models. Immunol Rev 202:115–138.
243. Sugimoto T, Ishikawa Y, Yoshimoto T, Hayashi N, Fujimoto J, Nakanishi K (2004) Interleukin 18 acts on memory T helper cells type 1 to induce airway inflammation and hyperresponsiveness in a naive host mouse. J Exp Med 199:535–545.
244. Kumano K, Nakao A, Nakajima H, Hayashi F, Kurimoto M, Okamura H, Saito Y, Iwamoto I (1999) Interleukin-18 enhances antigen-induced eosinophil recruitment into the mouse airways. Am J Respir Crit Care Med 160:873–878.
245. Wild JS, Sigounas A, Sur N, Siddiqui MS, Alam R, Kurimoto M, Sur S (2000) IFN-gamma-inducing factor (IL-18) increases allergic sensitization, serum IgE, Th2 cytokines, and airway eosinophilia in a mouse model of allergic asthma. J Immunol 164:2701–2710.
246. Wong CK, Ho CY, Ko FW, Chan CH, Ho AS, Hui DS, Lam CW (2001) Proinflammatory cytokines (IL-17, IL-6, IL-18 and IL-12) and Th cytokines (IFN-gamma, IL-4, IL-10 and IL-13) in patients with allergic asthma. Clin Exp Immunol 125:177–183.
247. Tanaka H, Miyazaki N, Oashi K, Teramoto S, Shiratori M, Hashimoto M, Ohmichi M, Abe S (2001) IL-18 might reflect disease activity in mild and moderate asthma exacerbation. J Allergy Clin Immunol 107:331–336.
248. Ho LP, Davis M, Denison A, Wood FT, Greening AP (2002) Reduced interleukin-18 levels in BAL specimens from patients with asthma compared to patients with sarcoidosis and healthy control subjects. Chest 121:1421–1426.
249. McKay A, Komai-Koma M, MacLeod KJ, Campbell CC, Kitson SM, Chaudhuri R, Thomson L, McSharry C, Liew FY, Thomson NC (2004) Interleukin-18 levels in induced sputum are reduced in asthmatic and normal smokers. Clin Exp Allergy 34:904–910.
250. Sheppard P, Kindsvogel W, Xu W, Henderson K, Schlutsmeyer S, Whitmore TE, Kuestner R, Garrigues U, Birks C, Roraback J, Ostrander C, Dong D, Shin J, Presnell S, Fox B, Haldeman B, Cooper E, Taft D, Gilbert T, Grant FJ, Tackett M, Krivan W, McKnight G, Clegg C, Foster D, Klucher KM (2003) IL-28, IL-29 and their class II cytokine receptor IL-28R. Nat Immunol 4:63–68.
251. Langer JA, Cutrone EC, Kotenko S (2004) The Class II cytokine receptor (CRF2) family: overview and patterns of receptor-ligand interactions. Cytokine Growth Factor Rev 15:33–48.
252. Dumoutier L, Leemans C, Lejeune D, Kotenko SV, Renauld JC (2001) Cutting edge: STAT activation by IL-19, IL-20 and mda-7 through IL-20 receptor complexes of two types. J Immunol 167:3545–3549.
253. Kotenko SV, Langer JA (2004) Full house: 12 receptors for 27 cytokines.Int Immunopharmacol 4:593–608.
254. Donnelly RP, Sheikh F, Kotenko SV, Dickensheets H (2004) The expanded family of class II cytokines that share the IL-10 receptor-2 (IL-10R2) chain. J Leukoc Biol 76:314–321.
255. Krause CD, Pestka S (2005) Evolution of the Class 2 cytokines and receptors, and discovery of new friends and relatives. Pharmacol Ther 106:299–346.
256. Uze G, Monneron D (2007) IL-28 and IL-29: newcomers to the interferon family.Biochimie 89:729–734.
257. Gallagher G, Eskdale J, Jordan W, Peat J, Campbell J, Boniotto M, Lennon GP, Dickensheets H, Donnelly RP (2004) Human interleukin-19 and its receptor: a potential role in the induction of Th2 responses. Int Immunopharmacol 4:615–626.
258. Gallagher G, Dickensheets H, Eskdale J, Izotova LS, O. Mirochnitchenko OV, Peat JD, Vazquez N, Pestka S, Donnelly RP, Kotenko SV (2000) Cloning, expression and initial characterization of interleukin-19 (IL-19), a novel homologue of human interleukin-10 (IL-10). Genes Immun 1:442.
259. Liao YC, Liang WG, Chen FW, Hsu JH, Yang MJJ, Chang S (2002) IL-19 induces production of IL-6 and TNF-α and results in cell apoptosis through TNF-α. J Immunol 169:4288.
260. Liao SC, Cheng YC, Wang YC, Wang CW, Yang SM, Yu CK, Shieh CC, Cheng KC, Lee MF, Chiang SR, Shieh JM, Chang MS (2004) IL-19 induced Th2 cytokines and was upregulated in asthma patients. J Immunol 173:6712–6718.

261. Zhong H, Wu Y, Belardinelli L, Zeng D (2006) A2B adenosine receptors induce IL-19 from bronchial epithelial cells, resulting in TNF-alpha increase. Am J Respir Cell Mol Biol 35:587–592.
262. Sivakumar PV, Foster DC, Clegg CH (2004) Interleukin-21 is a T-helper cytokine that regulates humoral immunity and cell-mediated anti-tumour responses. Immunology 112:177–182.
263. Habib T, Nelson A, Kaushansky K (2003) IL-21: a novel IL-2-family lymphokine that modulates B, T, and natural killer cell responses. J Allergy Clin Immunol 112:1033–1045.
264. Ozaki KR, Spolski CG, Feng C-F, et al. (2002) A critical role for IL-21 in regulating immunoglobulin production. Science 298:1630–1634.
265. Shang XZ, Ma KY, Radewonuk J, Li J, Song XY, Griswold DE, Emmell E, Li T (2006) IgE isotype switch and IgE production are enhanced in IL-21-deficient but not IFN-gamma-deficient mice in a Th2-biased response. Cell Immunol 241:66–74.
266. Kasaian MT, Whitters MJ, Carter LL, Lowe LD, Jussif JM, Deng B, Johnson KA, Witek JS, Senices M, Konz RF, Wurster AL, Donaldson DD, Collins M, Young DA, Grusby MJ (2002) IL-21 limits NK cell responses and promotes antigen-specific T cell activation: a mediator of the transition from innate to adaptive immunity. Immunity 16:559–569.
267. Curti BD (2006) Immunomodulatory and antitumor effects of interleukin-21 in patients with renal cell carcinoma. Expert Rev Anticancer Ther 6:905–909.
268. Fina D, Fantini MC, Pallone F, Monteleone G (2007) Role of interleukin-21 in inflammation and allergy. Inflamm Allergy Drug Targets 6:63–68.
269. Wolk K, Sabat R (2006) Interleukin-22: a novel T- and NK-cell derived cytokine that regulates the biology of tissue cells. Cytokine Growth Factor Rev 17:367–380.
270. Oral HB, Kotenko SV, Yilmaz M, Mani O, Zumkehr J, Blaser K, Akdis CA, Akdis M (2006) Regulation of T cells and cytokines by the interleukin-10 (IL-10)-family cytokines IL-19, IL-20, IL-22, IL-24 and IL-26. Eur J Immunol 36:380–388.
271. Whittington HA, Armstrong L, Uppington KM, Millar AB (2004) Interleukin-22: a potential immunomodulatory molecule in the lung. Am J Respir Cell Mol Biol 31:220–226.
272. Heijink IH, van Oosterhout AJM (2006) Strategies for targeting T-cells in allergic diseases and asthma. Pharmacol Ther 112:489–500.

Transgenic Rice for Mucosal Vaccine and Immunotherapy

Yoshikazu Yuki, Fumio Takaiwa, and Hiroshi Kiyono

Introduction

Allergic diseases are a form of immunological hypersensitivity that causes chronic illness. The hypersensitivity occurs through the interaction of innocuous environmental antigens such as allergens with antigen-specific IgE antibodies [1,2]. After allergen exposure via the aerodigestive tract, the formation of allergen–IgE immune complexes on mast cells and basophils via Fc receptor for IgE (FcεR) induces the release of chemical mediators of inflammation such as histamine, prostaglandins, cytokines, chemokines, and leukotrienes, which cause allergic inflammatory reactions [3,4]. Repeated contact with allergens not only induces strong rises in the level of allergen-specific IgE antibodies but also leads to progression of the hypersensitivity disease [5].

Current pharmacological treatments for allergic diseases, such as steroids and antihistamines, are palliative (i.e., they alleviate the symptoms without treating the underlying causes), although some may result in nonspecific immunosuppression [6]. However, allergen-specific immunotherapy (SIT) can affect the process by which allergen-specific IgE antibodies are produced [7]. Thus far, various forms of allergen-SIT have been developed and tested in both experimental animals and humans.

Y. Yuki and H. Kiyono (✉)
Division of Mucosal Immunology, Department of Microbiology and Immunology, The Institute of Medical Science, The University of Tokyo, 4-6-1 Shirokanedai, Minato-ku, Tokyo 108-8639, Japan; Core Research for Evolutional Science and Technology (CREST), Japan Science and Technology Corporation (JST), Saitama 332-0012, Japan
e-mail: kiyono@ims.u-tokyo.ac.jp

Y. Yuki
Creation and Support Program for Start-ups from Universities, Japan Science and Technology Corporation (JST), Saitama 332-0012, Japan

F. Takaiwa
Transgenic Crop Research and Development Center, National Institute of Agrobiological Sciences, Ibaraki 305-8602, Japan

R. Pawankar et al. (eds.), *Allergy Frontiers: Future Perspectives*,
DOI 10.1007/978-4-431-99365-0_9, © Springer 2010

These allergen-SITs include subcutaneous (intradermal) injection, and oral, nasal, or sublingual administration of allergen extracts or recombinant allergens [7,8]. Although subcutaneous injection is a common allergen-SIT, it is burdened with the risk of severe adverse reactions. Thus, the safer oral, nasal, bronchial, and sublingual routes of administration have been investigated and developed [9]. Recently, derivatives of several recombinant allergens, including synthetic peptides and variants of wild-type recombinant allergens, have been used to avoid the clinical complication of allergic anaphylaxis [10–12].

In this chapter, we review recent progress in the development of rice-based vaccines, specific for a pollen allergy, in which the vaccine expresses multiple T-cell epitopes of Japanese cedar (*Cryptomeria japonica*) pollen allergens. The rice-based oral immunotherapy possesses many practical advantages over most traditional treatments based on the concept of systemic immune system. The rice-based allergy vaccine is heat stable and can thus tolerate room-temperature storage and heat treatment (e.g., boiling). Oral administration of the transgenic rice seeds resulted in the inhibition of aberrant immunological responses and clinical symptoms associated with pollen allergy by reducing allergen-specific IgE as well as histamine levels in a mouse model of a pollen-induced allergic response [13,14]. The uniqueness and advantage of the rice transgenic (Tg) system as a new vaccine production and delivery vehicle will be discussed in this chapter. The rice-based vaccine offers a potentially practical strategy for the development of peptide-based mucosal vaccines or immunotherapy for the control of allergic diseases.

Mucosally Induced Immunity and Tolerance

The mucosal immune system is constantly exposed to a huge number and variety of food and microbial antigens that enter the body via the aerodigestive tract. Depending on the natures of the antigens and of the cells that process and present them, the animal model, and the immunological and environmental circumstances involved, oral administration of an antigen leads to an opposite phase of antigen-specific immune responses. Oral immunization has thus been shown to stimulate the induction of both mucosal and systemic antigen-specific immune responses or to result in the generation of a state of systemic unresponsiveness that is termed "mucosally induced tolerance" (e.g., oral tolerance) [15]. Thus, the mucosal immune system not only provides a front line of defense against invading pathogens by its induction of positive immune responses but also induces immunologic unresponsiveness as a negative immune response to food antigens and commensal bacteria, and then creates a cohabitant situation between the host's mucosal surfaces and the external environment [16].

The mucosal immune system consists of both inductive and effector sites and plays a key role in the induction of such dynamic immune responses as secretory IgA (SIgA) and mucosal CTL, and regulation of these responses by regulatory T cells representing active and quiescent phases of antigen-specific immune responses, respectively [17]. When foreign antigens and pathogens are encountered as a result of ingestion or inhalation, these antigens are taken up by the inductive tissues that lain on the digestive and respiratory tracts. Hosts have evolved a family of organized lymphoid tissues known as mucosa-associated lymphoid tissues (MALT) in the region [17]. Peyer's patches (gut-associated lymphoid tissue, GALT) and nasopharynx-associated lymphoid tissue (NALT) are well characterized members of the MALT family that are located in the intestinal and respiratory tracts, respectively [17]. In general, MALT is covered by unique follicle-associated epithelium (FAE) that contains professional antigen-sampling cells, known as M cells, that take up antigens from the lumen of the aerodigestive tract [18]. Immediately underneath the FAE, layers of dendritic cells (DC) capture and process antigens taken up by the M cells. The MALT contains a well organized microarchitecture of B and T lymphocyte zones that respond to antigens presented by the DC and the induce effector and memory B and T cells, leading to the execution of either active or quiescent immune responses at distant mucosal and systemic effector sites [19–21].

In addition to antigen presentation by DC in PP, recent studies have demonstrated an additional important biological role of mucosal DC for gut imprinting of antigen-primed B and T cells (e.g., CCR9 and a4β7) via the production of retinoic acids [20]. These gut-imprinted antigen-specific B and T cell population then emigrate from the site of induction via lymphatic drainage, circulate through the bloodstream, and migrate to distant mucosal effector sites [19]. It was also recently shown that lipid mediators are critically involved in the egress of antigen-primed lymphocytes from PP [22–24]. For example, IgA plasma blasts that developed in PP, expressed high levels of the sphingosine 1-phosphate receptor and responded to the corresponding lipid mediator by emigrating from the organized lymphoid tissue and entering the mucosal migration pathway [24]. The final destination of antigen-specific B and T lymphocytes that originated in PP, namely mucosal effector sites, include diffused tissues of the lamina propria region of the intestines, where they form a mucosal network with epithelial cells that execute their respective functions of productive immunity or tolerance via a series of IgA enhancing and regulatory cytokines (e.g., IL-5, IL-6, IL-10, and TGF-β) to create protective and cohabitant environments, respectively, at the mucosal surfaces [20].

Given the anatomical and physiological conditions of the digestive tract, the quantity of antigen loads in the gut is several orders of magnitude greater than the numbers of immunocompetent cells located in other immunological tissues and the level of antibodies produced per day. Therefore, the mucosal immune system is equipped with an immunologically unique regulatory system for the induction and maintenance of unresponsiveness or insensitivity to luminal antigens, and is referred to as "oral tolerance" [25]. In the harsh environment of the intestines, oral tolerance seems to be a more common immunological response than the generation of an antigen-specific active immune response [26]. In practice, oral tolerance is the default response to food antigens and commensal bacteria. Oral administration of large or continuous dosages of antigens has thus been shown to induce tolerance in all aspects of the subsequent systemic immune responses, including the production of IgM, IgG, and IgE antibodies as well as cell-mediated immune responses measured by lymphocyte proliferation and delayed-type hypersensitivity [15,25–27]. Thus, oral tolerance could be a potentially powerful tool for the control of immunological diseases, including autoimmunity and allergic conditions that include IgE-mediated hypersensitivities or type I allergic diseases [15].

Induction of Oral Tolerance and Its Application for the Development of Therapeutic Vaccines for Allergic Diseases

Oral administration of a single high dose of a protein or repeated oral delivery of low doses of a protein has been shown to induce a state of oral tolerance or systemic unresponsiveness [26]. In mice, oral tolerance was induced after gastric administration of either a single high dose (20–500 mg) or repeated low doses (20 μg mg) of protein antigens, with the ensuing responses referred to as high- and low-dose oral tolerance, respectively [26]. In general, autoreactive T cells that escape negative selection in the thymus but then encounter many self-antigens in the periphery, may be anergized or deleted in a process of peripheral tolerance [15,26]. In the case of high-dose oral antigens, deletion or anergy of antigen-specific effector T cells are thought to be responsible for the induction of a quiescent immune condition [26]. It has been shown that Fas(CD95)-dependent apoptosis is responsible for the deletion of effector T cells related to oral tolerance [28]. The anergy occurs through T-cell receptor ligation with inadequate costimulation by cognate interactions between CD80/86 on antigen presentation cells with CD28 on effector T cells. For example, the anergy was induced by means of TCR cross-linking in the absence of costimulation [29,30] (Fig. 1).

In contrast, orally administered low doses of antigen can induce active suppression by the induction of inhibitory immune responses mediated by regulatory T cells (Fig. 1). It has been confirmed that naïve mice that received T cells from mice in which tolerance was induced by low doses of antigen also exhibited oral tolerance [31]. Although both anergy and T-cell deletion associated with high-dose oral tolerance are known to contribute to the establishment of peripheral tolerance [26,31], it is now broadly accepted that natural regulatory T cells as well as an antigen-induced regulatory T cell population with a suppressive or inhibitory function also play a key role in inducing and maintaining quiescent immune responses [32]. These cells are heterogeneous and include naturally occurring $CD4^+$ $CD25^+$ ($CTLA4^+$ $Foxp3^+$) regulatory T cells, IL-10-producing Tr1 cells, TGF-β-producing Th3 cells, regulatory $CD8^+$ T cells, and antigen-induced regulatory T cells [15,26,31,33–35]. The regulatory T cell network has been shown to play an important role in low-dose tolerance, with the effector phenotype depending on the nature of the antigens and the antigen presenting cells [15]. For example, protein antigens tend to induce TGF-β-producing Th3 cells, whereas short peptide antigens elicit IL-10-producing Tr1 cells [28,36]. One of the unique properties of the regulatory

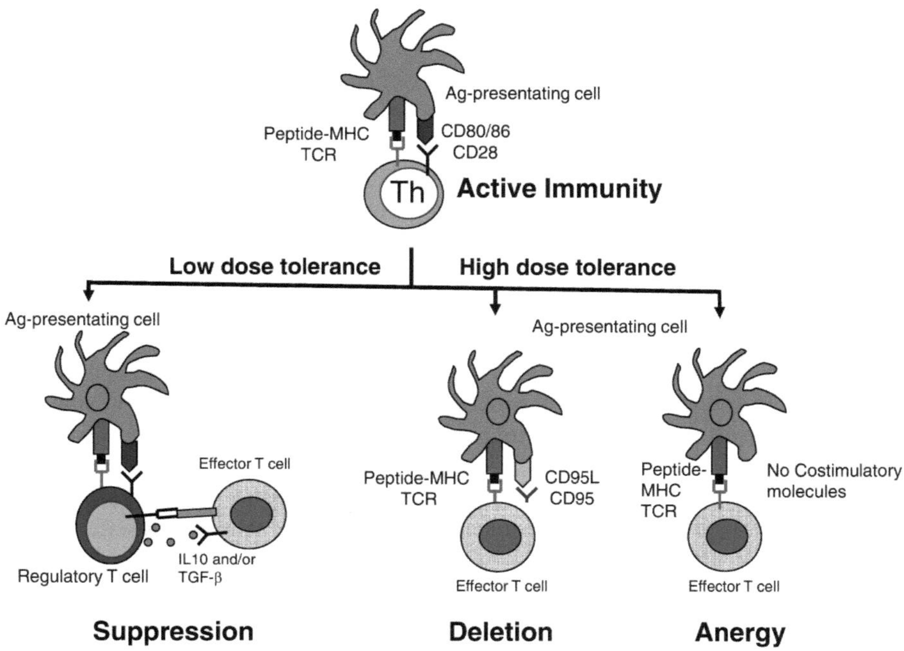

Fig. 1 Mechanisms of oral tolerance. The generation of an immune response requires cognition of appropriate co-stimulatory molecules (e.g., CD28 and CD80 or CD86) in addition to the ligation of the T cell receptor with a peptide-MHC complex. High doses of an antigen lead to deletion and anergy of antigen-specific T cells by means of Fas(CD95)-dependent apoptosis and TCR crosslinking in the absence of co-stimulation, respectively. In contrast, low doses of an antigen results in induction of regulatory T cells, which suppress immune responses by means of cognate interaction or production of inhibitory cytokines IL-10 and/or TGF-β. Ag, antigen; MHC, major histocompatibility complex; TCR, T-cell receptor

cells induced through mucosally induced tolerance (oral tolerance) is that these cells have been shown to mediate bystander suppression, a process through which regulatory T cells for a specific form of protein antigen suppress nearby effector cells even when those cells exhibit antigen specificity to another unrelated protein. Thus, regulatory T cells can be activated in an antigen-specific manner, but they can suppress aggressive immune responses in the area immediately surrounding them in a nonantigen-specific manner [31]. The bystander ability of the regulatory T cell network is a potentially powerful therapeutic tool for controlling aggravated inflammatory conditions [7].

In the adaptation of mucosally induced tolerance (oral tolerance) for the control of allergic responses, one can consider both preventive and therapeutic vaccine approaches. The former is intended to pre-educate or activate the mucosal regulatory network against an allergen, starting from a naïve condition. In contrast, a therapeutic vaccine is intended to introduce a negative signal under presensitized conditions and to achieve the suppression or inhibition of ongoing aggressive allergic responses via activation of the mucosal regulatory network [7]. The accumulated evidence from various experimental animal model systems suggests a general consensus that the state of oral tolerance can be easily induced under the naïve condition, but that inducing tolerance is more difficult under presensitized conditions in which an allergy response is already underway [15,25,26]. Given the existing social circumstances for pollen allergies (i.e., widespread presensitization in industrialized countries), researchers must consider the development of a therapeutic vaccine, despite the difficulty of this approach, in addition to devoting their efforts to the development of a preventive vaccine. Some research efforts have targeted the development of immunotherapy to control preexisting allergic conditions [37–40]. In this research, allergen exposure via inhalation or ingestion leads to the activation of a pool of allergen-specific effector cells that overcome the physiological control of regulatory T cells and lead to the development of immunological hypersensitivity. An ideal therapeutic vaccine must expand the regulatory pool, thereby allowing the immune system to downregulate the population and function of allergen-induced effector cells [6].

The allergen-SIT approach has been used for almost a century to redirect immunological hypersensitivity in patients with an allergy. It has proven to be efficacious in treating type I allergies to a variety of allergens [7]. Although parenteral approaches such as the subcutaneous route of immunization are effective, local routes such as nasal, oral, and sublingual routes have been preferred because of their safety and efficacy [9]. Sublingual immunotherapy has been shown to be efficacious if high doses of the allergen (i.e., 50–100 times the subcutaneous dose) are administered [8]. For oral administration of allergens such as dust mites and pollen, preventive and therapeutic effects resulting from the induction of oral tolerance have been shown in the murine model. In recent years, increasing amount of food allergens have been administered orally with the aim of achieving tolerance and desensitization in patients with IgE-mediated food allergies [37,40].

Administration of the intact allergen has successfully treated allergic diseases [41], but this treatment has always been associated with an increased risk of systemic anaphylaxis mediated by the crosslinking of preexisting allergen-specific IgE on FcεR-bearing mast cells and basophils [6,7]. To avoid this risk, molecular bioengineering strategies have been applied to modify the structure of allergens, including disruption of the tertiary structure of proteins and the use of synthetic peptides to represent MHC class II-restricted T cell epitopes [10–12]. As short linear peptide sequences generally lack the ability to crosslink adjacent native antigen-binding grooves of IgE molecules on mast cells and basophils, a particular advantage of using synthetic T cell epitopes in treating allergic diseases is that it avoids IgE-mediated activation of hypersensitivity [38,39,42–45]. For example, nasal administration with a low concentration of peptides containing the major T cell epitope of Der p1 (residues 111–139) induces tolerance not only in naïve mice but also in mice with ongoing immune responses to the allergen [38]. Oral administration of a dominant T cell determinant peptide (residues 246–259) to mice before or even after sensitization, induced immunologic tolerance against the whole allergen [45]. Sublingual administration of the T-cell epitope peptide P2–246–259 derived from Cry j 2, a major Japanese cedar pollen allergen, to mice that had been sensitized to Cry j 2, induced immunological tolerance [44]. In addition to therapy based on T-cell epitope peptides in experimental allergy models, the effect of overlapping Fel d1-derived T cell peptides have been reported in subjects allergic to cats [39]. Sixteen subjects received either Fel d1 peptides or a placebo nasally. There were significant decreases in the asthmatic reaction in the active group but not in the placebo group. Multiple short, overlapping fel d1 T cell peptides can thus potentially inhibit upper and lower airway constriction in these patients. These promising results demonstrate the potential for allergen-derived peptide mucosal immunotherapy to treat allergic diseases.

Rice Seeds as a New Vehicle for the Development of Oral Vaccines

Oral administration of protein antigens can induce antigen-specific immunological tolerance and is thus useful in treating allergic and autoimmune diseases [15]. For clinical application, a large quantity of antigen is generally thought to be required for mass administration in large population of patients who are suffering from allergic diseases. For example, it has been shown that a large amount of oral antigen was required for the establishment of oral tolerance in humans [15]. To overcome this concern, a practical approach based on the creation of an effective antigen-delivery system to the mucosal immune compartment is required. It has been shown that the administration of a chimeric form of a mucosal vaccine that consisted of an allergen peptide and the B subunit of the cholera toxin (CTB; the nontoxic portion of the toxin with a high affinity to epithelial cells) resulted in the induction of antigen-specific unresponsiveness with a low dose of vaccine antigen [46–48]. Although recombinant allergens, including peptides, can be produced by means of controlled procedures that yield defined molecules with specific immunological and biological characteristics, the clinical value of the resulting oral tolerance may be limited if the vaccine antigens or peptides cannot be effectively produced using an appropriate bioreactor and cannot be delivered via the mucosal surface in physiologically and immunologically reasonable doses [41]. For mucosal vaccines to be an effective treatment against allergic diseases, it is essential to create an innovative system that simultaneously serves as a vaccine antigen production system as well as a delivery vehicle.

Plants have been used as bio-reactors to express a number of recombinant proteins [49]. Transgenic plant expression systems offer some advantages compared to other systems of expression of foreign proteins, including prokaryotic and eukaryotic cell cultures [50,51]. These include cost effective production, rapid scaling up of production to produce large quantities of the proteins, posttranslational modifications to other higher eukaryotes, a low risk of contamination by human pathogens, and resistance to enzymatic digestion in the gastrointestinal tract. In addition, plants can express multiple genes simultaneously. Thus, one suitable vaccine formulation could be a plant that expresses multiple antigen peptides.

Furthermore, plant-based vaccines offer the additional advantage of achieving a simple method for mucosal delivery of a vaccine without the necessity for purification steps or the requirement to use syringes or needles [49]. Among the various transgenic plant expression systems that have been considered, the use of transgenic rice offers several benefits over other plants for production of a mucosal vaccine, as shown in Table 1 [13,52]. Although several plants have been proposed for the creation of oral vaccines, seed crops such as soybean, maize, wheat, or rice seem to be most suitable species based on the criteria in Table 1 [52]. Although maize has been shown to be a useful crop for transgenic expression and the generation of vaccines against antigens from bacterial toxins [53], the long distance transport of pollen in this species is a major environmental concern because of the risk of transgene escape. The difficulty of transformation of wheat via inserted genes in the current wheat vector systems has unfortunately disqualified this species from oral vaccine development.

On the other hand, rice undergoes considerable self-fertilization and its pollen is considered to be transported generally no more than a few meters [52]. In addition, rice plants have unique features for the efficient production and storage of proteins using two types of protein body, PB-I and PB-II [54,55], which are thought to be a suitable natural form of storage for the accumulation of vaccine antigens. According to our recent study of rice-based vaccines, which used CTB as a prototype vaccine antigen, the vaccine that accumulated in rice protein bodies was protected from a digestive enzyme (pepsin) *in vitro* and was taken up by antigen-sampling cells (M cells located in the FAE of the mucosal inductive tissues such as PP); these results demonstrated the viability of a rice-expressed antigen system for the delivery of vaccine antigens to the inductive tissues of the mucosal immune system to initiate active or quiescent immune responses [13,52]. Furthermore, the rice-based vaccine was stable at room temperature for more than 18 months without affecting its oral immunogenicity, thereby permitting vaccine management and administration without the need for refrigeration or syringes [13,52]. These features suggest that the use of rice as a delivery mechanism could be a highly practical and cost effective strategy for orally vaccinating large populations against mucosal infections and allergic diseases.

Table 1 Potential advantages of rice-based vaccine immunotherapy

Low cost of production
Rapid scale-up of production
Multiple vaccines may be produced simultaneously
Increased resistant to enzyme digestion in gastrointestinal tract
No need for cold chain during transport and storage
No need medical assistance in administration/self administration
No purification requirement
Reduced concern over human pathogen contamination during the vaccine preparation
Eliminate concern over blood bone disease through needle reuse
Eliminate cost of syringes and needles

A Rice-Based Pollen Allergy Vaccine

Japanese cedar pollinosis is the most common seasonal allergic disease in Japan. Approximately 20% of Japanese suffer from this pollinosis, which causes rhinitis and conjunctivitis [56]. As discussed above, immunotherapy using synthetic T cell epitope peptides or denatured allergens has been proposed as an alternative treatment to avoid this severe side effect [11,12]. In the case of Japanese cedar pollinosis, two major allergens (Cry j 1 and Cry j 2) have been isolated from the pollen, and multiple T cell epitopes for mice and humans have been identified [45,57–59]. Oral administration of a dominant T cell epitope, the synthesized peptide p246–p259, inhibited allergen-specific Th1- and Th2-mediated hypersensitivity responses, including an allergen-specific IgE antibody response [45]. The result showed the potential for developing oral immunotherapy based on allergen peptides to control Japanese cedar pollinosis.

To develop a new peptide-based mucosal immunotherapy, rice seeds that accumulated major T cell epitope peptides from pollen allergens were tested as a vaccine-delivery vehicle for inducing a state of oral tolerance [60]. To establish a proof of concept for the rice-based allergy vaccine, transgenic rice seeds were developed that contained Cry j 1 p277–p290 (Crp1) and Cry j 2 p246–p259 (Crp2), two major T cell epitope peptides of Balb/c mice [13]. These epitope peptides were expressed as a fusion protein of highly variable regions of the soybean seed storage protein glycinin A1aB1b (Fig. 2a). After ligation of the fusion protein gene between the endosperm-specific 2.3-kb glutelin *GluB-1* promoter and 0.6-kb GluB-1 terminator, the product was inserted into the pGPTV-35S-HPT binary vector, and was then transformed into the rice genome by means of *Agrobacterium*-mediated transformation [13]. The accumulation level of the AlaB1b-Crp1 and AlaB1b-Crp2 fusion protein reached 7 μg grain^{-1} in the rice seeds (0.5% of total seed protein). Daily oral

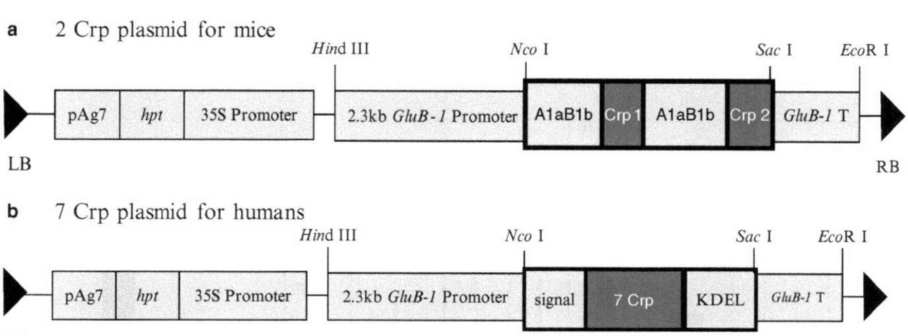

Fig. 2 Schematic representation of the transformation plasmids used to develop a rice-based vaccine against Japanese cedar pollinosis. The DNA fragments encoding the A1aB1b-Crp1 and A1aB1b-Crp2 protein (**a**) and signal-7Crp-KDEL (**b**) were placed under the control of the major rice seed storage protein glutelin 2.3-kb *GluB-1* promoter. *35S promoter* Cauliflower mosaic virus 35S promoter; *hpt* hygromycin phosphotransferase gene; *LB* left border; *pAg7* agropine synthase polyadenylation signal sequence; *RB* right border

feeding of naïve mice with 2 μg of rice-expressed epitope peptide (200 mg total rice powder) for 4 weeks before the systemic challenge with the total protein of cedar pollen inhibited the production of allergen-specific serum IgE and IgG antibodies, indicating the induction of oral tolerance by the rice-based vaccine (Fig. 3) [13]. Both allergen-specific $CD4^+$ T cell proliferative responses and levels of Th2 cytokines such as IL-4, IL-5, and IL-13 were inhibited by the oral administration of rice-expressed T cell epitope peptides [13]. It should be noted that histamine release from mast cells and clinical symptoms of allergy symptoms such as sneezing were also suppressed in mice that developed allergen-specific tolerance as a result of the continuous oral administration of rice grains expressing the T cell epitope peptides (Fig. 3) [13,61]. These results showed that a rice-based oral vaccine expressing T cell epitopes can induce oral tolerance in the naive condition for the inhibition of Th2-mediated IgE responses and suppress pollen-induced clinical symptoms such as sneezing.

The mechanism for the induction of oral tolerance may involve the generation and activation of an inhibitory network mediated by antigen-specific regulatory T cells [31]. In this regard, the plant-based vaccine has been shown to induce a regulatory network that can control asthma development. A report of using sunflower seed albumin expressed by narrow-leaf lupin as a form of plant-based allergen vaccine showed the vaccine to effectively induce oral tolerance via the induction of

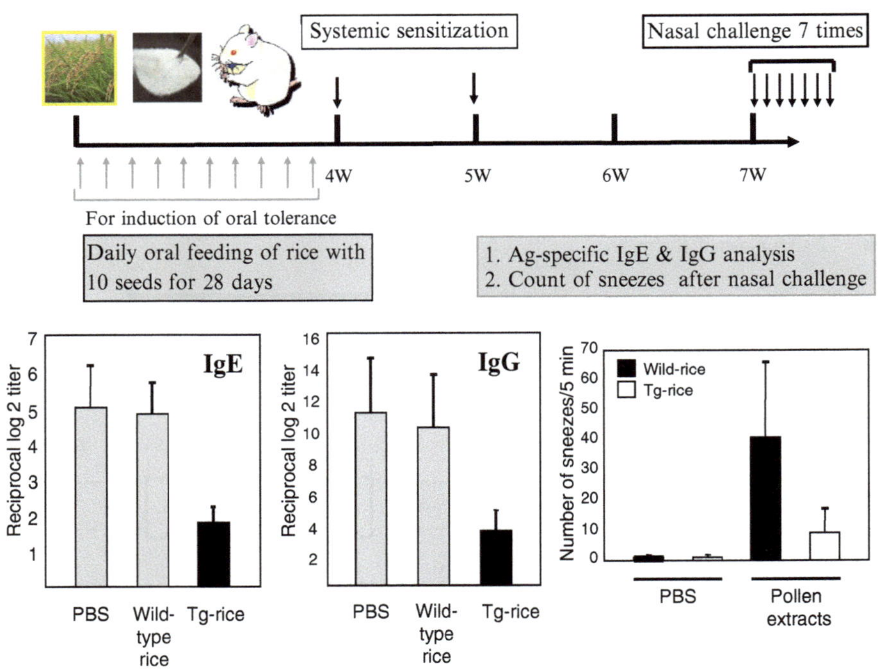

Fig. 3 Inhibition of allergen-specific serum IgE, IgG, and sneezing by oral administration of transgenic (Tg) rice seeds after nasal challenging the mice with cedar pollen allergens

regulatory cells [62]. Oral administration of lupin-expressed sunflower seed albumin to mice promoted the induction of an antigen-specific IgG2a antibody response, and attenuated the induction of DTH responses and pathological features of experimental asthma, suggesting that the plant-based vaccine may have therapeutic potential for protection against allergic diseases [62]. Importantly, suppression of the experimental asthma was associated with the development of a $CD4^+$ $CD45RB^{Low}$ suppressor T cell population and IFN-γ production, but not the development of a typical regulatory phenotype of $CD4^+$ $CD25^+$ T cells and TGF-β [62,63].

Human T-cell epitopes of the Cry j 1 and Cry j 2 allergens have been mapped using in vitro peripheral blood mononuclear cells from individual patients suffering from Japanese cedar pollinosis [58]. Although the sequences recognized by individual patients were highly variable, the use of hybrid peptides comprising multiple predominant T cell epitopes derived from Cry j 1 and Cry j 2 for the peptide immunotherapy was considered to overcome difficulties arising from the genetic diversity of the patients [59]. When a recombinant seven-linked epitope peptide (7Crp) was designed and produced in an *E. coli* expression system, 7Crp was approximately 100 times as effective for the induction of T cell proliferation as a mixture of the individual seven-epitope peptides. In addition, 7Crp did not show any binding activity to allergen-specific IgE antibodies [59]. These results suggested that 7Crp could be used as a peptide immunotherapy or vaccine. To explore this possibility, a 7Crp gene encoding a peptide with 96 amino acids was constructed and synthesized using a codon optimized for expression in rice seeds [14]. To maximize the expression and accumulation of 7Crp, a DNA-encoding N-terminal *GluB-1* signal peptide and a C-terminal KDEL ER retention signal were ligated to 7Crp. Then, the endosperm-specific 2.3-kb glutelin *GluB-1* promoter and 0.6-kb *GluB-1* terminator were further ligated to the chimeric 7Crp gene and introduced into the pGPTV-35S-HPT binary vector (Fig. 2b), which was then transformed into the rice genome by means of *Agrobacterium*-mediated transformation [14]. As shown in Fig. 4, 7Crp accumulated in large quantities (up to $60\,\mu g\ grain^{-1}$) in rice seeds (4% of total seed protein) [14]. The 7Crp accumulated in both PB-I and PB-II in the endosperm cells of the rice seeds, suggesting that rice-expressed 7Crp will be protected from digestive enzymes, as mentioned above [52].

A mouse model has been developed to evaluate the effectiveness of rice-expressed 7Crp against the cedar pollen allergy using B10.S mice, which recognized Cry j 1 p211–p225 as a dominant human T cell epitope in 7Crp [64]. When the rice-expressed 7Crp (560 μg total dose of 7Crp) was orally administered to B.10S mice once per day for 32 consecutive days, both the T-cell proliferative response and IgE levels against Cry j 1 were depressed, indicating the efficacy of oral immunotherapy using rice-expressed 7Crp [14]. It should be noted that the inhibition of the T cell proliferative responses by rice expressing 7Crp was retained even after boiling of the transgenic rice for 20 min at 100°C or autoclaving the rice for 20 min, indicating that the peptide expressed in the PB of rice seeds was highly resistant to heat [14]. Furthermore, the biochemical properties of rice-expressed 7Crp were characterized in a safety evaluation of the transgenic rice [65]. The levels of chemical components such as carbohydrates, proteins, amino acids, lipids, fatty acids, minerals, and

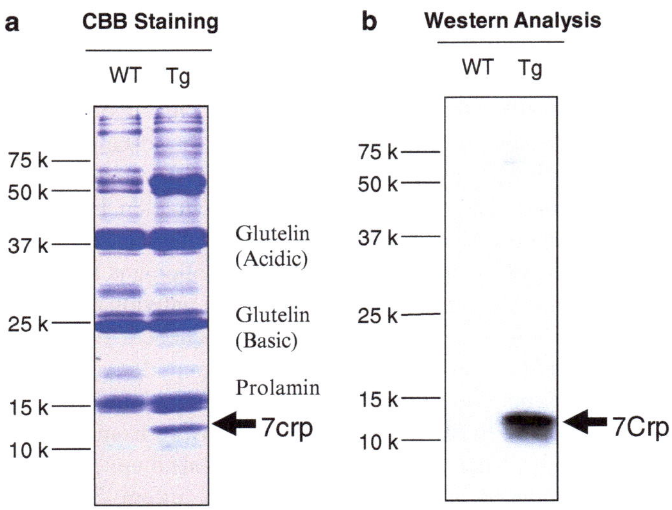

Fig. 4 Accumulation of 7Crp in transgenic (Tg) and wild-type (WT) rice seeds. (**a**) Coomassie brilliant blue (CBB) staining on SDS-PAGE. (**b**) Western blot analysis with anti-7Crp

vitamins were substantially equivalent between the transgenic and wild-type rice. No sign of N-glycosylation was observed in rice that expressed 7Crp [65]. These results indicate that the transgenic rice maintained the biochemical characteristics of the wild-type rice except for the presence of the inserted antigen. Before the vaccine will be suitable for human use, the selective marker genes that confer resistance to antibiotics must be removed from the transgenic rice. To this end, marker-free transgenic rice harboring the 7Crp gene has already been established using only the multi-auto-transformation vector system [60]. Thus, the transgenic rice system is undergoing continuous technical progress towards translating the approach into a clinical setting. At the current stage, the accumulated evidence obtained in the experimental animal system indicate that oral administration of the transgenic rice that expresses Cry peptides effectively induced oral tolerance in naïve mice [13,14]. However, it is still necessary to carefully examine whether oral administration of the transgenic rice can effectively and safely induce allergen-specific unresponsiveness in patients who have been presensitized or who have an ongoing accelerated allergic condition.

Future Perspectives and Concluding Remarks

Seeds are ideal plant production vessels because they are natural storage organs that produce and accumulate proteins, starches, and lipids, and thus offer an ample storage environment even for foreign recombinant proteins [60]. As a vaccine antigen production system, rice seed has several advantages over other crops, including its easier storage and processing, greater yield, and low risk of transgene escape due to the rice's tendency to self-pollinate [52]. In addition, the rice transformation system has been established and the full genome sequence of the species has been elucidated, so this genetic information can be easily applied for the creation of gene manipulation products [13,52]. As a new form of peptide vaccine or immunotherapy, rice seeds that accumulate major T cell epitopes derived from pollen allergens can be used as a vehicle to deliver mucosal tolerogens. When the rice-based peptide vaccine for the Japanese cedar pollen allergy was orally administered to mice, immunological and biochemical responses associated with the pollen-induced allergy, including the production of antigen-specific IgE antibodies, $CD4^+$ T cell proliferation, and histamine release, were all inhibited [13,14]. Clinical symptoms of the allergy, including sneezing and nose scratching, were also alleviated in the mice vaccinated with the transgenic rice after exposure to cedar pollen.

These results have important implications for the development of oral vaccines based on T cell epitope peptides and for immunotherapy against type I allergies, especially in naïve populations [13]. A human T-cell epitope version of 7Crp is also produced and stably accumulated only in the seeds of transgenic rice, and its yield amounts to 4% of total soluble protein [14]. Although the rice-based vaccine is protected against enzymatic degradation in the gastrointestinal tract and delivers the incorporated vaccine antigens to the mucosal epithelium (which consists of professional antigen-sampling cells, M cells, and columnar epithelial cells covering the gut-associated lymphoid tissue) [52], a rice-based vaccine equipped with a targeting vehicle specific to M cells or epithelial cells will be more effective for the induction of immune tolerance. It may be possible to induce oral tolerance at much lower concentrations of inserted peptide antigens if CTB or the heat labile enterotoxin B subunit is introduced in the transgenic rice as the epithelium-targeting molecule, since the B subunit has been shown to possess high affinity for the GM1 ganglioside expressed on cells at the mucosal surface [46,47,66,67].

Two guidelines for transgenic plant-derived substances intended for parenteral administration have been published as draft versions by the European Medicines Agency (EMEA) and the US Food and Drug Administration (FDA) [68,69]. A rice-based oral vaccine, which is intended for nonparenteral administration, may not be governed by these guidelines, but similar fundamental principles will apply to the use of the rice system for production of vaccine antigens and subsequent application as a natural form of mucosal delivery of vaccine antigens. Thus, the rice-based vaccine should be categorized and developed not as a medical food but rather as a medical drug [69].

From the standpoint of further development of the rice-based vaccine as a new form of medical drug, many regulatory issues must be identified and resolved before considering the phase of translational research, including safety and stability studies. Transgenic plant technology has emerged as a new and innovative strategy for producing pharmacologically active compounds, including proteins and peptides, including those associated with allergens. However, unlike systems based on prokaryotic, yeast, and mammalian cells, certain considerations specific to transgenic plants must be taken into account for the effective expression and production of vaccine antigens [68,69]. For example, N-linked glycans lack terminal sialic acid residues, and many complex plant glycans contain either fucose or xylose residues with linkages that do not occur in humans, which may affect the safety and efficacy, including the immunogenicity, of the active substance produced by plants [70]. In the transgenic rice-expressed T cell epitopes, there is no evidence for the appearance of putative N-linked glycosylation motifs, but O-glycosylation sometimes occurred in the Golgi apparatus of plant systems [70]. Thus, vaccine antigens expressed in plants, including rice, must be carefully analyzed to determine their amino acid sequence as well as their sugar chain expression.

The other major issue related to the expression of vaccine antigens in plants is the variation in protein expression levels in transgenic plants [50,51,71]. Since a vaccine is a form of medical drug, the content and quality of the vaccine expressed by the plants must not be influenced by variations in the natural environment of the plants. In order to maintain consistent expression and quality levels, the plant culture system, including factors such as the levels of light, carbon dioxide, water, temperature, and fertilization, must be carefully and stably controlled to prevent variations in these factors from affecting vaccine production. Soil for rice plantation may not be appropriate culture for Good Agriculture Practice which regulated by US Department of Agriculture [68] because it is technically difficult to use as a recycle platform with a controlled fertilization. In contrast, hydroponics with high recycling efficiency can be easy to control fertilization for the rice plant, thus is one candidate system for the establishment of pharmacological transgenic rice plantations. Taken together, semi- or fully-closed molecular farming factories based on hydroponics and controlled environmental conditions is recommended for the production of rice-based vaccines. Such a molecular farming factory could be operated year-round, with three harvests per year, and is thus a cost effective system. Production of transgenic rice in the well protected and controlled environment of a molecular farming factory should also be more publicly acceptable because the risk of biological contamination, including pollen scattering into the environment (i.e., transgene escape), is greatly reduced. Continuing co-operation among different areas of the biological sciences, including immunology, allergology, plant biology, and genetic engineering, will lead to sharing of concepts and technologies, increasing the likelihood of creating an attractive new rice-based strategy for the prevention and control of immunological diseases.

Acknowledgments This work was supported by grants from Core Research for Evolutional Science and Technology (CREST) and the Creation and Support Program for Start-ups from Universities of the Japan Science and Technology Corporation (JST), the Ministry of Education, Science, Sports and Culture, the Ministry of Health and Labor, the Ministry of Agriculture, Forestry and Fisheries and the Ministry of Economy, Trade and Industry in Japan.

References

1. Kay, A. B., Allergy and allergic diseases. First of two parts. *N Engl J Med* 2001. 344: 30–37.
2. Kay, A. B., Allergy and allergic diseases. Second of two parts. *N Engl J Med* 2001. 344: 109–113.
3. Reischl, I. G., Coward, W. R. and Church, M. K., Molecular consequences of human mast cell activation following immunoglobulin E-high-affinity immunoglobulin E receptor (IgE-FcepsilonRI) interaction. *Biochem Pharmacol* 1999. 58: 1841–1850.
4. Umetsu, D. T., McIntire, J. J., Akbari, O., Macaubas, C. and DeKruyff, R. H., Asthma: an epidemic of dysregulated immunity. *Nat Immunol* 2002. 3: 715–720.
5. Simons, F. E., Allergic rhinobronchitis: the asthma-allergic rhinitis link. *J Allergy Clin Immunol* 1999. 104: 534–540.
6. Larche, M. and Wraith, D. C., Peptide-based therapeutic vaccines for allergic and autoimmune diseases. *Nat Med* 2005. 11: S69–S76.
7. Larche, M., Akdis, C. A. and Valenta, R., Immunological mechanisms of allergen-specific immunotherapy. *Nat Rev Immunol* 2006. 6: 761–771.
8. Moingeon, P., Batard, T., Fadel, R., Frati, F., Sieber, J. and Van Overtvelt, L., Immune mechanisms of allergen-specific sublingual immunotherapy. *Allergy* 2006. 61: 151–165.
9. Canonica, G. W. and Passalacqua, G., Noninjection routes for immunotherapy. *J Allergy Clin Immunol* 2003. 111: 437–448; quiz 449.
10. Niederberger, V., Horak, F., Vrtala, S., Spitzauer, S., Krauth, M. T., Valent, P., Reisinger, J., Pelzmann, M., Hayek, B., Kronqvist, M., Gafvelin, G., Gronlund, H., Purohit, A., Suck, R., Fiebig, H., Cromwell, O., Pauli, G., van Hage-Hamsten, M. and Valenta, R., Vaccination with genetically engineered allergens prevents progression of allergic disease. *Proc Natl Acad Sci U S A* 2004. 101 Suppl 2: 14677–14682.
11. Wallner, B. P. and Gefter, M. L., Peptide therapy for treatment of allergic diseases. *Clin Immunol Immunopathol* 1996. 80: 105–109.
12. Haselden, B. M., Kay, A. B. and Larche, M., Peptide-mediated immune responses in specific immunotherapy. *Int Arch Allergy Immunol* 2000. 122: 229–237.
13. Takagi, H., Hiroi, T., Yang, L., Tada, Y., Yuki, Y., Takamura, K., Ishimitsu, R., Kawauchi, H., Kiyono, H. and Takaiwa, F., A rice-based edible vaccine expressing multiple T cell epitopes induces oral tolerance for inhibition of Th2-mediated IgE responses. *Proc Natl Acad Sci U S A* 2005. 102: 17525–17530.
14. Takagi, H., Saito, S., Yang, L., Nagasaka, S., Nishizawa, N. and Takaiwa, F., Oral immunotherapy against a pollen allergy using a seed-based peptide vaccine. *Plant Biotechnol J* 2005. 3: 521–533.
15. Mayer, L. and Shao, L., Therapeutic potential of oral tolerance. *Nat Rev Immunol* 2004. 4: 407–419.
16. McGhee, J. R., Michalek, S. M., Kiyono, H., Eldridge, J. H., Colwell, D. E., Williamson, S. I., Wannemuehler, M. J., Jirillo, E., Mosteller, L. M., Spalding, D. M., et al., Mucosal immunoregulation: environmental lipopolysaccharide and GALT T lymphocytes regulate the IgA response. *Microbiol Immunol* 1984. 28: 261–280.
17. Yuki, Y. and Kiyono, H., New generation of mucosal adjuvants for the induction of protective immunity. *Rev Med Virol* 2003. 13: 293–310.
18. Yuki, Y., Nochi, T. and Kiyono, H., Progress towards an AIDS mucosal vaccine: an overview. *Tuberculosis (Edinb)* 2007. 87 Suppl 1: S35–S44.
19. Neutra, M. R. and Kozlowski, P. A., Mucosal vaccines: the promise and the challenge. *Nat Rev Immunol* 2006. 6: 148–158.
20. Kunisawa, J. and Kiyono, H., A marvel of mucosal T cells and secretory antibodies for the creation of first lines of defense. *Cell Mol Life Sci* 2005. 62: 1308–1321.
21. Kiyono, H. and Fukuyama, S., NALT- versus Peyer's-patch-mediated mucosal immunity. *Nat Rev Immunol* 2004. 4: 699–710.

22. Kunisawa, J., Kurashima, Y., Gohda, M., Higuchi, M., Ishikawa, I., Miura, F., Ogahara, I. and Kiyono, H., Sphingosine 1-phosphate regulates peritoneal B-cell trafficking for subsequent intestinal IgA production. *Blood* 2007. 109: 3749–3756.
23 Kunisawa, J., Gohda, M., Kurashima, Y., Ishikawa, I., Higuchi, M. and Kiyono, H., Sphingosine 1-phosphate-dependent trafficking of peritoneal B cells requires functional NF{kappa}B-inducing kinase in stromal cells. *Blood* 2008. 111: 4646–4652.
24. Kunisawa, J., Kurashima, Y., Higuchi, M., Gohda, M., Ishikawa, I., Ogahara, I., Kim, N., Shimizu, M. and Kiyono, H., Sphingosine 1-phosphate dependence in the regulation of lymphocyte trafficking to the gut epithelium. *J Exp Med* 2007. 204: 2335–2348.
25. Czerkinsky, C., Anjuere, F., McGhee, J. R., George-Chandy, A., Holmgren, J., Kieny, M. P., Fujiyashi, K., Mestecky, J. F., Pierrefite-Carle, V., Rask, C. and Sun, J. B., Mucosal immunity and tolerance: relevance to vaccine development. *Immunol Rev* 1999. 170: 197–222.
26. Weiner, H. L., Friedman, A., Miller, A., Khoury, S. J., Sabbagh, A., Santos, L., Sayegh, M., Nussenblatt, R. B., Trentham, D. E. and Hafler, D. A. Oral tolerance: immunologic mechanisms and treatment of animal and human organ-specific autoimmune diseases by oral administration of autoantigens. *Annu Rev Immunol* 1994. 12: 809–837.
27. Kiyono, H., Kunisawa, J., McGhee, J. R. and Mestecky, J. *The mucosal immune system*: In Fundamental Immunology, Paul, W.E (ed). Lippincott, Williams & Wilkins, Philadelphia, 2008, pp 983–1030
28. Chen, Y., Kuchroo, V. K., Inobe, J., Hafler, D. A. and Weiner, H. L., Regulatory T cell clones induced by oral tolerance: suppression of autoimmune encephalomyelitis. *Science* 1994. 265: 1237–1240.
29. Marth, T., Zeitz, Z., Ludviksson, B., Strober, W. and Kelsall, B., Murine model of oral tolerance. Induction of Fas-mediated apoptosis by blockade of interleukin-12. *Ann N Y Acad Sci* 1998. 859: 290–294.
30. Chen, Y., Inobe, J., Marks, R., Gonnella, P., Kuchroo, V. K. and Weiner, H. L., Peripheral deletion of antigen-reactive T cells in oral tolerance. *Nature* 1995. 376: 177–180.
31. Robinson, D. S., Larche, M. and Durham, S. R., Tregs and allergic disease. *J Clin Invest* 2004. 114: 1389–1397.
32. Zhang, X., Izikson, L., Liu, L. and Weiner, H. L., Activation of CD25(+) CD4(+) regulatory T cells by oral antigen administration. *J Immunol* 2001. 167: 4245–4253.
33. Sakaguchi, S., Regulatory T cells: key controllers of immunologic self-tolerance. *Cell* 2000. 101: 455–458.
34. Sakaguchi, S., Ono, M., Setoguchi, R., Yagi, H., Hori, S., Fehervari, Z., Shimizu, J., Takahashi, T. and Nomura, T., Foxp3+ CD25+ CD4+ natural regulatory T cells in dominant self-tolerance and autoimmune disease. *Immunol Rev* 2006. 212: 8–27.
35. Sakaguchi, S., Naturally arising CD4+ regulatory T cells for immunologic self-tolerance and negative control of immune responses. *Annu Rev Immunol* 2004. 22: 531–562.
36. Sundstedt, A., O'Neill, E. J., Nicolson, K. S. and Wraith, D. C., Role for IL-10 in suppression mediated by peptide-induced regulatory T cells in vivo. *J Immunol* 2003. 170: 1240–1248.
37. Patriarca, G., Nucera, E., Roncallo, C., Pollastrini, E., Bartolozzi, F., De Pasquale, T., Buonomo, A., Gasbarrini, G., Di Campli, C. and Schiavino, D., Oral desensitizing treatment in food allergy: clinical and immunological results. *Aliment Pharmacol Ther* 2003. 17: 459–465.
38. Hoyne, G. F., O'Hehir, R. E., Wraith, D. C., Thomas, W. R. and Lamb, J. R., Inhibition of T cell and antibody responses to house dust mite allergen by inhalation of the dominant T cell epitope in naive and sensitized mice. *J Exp Med* 1993. 178: 1783–1788.
39. Alexander, C., Tarzi, M., Larche, M. and Kay, A. B., The effect of Fel d 1-derived T-cell peptides on upper and lower airway outcome measurements in cat-allergic subjects. *Allergy* 2005. 60: 1269–1274.
40. Meglio, P., Bartone, E., Plantamura, M., Arabito, E. and Giampietro, P. G., A protocol for oral desensitization in children with IgE-mediated cow's milk allergy. *Allergy* 2004. 59: 980–987.

41. Valenta, R. and Niederberger, V., Recombinant allergens for immunotherapy. *J Allergy Clin Immunol* 2007. 119: 826–830.
42. Oldfield, W. L., Kay, A. B. and Larche, M., Allergen-derived T cell peptide-induced late asthmatic reactions precede the induction of antigen-specific hyporesponsiveness in atopic allergic asthmatic subjects. *J Immunol* 2001. 167: 1734–1739.
43. Oldfield, W. L., Larche, M. and Kay, A. B., Effect of T-cell peptides derived from Fel d 1 on allergic reactions and cytokine production in patients sensitive to cats: a randomised controlled trial. *Lancet* 2002. 360: 47–53.
44. Yoshitomi, T., Nakagami, Y., Hirahara, K., Taniguchi, Y., Sakaguchi, M. and Yamashita, M., Intraoral administration of a T-cell epitope peptide induces immunological tolerance in Cry j 2-sensitized mice. *J Pept Sci* 2007. 13: 499–503.
45. Hirahara, K., Saito, S., Serizawa, N., Sasaki, R., Sakaguchi, M., Inouye, S., Taniguchi, Y., Kaminogawa, S. and Shiraishi, A., Oral administration of a dominant T-cell determinant peptide inhibits allergen-specific TH1 and TH2 cell responses in Cry j 2-primed mice. *J Allergy Clin Immunol* 1998. 102: 961–967.
46. Sun, J. B., Raghavan, S., Sjoling, A., Lundin, S. and Holmgren, J., Oral tolerance induction with antigen conjugated to cholera toxin B subunit generates both Foxp3+CD25+ and Foxp3-CD25- CD4+ regulatory T cells. *J Immunol* 2006. 177: 7634–7644.
47. Sun, J. B., Rask, C., Olsson, T., Holmgren, J. and Czerkinsky, C., Treatment of experimental autoimmune encephalomyelitis by feeding myelin basic protein conjugated to cholera toxin B subunit. *Proc Natl Acad Sci U S A* 1996. 93: 7196–7201.
48. Rask, C., Holmgren, J., Fredriksson, M., Lindblad, M., Nordstrom, I., Sun, J. B. and Czerkinsky, C., Prolonged oral treatment with low doses of allergen conjugated to cholera toxin B subunit suppresses immunoglobulin E antibody responses in sensitized mice. *Clin Exp Allergy* 2000. 30: 1024–1032.
49. Streatfield, S. J. and Howard, J. A., Plant-based vaccines. *Int J Parasitol* 2003. 33: 479–493.
50. Walmsley, A. M. and Arntzen, C. J., Plant cell factories and mucosal vaccines. *Curr Opin Biotechnol* 2003. 14: 145–150.
51. Walmsley, A. M. and Arntzen, C. J., Plants for delivery of edible vaccines. *Curr Opin Biotechnol* 2000. 11: 126–129.
52. Nochi, T., Takagi, H., Yuki, Y., Yang, L., Masumura, T., Mejima, M., Nakanishi, U., Matsumura, A., Uozumi, A., Hiroi, T., Morita, S., Tanaka, K., Takaiwa, F. and Kiyono, H., From the cover: rice-based mucosal vaccine as a global strategy for cold-chain- and needle-free vaccination. *Proc Natl Acad Sci U S A* 2007. 104: 10986–10991.
53. Streatfield, S. J., Jilka, J. M., Hood, E. E., Turner, D. D., Bailey, M. R., Mayor, J. M., Woodard, S. L., Beifuss, K. K., Horn, M. E., Delaney, D. E., Tizard, I. R. and Howard, J. A., Plant-based vaccines: unique advantages. *Vaccine* 2001. 19: 2742–2748.
54. Yamagata, H. and Tanaka, K., The site of synthesis and accumulation of rice storage proteins. *Plant Cell Physiol* 1986. 27: 135–145.
55. Katsube, T., Kurisaka, N., Ogawa, M., Maruyama, N., Ohtsuka, R., Utsumi, S. and Takaiwa, F., Accumulation of soybean glycinin and its assembly with the glutelins in rice. *Plant Physiol* 1999. 120: 1063–1074.
56. Kaneko, Y., Motohashi, Y., Nakamura, H., Endo, T. and Eboshida, A., Increasing prevalence of Japanese cedar pollinosis: a meta-regression analysis. *Int Arch Allergy Immunol* 2005. 136: 365–371.
57. Yoshitomi, T., Hirahara, K., Kawaguchi, J., Serizawa, N., Taniguchi, Y., Saito, S., Sakaguchi, M., Inouye, S. and Shiraishi, A., Three T-cell determinants of Cry j 1 and Cry j 2, the major Japanese cedar pollen antigens, retain their immunogenicity and tolerogenicity in a linked peptide. *Immunology* 2002. 107: 517–522.
58. Sone, T., Morikubo, K., Miyahara, M., Komiyama, N., Shimizu, K., Tsunoo, H. and Kino, K., T cell epitopes in Japanese cedar (*Cryptomeria japonica*) pollen allergens: choice of major T cell epitopes in Cry j 1 and Cry j 2 toward design of the peptide-based immunotherapeutics for the management of Japanese cedar pollinosis. *J Immunol* 1998. 161: 448–457.

59. Hirahara, K., Tatsuta, T., Takatori, T., Ohtsuki, M., Kirinaka, H., Kawaguchi, J., Serizawa, N., Taniguchi, Y., Saito, S., Sakaguchi, M., Inouye, S. and Shiraishi, A., Preclinical evaluation of an immunotherapeutic peptide comprising 7 T-cell determinants of Cry j 1 and Cry j 2, the major Japanese cedar pollen allergens. *J Allergy Clin Immunol* 2001. 108: 94–100.
60. Takaiwa, F., A rice-based edible vaccine expressing multiple T-cell epitopes to induce oral tolerance and inhibit allergy. *Immunol Allergy Clin North Am* 2007. 27: 129–139.
61. Iwasaki, M., Saito, K., Takemura, M., Sekikawa, K., Fujii, H., Yamada, Y., Wada, H., Mizuta, K., Seishima, M. and Ito, Y., TNF-alpha contributes to the development of allergic rhinitis in mice. *J Allergy Clin Immunol* 2003. 112: 134–140.
62. Smart, V., Foster, P. S., Rothenberg, M. E., Higgins, T. J. and Hogan, S. P., A plant-based allergy vaccine suppresses experimental asthma via an IFN-gamma and CD4+CD45RBlow T cell-dependent mechanism. *J Immunol* 2003. 171: 2116–2126.
63. Zuany-Amorim, C., Sawicka, E., Manlius, C., Le Moine, A., Brunet, L. R., Kemeny, D. M., Bowen, G., Rook, G. and Walker, C., Suppression of airway eosinophilia by killed Mycobacterium vaccae-induced allergen-specific regulatory T-cells. *Nat Med* 2002. 8: 625–629.
64. Ohno, N., Ide, T., Sakaguchi, M., Inouye, S. and Saito, S., Common antigenicity between Japanese cedar (*Cryptomeria japonica*) pollen and Japanese cypress (*Chamaecyparis obtusa*) pollen, II. Determination of the cross-reacting T-cell epitope of cry j 1 and cha o 1 in mice. *Immunology* 2000. 99: 630–634.
65. Takagi, H., Hirose, S., Yasuda, H. and Takaiwa, F., Biochemical safety evaluation of transgenic rice seeds expressing T cell epitopes of Japanese cedar pollen allergens. *J Agric Food Chem* 2006. 54: 9901–9905.
66. Yuki, Y., Byun, Y., Fujita, M., Izutani, W., Suzuki, T., Udaka, S., Fujihashi, K., McGhee, J. R. and Kiyono, H., Production of a recombinant hybrid molecule of cholera toxin-B-subunit and proteolipid-protein-peptide for the treatment of experimental encephalomyelitis. *Biotechnol Bioeng* 2001. 74: 62–69.
67. Yuki, Y., Hara-Yakoyama, C., Guadiz, A. A., Udaka, S., Kiyono, H. and Chatterjee, S., Production of a recombinant cholera toxin B subunit-insulin B chain peptide hybrid protein by Brevibacillus choshinensis expression system as a nasal vaccine against autoimmune diabetes. *Biotechnol Bioeng* 2005. 92: 803–809.
68. online, F. F. a. D. A., Guidance for Industry: Drug. Biologics, and Medical Deivices Derived from Bioengineered Plants for Use in Humans and Animals. http://www.fda.gov/cder/guidance/index.htm 2001.
69. online, E. M. A. E., Guideline on the quality of biological active substances produced by stable transgene expression in higher plants. http://www.emea.europa.eu 2006.
70. Twyman, R. M., Stoger, E., Schillberg, S., Christou, P. and Fischer, R., Molecular farming in plants: host systems and expression technology. *Trends Biotechnol* 2003. 21: 570–578.
71. Stoger, E., Sack, M., Fischer, R. and Christou, P., Plantibodies: applications, advantages and bottlenecks. *Curr Opin Biotechnol* 2002. 13: 161–166.

Targeting STAT6 in Atopic Eczema/Dermatitis

Ichiro Katayama, Hiroyuki Murota, Ken Igawa, Takahiro Satoh, Kiyoshi Nishioka, and Hiroo Yokozeki

Introduction

We previously demonstrated that in murine atopic eczema/dermatitis (AD)-model, mast cells and inflammatory cells other than T cells are thought to play an important role in IgE-mediated biphasic reactions [1], however, it remains unclear as to whether Th2 type cytokines; IL-4, IL-5, or IL-13 play a role in the induction of the IgE-mediated reaction. Recently, STAT6 signalling has been demonstrated to play an essential role in the induction of contact hypersensitivity [2].

We also recently established STAT6 deficient (STAT6–/–) mice [3] and demonstrated that STAT6 plays a central role in IL-4 and IL-13 mediated biological responses [3,4]. In an attempt to clarify a role of Th2 cytokines, especially IL-4 and IL-13 in the IgE-mediated biphasic reaction, we examined the IgE-mediated response in the STAT6–/– mice in which the IL-4 and IL13 signaling pathways are completely abolished. Furthermore, there are currently no effective therapies for severe AD except for the administration of glucocorticoid or immunosuppressant (such as tacrolimus or pimecrolimus) which have several side effects after long time application. The transfection of cis-element double-stranded oligodeoxynucleotides (ODNs), referred to as "decoy," has been reported to be a powerful tool and a new type of antigen treatment strategy, for gene therapy and for study gene transfection. Systemic ODNs act as decoy *cis* elements to block the binding of nuclear factors to the promoter regions of targeted genes, thus resulting in the inhibition of

I. Katayama (✉) and H. Murota
Department of Dermatology, Integrated Medicine, Graduate School of Medicine, Osaka University, 2-2 Yamada-oka, Suita-shi, Osaka 565-0871, Japan
e-mail: katayama@derma.med.osaka-u.ac.jp

K. Igawa, T. Satoh, K. Nishioka, and H. Yokozeki
Department of Dermatology, Graduate School of Medicine, Tokyo Medical and Dental University, 1-5-45 Yushima, Bunkyo-ku, Tokyo 113-8519, Japan

R. Pawankar et al. (eds.), *Allergy Frontiers: Future Perspectives*,
DOI 10.1007/978-4-431-99365-0_10, © Springer 2010

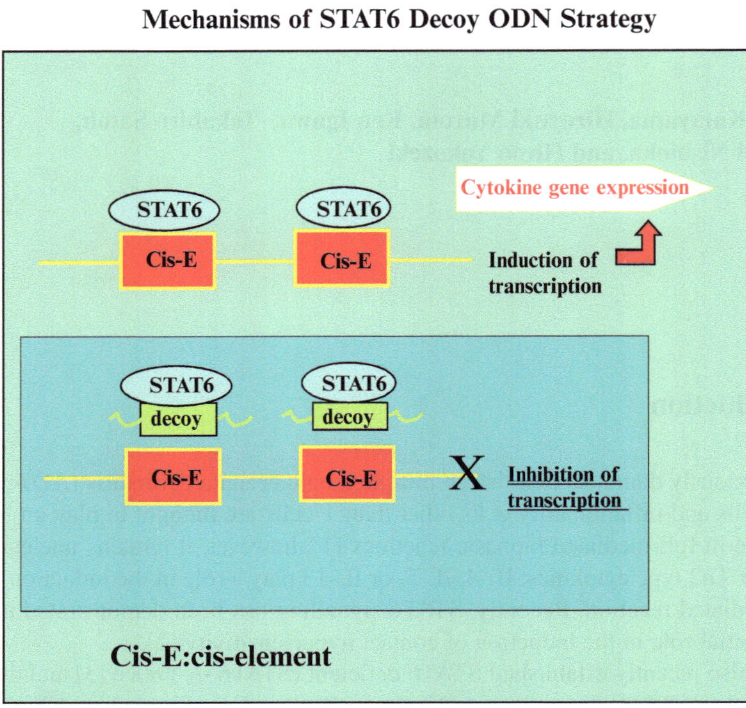

Fig. 1 Mechanisms of STAT6 decoy ODN strategy
Synthetic double-stranded DNA with a high affinity for STAT6 could be introduced in vivo decoy cis elements to bind the transcriptional factor and to block the gene activation of contributing the onset and progression of AD such as STAT6 in this study

gene transactivation both in vitro and in vivo. For example, an NF-κB decoy has been shown to reduce both myocardial reperfusion injury by inhibiting the protein expression (IL-6, IL-8) and adhesion molecules expressed by aortic endothelial cells [5–7], while also preventing AD[8] and sunburn [9]. Recently, a targeted disruption of the STAT6 DNA binding activity by a STAT6 decoy has been reported to block IL-4-driven Th2 cell response in vitro as shown in Fig. 1 [10] We therefore, examine the inhibitory effect of a STAT6 Decoy ODN on the induction of the IgE medicated late phase reaction in an AD mouse model in vivo system.

Pathogenesis of Atopic Dermatitis

As well known, the skin of a patient with AD is often very susceptible to allergy and is called atopic skin. Such vulnerability of the skin may result in a combination of genetic and environmental factors. Environmental allergens involved in atopic disease such as house dust mites, referred to as atopens, trigger the over production of IgE antibody when they come in contact with sensitive, atopic skin, while irritants induce epidermal keratinocytes and fibroblasts to release various types of cytokines and predispose skin to inflammation. External ointments, cosmetics, and shampoos can also cause allergic contact dermatitis in some people in addition to irritation to atopic skin. Very recently, filaggrin (keratohyaline granule-related small protein controlling skin barrier function) mutations have been reported to be closely associated with the risk of the development of AD and bronchial asthma in Iceland and Japanese populations [11].

Ever since the suggestion was made by Sulzberger that AD might be associated with the overproduction of IgE antibodies, IgE has been considered to play an important role in the pathogenesis of AD. However, the details of the involvement of IgE antibodies in the onset of AD remain unknown. Clinical observations have revealed elevation of IgE levels in aggravated AD and elevated IgE titers in proportion to the disease duration in AD. Experimental studies have shown that Fc epsilon Rl(+)Langerhans cells in the skin of patients of AD are more active in presenting antigens inducing the production of Th2 cytokines from T cells. These findings indicate that IgE contributes to the development and progression of AD in many ways [12–14].

The appearance of Th2 cells is tightly regulated through the IL-4-mediated STAT6 activation pathway; through GATA3. Thus, STAT6 is a critical transcriptional factor that regulates Th2-mediated immune responses [15,16]. This STAT6 induced -Th2 polarization is regulated by the SOCS proteins as negative regulators of cytokines (Fig. 2). In T cells, SOCS3 is selectively induced under Th2 culture conditions in the presence of IL-4. The induced SOCS3 specifically binds to the cytoplasmic region of IL-12R and inhibits IL-12-mediated STAT4 activation. Such SOCS3-mediated Th1 inhibition subsequently enhances Th2 development and increases the incidence of allergic inflammations of the skin or airway [17].

In the lesional skin of AD, strong expression of SOCS3 was observed in the epidermis and cellular infiltrates in the dermis (Fig. 3) in contrast to weak or virtually the same as for normal skin expression in patients with psoriasis [17]. Like the immunochemical results, in situ hybridization showed SOCS3 mRNA to be strongly expressed in lesional epidermis, where many infiltrated cells were present.

Establishment of Mouse Atopic Dermatitis Model

Several animal models of AD including rodents, such as Nc/Nga mouse [18], IL4 trasgenic mouse [19], keratinocyte specific IL18 transgenic mouse [20] or repeated hapten-challenge model [21] have been reported in the literatures, and provided new information for the understanding of the pathomechanisms of human AD.

Among these animal models, we reported for the first time that eczematous skin reactions mimicking human atopic dermatitis skin lesions can be induced in retinoic acid pretreated mouse skin by intravenous monoclonal – anti-DNP IgE antibody

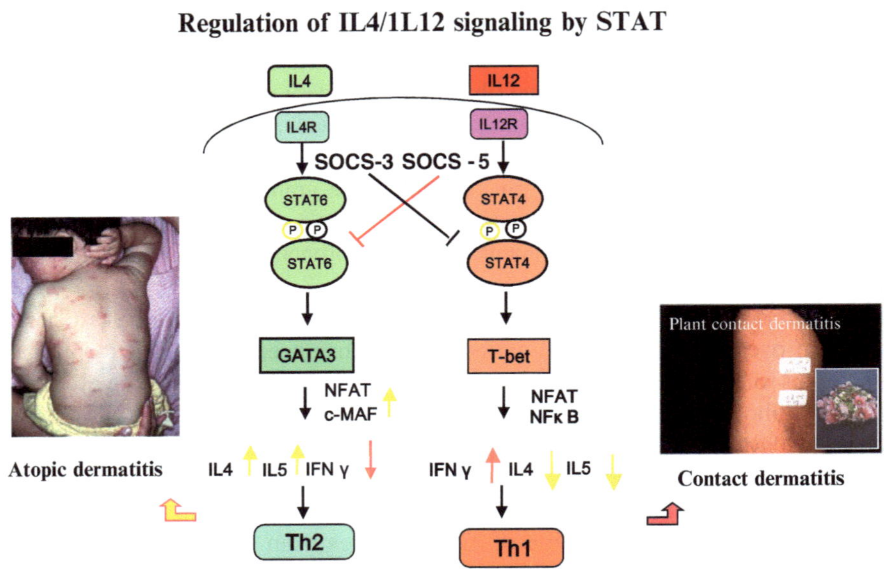

Fig. 2 Regulation of IL4/1L12 signaling by STAT
The appearance of Th2 cells is tightly regulated through the IL-4-mediated STAT6 activation pathway; through GATA3. Thus, STAT6 is a critical transcriptional factor that regulates Th2-mediated immune responses. This STAT6 induced -Th2 polarization is regulated by the SOCS proteins as negative regulators of cytokines. In T cells, SOCS3 is selectively induced under Th2 culture conditions in the presence of IL-4. The induced SOCS3 specifically binds to the cytoplasmic region of IL-12R and inhibits IL-12-mediated STAT4 activation. Such SOCS3-mediated Th1 inhibition subsequently enhances Th2 development and increases the incidence of allergic inflammations of the skin or airway

application and subsequent skin test with dinitronuorobenzene (DNFB) [1]. Female Balb/c mice were used in this experiment and biphasic skin reaction with peak response at immediate (1 h) and delayed (24 h) time space with prominent mast cell degranulation was induced by the method described above (Fig. 4). This reaction was hapten-specific and mast-cell dependent because no reaction was observed when oxasolone was used as an elicitation antigen or skin test was elicited in genetically mast cell deficient mice (W/Wvv). A partial spongiotic reaction and mononuclear cell infi1tration into the epidermis were observed in mice with hyperplastic epidermis induced by topical retinoic acid pre-treatment and subsequent IgE antibody treatment and challenge test. Co-transfer of DNFB-sensitized lymph node cells with anti-DNP IgE antibodies, failed to enhance the skin test reaction in unsensitized mice. These results suggest that, to some degree, IgE antibody may play some role in the development of eczematous skin lesions in the rodent system without the involvement of cellular hypersensitivity.

SOCS3 expressions inatopic derrmatitis

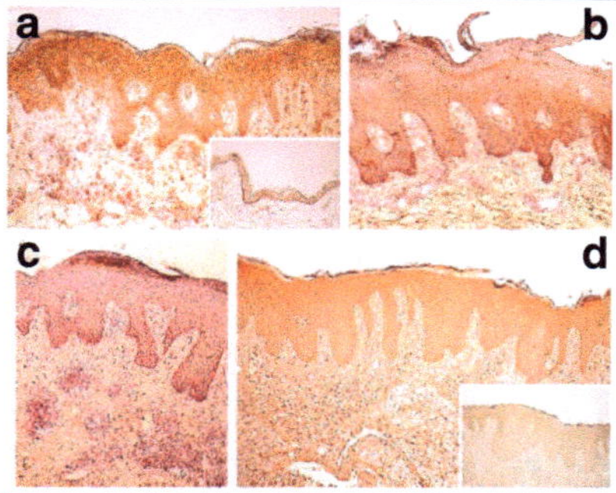

a Atopic dermatitis (lesional skin, x100)

b Psoriasis (lesional skin, x100)

c Normal control (x100)

d Atopic dermatitis (lesional skin, x100) (in situ hybridization) Anti-sense probe sense-probe (inset)

Number/Age/sex/SOCS3 intensity

Patient	AD		Psoriasis			Normal subjects		
1	42M	+3	8	58M	+1	13	68F	+1
2	33M	+3	9	28F	+1	14	54F	+1
3	26F	+3	10	74F	+1	15	29M	+1/-
4	29M	+3	11	52M	+1			
5	45M	+3	12	54M	+1			
6	28M	+3						
7	19M	+3						
+3, Very strong; +2, strong; +1, weakly positive; -, negative.								

Fig. 3 SOCS3 expressions in atopic derrmatitis
Immunohistochemistry and in situ hybridization of SOCS3. Very intense staining of SOCS3 evident in the epidermis and dermal infiltrates in the lesional skin of atopic dermatitis (**a**). Very weak staining of SOCS3 in epidermis and some positive dermal infiltrates in the patient with psoriasis; (**b**). Negative control specimens (with no second antibody application) of the same lesions in patient (**d**) show acanthosis and intense inflammatory mononuclear cells in the dermis; which is contrasted with the very weak staining of the normal skin from normal control (**c**) *inset*. Quite strong in situ expression of SOCS3 mRNA in the epidermis and dermal infiltrates of patient with AD which is contrasted with the sense negative control of SOCS3 in situ in the same patient (**d**). Immunohistochemical antibody sites and mRNA in situ expression were determined with diaminobenzidine solution and counterstaining was carried out lightly with haematoxylin

Synthesis of ODN and Selection of Target Sequences

Sequences of the phosphorothioate ODN utilized were as follows: [10]
[STAT6 decoy ODN]

- 5' – GATCAAGACCTTTTCCCAAGAAATCTAT – 3'
  3' – ATAGATTTCTTGGGAAAAGGTCTTGATC – 5'
  [Scrambled decoy ODN]
- 5' – CGAAAATTCGTTAAATCACTAGCTTACC – 3'
  3' – GGTAAGCTAGTGATTTAACGAATTTTCG – 5'

Induction of biphasic skin reaction by anti-DNP IgE antibody and skin challenge test

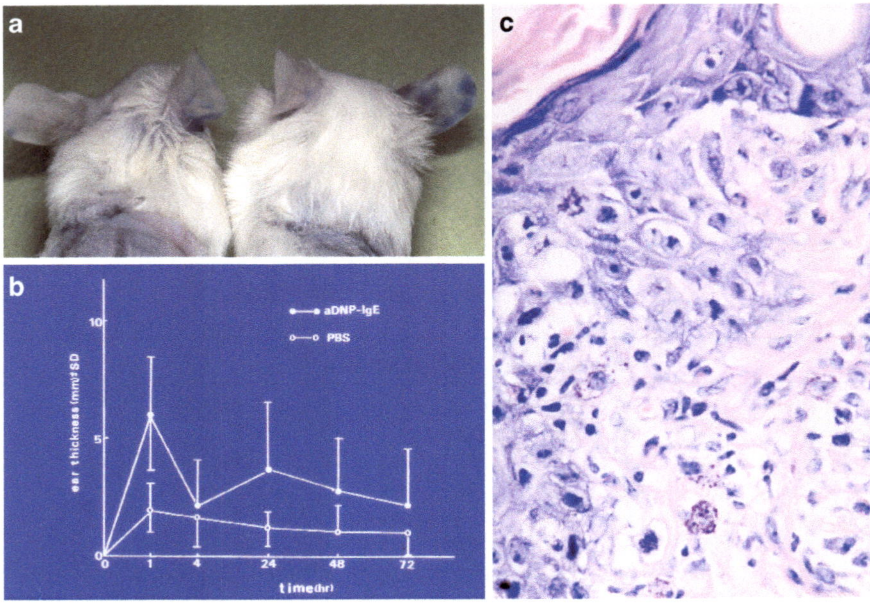

Fig. 4 Induction of biphasic skin reaction by anti-DNP IgE antibody and skin challenge test (**a**) Right ear of the each mouse shows increased vascular permeability response by intravenous anti-DNP IgE antibody and subsequent challenge test by Evance blue dye extravasation (**b**) Biphasic inflammatory skin responses were induced in Balb/C mouse (**c**) Inflammatory cell infiltrations were demonstrated in challenged ear skin with epidermal spongiosis and mast cell degranulation

The STAT6 decoy ODN is a double-stranded phosphorothioate 28 mer that exhibits a high sequence-specific binding affinity to the transcription factor STAT6. Synthetic ODNs were dissolved in sterile Tris-EDTA buffer (10 mM Tris, 1 mM EDTA pH 8.0), purified by high-performance liquid chromatography and quantitated by spectrophotometry. Each pair of single-stranded ODN was annealed for 3 h, during which time the temperature was reduced from 90 to 25°. These decoy ODNs were then stored at –20°C until use.

Preparation of the HVJ-E Vector

HVJ (also known as Sendai virus) was amplified as described previously [22]. The virus was inactivated by β-propiolactone (0.0075–0.001%) treatment or by UV irradiation. In both cases, the virus preparation lost the ability to replicate. The aliquots of the virus (3×10^{10} particles/1.5 μl tube) were centrifuged (18,500*g*, 15 min) at 4°C, and the viral pellet was stored at –20°C [22]. The inactivated virus suspension (10,000 haemagglutinating activity units) (HAU) was mixed with STAT6 decoy OND or scrambled decoy ODN (800 μg of DNA), 8 μl of 3% Triton/TE and balanced salt solution (BSS; 10 nM Tris-HCl (pH 7.5), 137 mM NaCl and 5.4 mM KCl), to yield a final volume of 100 μl. The mixture was centrifuged at 18,500*g* for 15 min at 4°C. After the pellet was washed with 1 ml of human tubal fluid (HTF) medium (Nippon Medical and Chemical Instrument Co. Ltd, Osaka, Japan) to remove the detergent and un-incorporated DNA, the envelope vector was suspended in 250 μl of HTF medium. Approximately 15–20% of DNA was incorporated into the vector. The HVJ-E vector was stored at 4°C until use. HVJ-E vector is also commercially available from Ishihara Sangyo Co. Ltd (Osaka, Japan).

Inhibition of the Late Phase Response but Not the Early Phase Response Induced by Anti-DNP-IgE Antibody

To determine the inhibition of decoy ODN against STAT6 in view of the response induced by anti-DNP-IgE antibody, the ear swelling response challenged by DNFB was examined with or without STAT6 decoy ODN or scrambled decoy ODN. STAT6 Decoy ODN weakly inhibited the early phase response but not significantly, while the late phase response was inhibited dramatically by STAT6 decoy ODN significantly (Fig. 5a), in line with Kaneda's report [23]. Next, we compared the effect of STAT6 decoy ODN in between several routes of the injection. Interestingly, both the subcutaneous and intramuscular injection of STAT6 decoy ODN was effective; however, neither the intraperitoneal injection nor intravenous injection (data not shown) of that was effective. In the inhibitory study of STAT6 Decoy ODN in various mice strains, STAT6 Decoy ODN suppressed the late phase response in Balb/c, C3H/He and C57BL/6 mice. It was, however, inhibited most strongly in Balb/c mice since Balb/c mice may be Th2-dominant mice. These data are consistent with the response of the late phase reaction in STAT6–/– mice.

Histopathology of Skin Reactions in Mice with or Without STAT6 Decoy ODN-Liposomes

Since the anti-DNP-IgE antibody induced decreased late phase response to DNFB in mice transfected with STAT6 decoy ODN, we performed a histological analysis in mice injected with or without STAT decoy ODN or scrambled decoy ODN sensitized by anti-DNP-IgE antibody. As shown in Fig. 5b a histological examination revealed edema and intense infiltration of eosinophils, neutrophils, and mononuclear cells in non-transfected or scramble decoy ODN transfected mice at 24 h after challenge but not in the mice transfected with STAT6 decoy ODN (Fig. 5c).

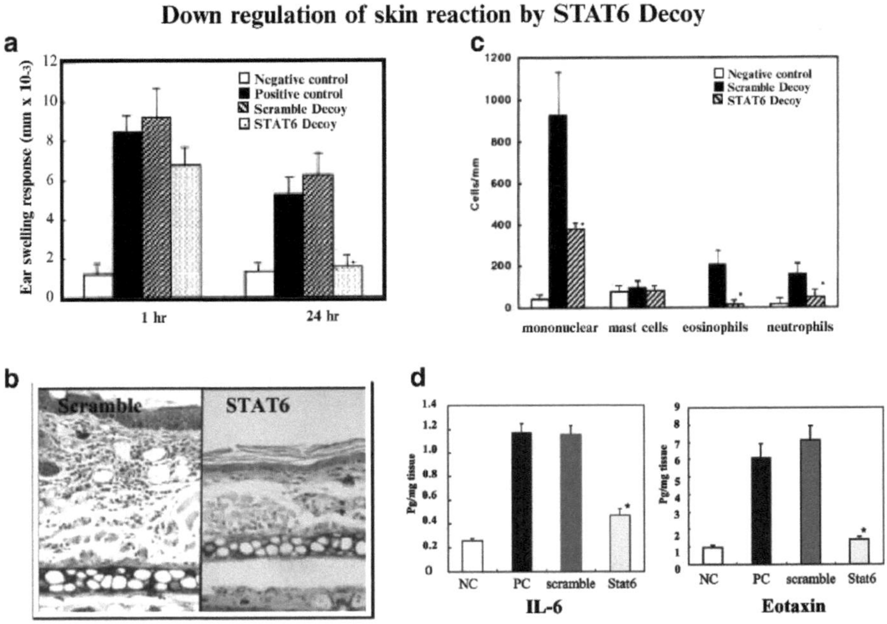

Fig. 5 Down regulation of skin reaction by STAT6 Decoy
(**a**) Balb/c mice were sensitized with anti-DNP-IgE antibody, and then 6 h after sensitization STAT6 decoy ODN or scrambled decoy ODN were injected subcutaneously. One day after, each mouse was challenged with DNFB. STAT6 decoy ODN inhibited the ear swelling at 24 h after challenge test but not scrambled decoy, however, neither STAT6 decoy nor the scrambled decoy inhibited significantly the ear swelling at 1 hr after challenge (**b**) The histologic features of 24 h ear skin reaction challenged by DNFB in mice injected scramble Decoy or in mice injected with STAT6 decoy stained with Giemsa's solution. An extremely large degree of edema was detected in the DNFB-challenged skin in the mice treated with scramble decoy but not in the mice treated with the STAT6 decoy (**c**) The columns represent the number of eosinophils, neutrophils, monocytes/macrophages and mast cells which infiltrated the challenged skin with scramble or STAT6 decoy ODN treatment (**d**) The cytokine levels in the skin tissue supernatants in olive oil and DNFB-challenged, sensitized Balb/c mice pretreated with STAT6 decoy ODN or scrambled decoy ODN. The cytokine levels of IL-4 and IL-5 were measured by comparing them with all other groups. The cytokine levels of IL-6 and eotaxin were measured by comparing them with all other groups

Local Production of Cytokines in Mice with or Without STAT6 Decoy ODN

In the supernatant from skin tissue obtained from DNFB-challenged mice after anti-DNP-IgE antibody sensitization, the levels of both IL-4 and IL-5 were significantly higher than those in the supernatant from olive oil-challenged mice (Fig. 5d). In contrast, these Th2 cytokine levels in the supernatant from DNFB-challenged mice with STAT6 decoy ODN, transfection decreased. The level of IFN-γ in the mice with STAT6 transfection was comparable to that in the non-transfected or scrambled decoy ODN transfected mice. Furthermore, not only Th2 cytokines but also the IL-6 and Eotaxin levels decreased in the supernatant from skin tissue obtained from STAT6 decoy transfected mice, however IL-13 level decreased weakly but not significantly [24].

Current Understanding of STAT6 Decoy ODN on Murine Model of AD

Recently, Yagi et al. demonstrated that the development of AD-like skin lesion in STAT6-deficient NC/Nga mice and Th2-mediated immune response is not necessary for the development of AD-like skin disease [25]. Their report is not consistent with our results, However, there are several mechanisms except for late phase reaction in the pathogenesis of AD. A histological analysis revealed a tremendous reduction in both the infiltration of eosinophils and neutrophils in DNFB challenged skin of STAT6–/– mice. In addition, the antigen induced edematous changes in the dermis, was also completely dependent on the STAT6 signaling. So far, the exact roles of these polymorphonuclear cells in the late phase response are still unclear, however, our data indicate that polymorphonuclear cells, including eosinophils and neutrophils dependent on STAT6 signaling, may play a major role in the induction of the late phase response induced by anti-DNP-IgE antibody. STAT6 signaling is essential for hapten-induced late phase reaction in Th2 cytokines production in vivo. The hapten challenged wt mice demonstrated significant elevations in the Th2 cytokines (i.e., IL-4 and IL-5). In marked contrast, STAT6–/– mice were unable to produce IL-4 or IL-5 in response to the skin challenge (Fig. 1d). Consistent with a recent report [26], no detectable TNF-α nor Eotaxin in supernatants of mast cells was observed upon the cross-linking of their IgE receptor/Fc epsilon RI on their surface in a hapten specific manner, in STAT6–/– mice (data not shown). These data indicated that STAT6 signal is essential in the production of Th2 cytokine, chemokine of neutorophils and eosinophils by mast cells [24]. These results of the response induced by anti-DNP-IgE antibody and antigen in STAT6–/– mice suggested to us that blocking of STAT6 signaling can be a therapeutic approach for AD.

Clinical Effect of STAT6 Decoy Ointment in Refractory Adult Type Atopic Dermatitis

In a preliminary study, we applied STAT6 decoy ointment to the refractory AD after ethical approval. Significant improvements of skin scores and pruritis were obtained in four cases (Fig. 6). Large scale clinical studies are under way and will provide much more information about the proper clinical use, indications and side effects and usefulness in daily clinical practice in the near future [30].

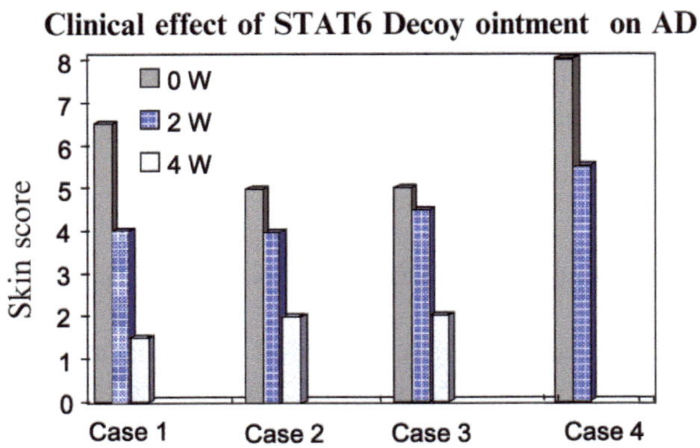

Fig. 6 Clinical effect of STAT6 Decoy ointment on adult patients with atopic dermatitis
In a preliminary study, we applied STAT6 decoy ointment to the refractory adult type AD after ethical approval. Significant improvements of skin scores and pruritis were obtained in four cases. Large scale of clinical studies are under way and will provide much more information about the appropriate clinical use, indications and side effect

Conclusions

Although considerable progress has been made in elucidating the mechanism of AD, the cellular and molecular mechanisms regulating AD still remains obscure. Recently, IgE mediated late phase reaction is thought to be mainly associated with the pathogenesis of AD [27–39]. We have established the eczematous skin reaction induced by anti-DNP-IgE antibody and DNFB in AD model mouse [1,2]. STAT6 is known as a regulator of IL-4-dependent immune responses. We have also established STAT6 deficient mice and concluded that STAT6 plays a crucial role in exerting IL-4 and IL-13 mediated biological responses [3,4]. On the basis of these earlier studies, we have developed novel therapy for AD using STAT6 Decoy ODN that clearly downregulated late phase cutaneous response of IgE mediated biphasic reactions, which is now thought to be closely related to skin reactions seen in human AD [24]. Additionally, this study demonstrated that the transcriptional factor, STAT6, is one of the key regulators promoting IgE induced late phase reaction. Although a number of important issues, such as the safety and side effects, have not yet been addressed in this study, the decoy strategy against STAT6 may provide a new therapeutic modality as gene therapy against AD. Since STAT6 has been postulated to play an important role in the pathogenesis of numerous diseases, for example, contact dermatitis, atopic asthma and allergic rhinitis, the development of STAT6 decoy strategy may also prove to be a useful therapeutic tool for treating these diseases.

References

1. Katayama I, Tanei R, Nishioka K, et al. (1990). Induction of eczematous skin reaction in experimentally induced hyperplastic skin of Balb/c mice by monoclonal anti-DNP-IgE antibody: Possible implication for skin lesion formation in atopic dermatitis. Int Arch Allergy Appl Immunol 93, 148–154
2. Yokozeki H, Ghoreishi M, Takagawa S, et al. (2000). Signal transduccer and activator of Transcription 6 is essential in the induction of contact hypersensitivity. J Exp Med 191, 995–1004
3. Takeda K, Tanaka T, Shi W, et al. (1996). Essential role of Stat6 in IL-4 signaling. Nature 380, 627–630
4. Taked K, Tanaka M, Tanaka T, et al. (1996). Impaired IL-13-mediated functions of macrophages in STAT6-deficient mice. J Immunol 157, 3220–3222
5. Morishita R, Gibbons GH, Horiuchi M, et al. (1995). A gene Therapy strategy using a transcription factor decoy of the E2F binding site inhibits smooth proliferation in vivo. Proc Natl Acad USA 92, 5855–5859
6. Morishita R, Higaki J, et al. (1996). Role of transcriptional cis-elements, angiotensinogen gene-activating element, of angiotensinogen genein blood pressure regulation. Hypertension 27, 502–507
7. Morishita R, Sugimoto T, Aoki M, et al. (1997). On vivo transfection of cis element decoy against nuclear factor-kB binding site prevents myocardial infection. Nature Med 3, 894–899
8. Nakamura H, Aoki M, Tamai K, et al. (2002). Prevention and regulation of atopic dermatitis by ointment containing NF-kB decoy oligodeoxynucleotides in NC/Nga atopic mouse model. Gene Ther 9, 1221–1229
9. Abeyama K, Eng W, Jester JV, Vink AA (2000). A role for NF-kB dependent gene transaction in sunburn. J Clin Invest 105, 1751–1759
10. Wang LH, Yang XY, Kirken RA, et al. (2000). Targeted disruption of Stat6 DNA binding activity by an oligonucleotide decoy blocks IL-4-deriven Th2 cell response. Blood 95, 1249–1257
11. McLean WH, Hull PR (2007). Breach delivery: increased solute uptake points to a defective skin barrier in atopic dermatitis. J Invest Dermatol 127, 8–10
12. Bieber T (1994). Fc epsilon RI on human Langerhans cells: a receptor in search of new functions. Immunol Today 15, 52–53
13. Yokozeki H, Takayama K, Ohki O, et al. (1998). Comparative analysis of CD80 and CD86 on human Langerhans cells: expression and function. Arch Dermatol Res 290, 547–552
14. Ohki O, Yokozeki H, Katayama I, et al. (1997). Functional CD86 (B7-2/B70) is predominantly expressed on Langerhans cells in atopic dermatitis. Br J Dermatol 136, 838–845
15. Agnello D, Lankford CS, Bream J, et al. (2003). Cytokines and transcription factors that regulate T helper cell differentiation: new players and new insights. J Clin Immunol 23, 147–161
16. Ozaki A, Ishida WK, Fukata K, et al. (2004). Detection of antigen-specific T cells in experimental immune-mediated blepharoconjunctivitis in DO11.10 T cell receptor transgenic mice. Microbiol Immunol 48, 39–48
17. Horiuchi Y, S-J Bae, Katayama I (2005). Overexpression of the suppressor of cytokine signalling 3 (SOCS3) in severe atopic dermatitis. Clin Exp Dermatol 31, 100–104
18. Horiuchi Y, Bae S, Katayama I, et al. (2006). Lipoteichoic acid-related molecule derived from the streptococcal preparation, OK-432, which suppresses atopic dermatitis-like lesions in NC/Nga mice. Arch Dermatol Res 298, 163–173
19. Elbe-Burger A, Egyed A, Olt S, et al. (2002). Overexpression of IL-4 alters the homeostasis in the skin. J Invest Dermatol 118, 767–778
20. Konishi H, Tsutsui H, Murakami T, et al. (2002). IL-18 contributes to the spontaneous development of atopic dermatitis-like inflammatory skin lesion independently of IgE/stat6 under specific pathogen-free conditions. Proc Natl Acad Sci USA 99, 11340–11345

21. Shiohara T, Hayakawa J, Mizukawa Y (2004). Animal models for atopic dermatitis: are they relevant to human disease? J Dermatol Sci 36, 1–9
22. Molitor JA, Walker WH, Doerre S, et al. (1990). NF-kB: a family of inducible and differentially expressed enhancer-binding proteins in human T cells. Proc Natl Acad Sci USA 1990 87, 10028–10032
23. Kaneda Y, Iwaki K, Uchida T (1989). Introduction of the human insulin gene in adult rat liver. J Biol Chem 264, 12126–12129
24. Yokozeki H, Wu MH, Sumi K, et al. (2004). In vivo transfection of a cis element decoy against signal transducers and activators of transcription 6 (STAT6)-binding site ameliorates IgE-mediated late-phase reaction in an atopic dermatitis mouse model. Gene Ther 11, 1753–1762
25. Yagi R, Nagai H, Iigo Y, et al. (2002). Development of atopic dermatitis-like lesions inSTAT6-deficient NC/Nga mice. J Immunol 168, 2020–2027
26. Malaviya R and Uckun MF (2002). Role of STAT6 in IgE receptor/FceRI- mediated late phase allegic response of mast cells. J Immunol 168, 421–426
27. Bruijnzeel PL, Kuijper PH, Kapp A, et al. (1993). The involvement of eosinophils in the patch test reaction to aeroallergens in atopic dermatitis: its relevance for the pathogenesis of atopic dermatitis. Clin Exp Allergy 23, 97–109
28. Sampson HA (1988). The role of food allergy and mediator release in atopic dermatitis. J Allergy Clin Immunol 81, 635–645
29. Rajka G (1988) Pathomechanism. Genetic and immunological factors, In Essential Aspects of Atopic Deramatitis. Tokyo, Springer, pp 108–111
30. Igawa K, Satoh T, Yokozeki H (2009). A therapeutic effect of STAT6 decoy oligodeoxynucleotide ointment in atopic dermatitis: a pilot study in adults. Br J Dermatol 160, 1124–1126

Mast Cell-Specific Genes as New Drug Targets

Hirohisa Saito

Introduction

By complete reading of the genome sequence, it became possible to understand the total function of various types of a single cell at least at the transcriptome level by using rapidly developed tools for functional genomics such as microarray technology [1].

Allergies such as bronchial asthma are complicated and diverse disorders affected by genetic and environmental factors. It is widely accepted that allergy is a Th2-type inflammation originating in the tissue and caused by invasion of ubiquitous allergens. Several attempts to clarify the pathogenesis of asthma and other allergic diseases have been carried out using microarray technology, providing us some novel biomarkers for diagnosis, therapeutic targets or understanding pathogenic mechanisms of asthma and allergies [2].

Mast cells are known to be the primary responders in allergic reactions, most of which are triggered by cross-linking of a high-affinity IgE receptor, FcεRI. After activation, mast cells exert their biological effects by releasing preformed and de novo-synthesized mediators, such as histamine, leukotrienes, proteases, and various cytokines/chemokines [3]. Biogenic amines and lipid mediators cause rapid leakage of plasma from blood vessels, vasodilation, and bronchoconstriction. Proteases cause tissue damage and airway herperresponsiveness in asthma. Cytokines mediate the late phase reaction characterized by an inflammatory infiltrate composed of eosinophils, basophils, neutrophils, and lymphocytes [3]. However, functions of a substantial number of genes or molecules present in mast cells remain undiscovered. In this chapter, various genes preferentially expressed by mast cells are discussed regarding the possibility of future drug targets for asthma and other allergic diseases. Here, molecules specifically or preferentially expressed by mast cells are discussed about the possibility of therapeutic targets or understanding pathogenic mechanisms of asthma and allergies by referring to the previous reports and public microarray database shown in Table 1 [4–13].

H. Saito
Department of Allergy and Immunology, National Research Institute for Child Health and Development, Setagaya, Tokyo, Japan
e-mail: hsaito@nch.go.jp

R. Pawankar et al. (eds.), *Allergy Frontiers: Future Perspectives*,
DOI 10.1007/978-4-431-99365-0_11, © Springer 2010

Table 1 Public database regarding gene expression profiles of human mast cells

1.Website	http://www.ncbi.nlm.nih.gov/geo/gds/gds_browse.cgi?gds=1775
Summary	Expression profiling of various major leukocyte types. Gene profiles for activated effector cells such as macrophages, neutrophils, and mast cells were also generated. Results establish expression signatures unique to each major leukocyte type.
Platform	Affymetrix GeneChip Human Genome U133 Array Set HG-U133A
Citation	Jeffrey KL, et al. Nat Immunol 2006 (ref. #4)
2.Website	http://www.ncbi.nlm.nih.gov/projects/geo/gds/gds_browse.cgi?gds=1520
Summary	Analysis of umbilical cord blood-derived mast cells 2 h post-stimulation by high-affinity IgE receptor (FcεRI). Cells incubated with myeloma IgE and IL-4 prior to stimulation. Cells activated via FcεRI with anti-IgE antibody to induce release of antihistamines and other inflammation mediators.
Platform	GPL2824: LC-13 (cDNA microarray)
Citation	Sayama K, et al. BMC Immunol 2002 (ref. #5)
3. Web sites	http://www.ncbi.nlm.nih.gov/geo/query/acc.cgi?acc=GSE1933
Summary	Human umbilical cord blood-derived mast cells IgE sensitized followed by crosslinking receptor at different time points.
Platform	Affymetrix GeneChip Human HG-Focus Target Array
Citation	Jayapal M, et al. BMC Genomics 2006 (ref #6)
4. Website	http://www.ncbi.nlm.nih.gov/geo/query/acc.cgi?acc=GSE4906
Summary	Cord blood-derived stem cells were in vitro cultured in the presence of 40 ng/ml SCF, 20 ng/ml IL6 and 2 microM lysophosphatidic acid for 5 week. Then mast cells were magnetically isolated and further cultured for 4 days in the presence or absence of 2 ng/ml TGF-β1. Total RNA was isolated and processed according to the Agilent Low-input RNA Linear Amplification Kit and microarray hybridization protocol.
Platform	Agilent-012391 Whole Human Genome Oligo Microarray G4112A
Citation	Wiener Z, et al. J Invest Dermatol 2007 (ref. #7)
5. Website	http://www.ncbi.nlm.nih.gov/geo/query/acc.cgi?acc=GSE1848
Summary	GeneChip Data of human lung mast cells and tonsillar mast cells.
Platforms	Affymetrix GeneChip Human Genome U133 Array Set HG-U133A & Affymetrix GeneChip Human Genome U133 Array Set HG-U133B
Citation	Kashiwakura J, et al. J Immunol 2004 (ref. #8)
6.Website	http://www.nch.go.jp/imal/GeneChip/public.htm
Summary	GeneChip Data of human Eosinophils, Neutrophils, CD4+ cells, CD14+ cells, Mast cells derived from adult peripheral blood-progenitors.
Platforms	Affymetrix GeneChip U95A
Citation	Nakajima T, et al. Blood 2001 (ref. #9)
7.Website	http://bio.mki.co.jp/en/results/comparativeDB/comparativeDB_index.html
Summary	GeneChip data of human mast cells derived from adult peripheral blood-progenitors and mouse bone marrow-derived mast cells were comparatively examined. These cells were examined before and after Fcε receptor aggregation.
Platforms	Affymetrix GeneChip Human Genome U133 Array Set HG-U133A & Mouse Genome MO430A
Citation	Nakajima T, et al. Blood 2002 (ref. #10)
8.Website	http://www.nch.go.jp/imal/GeneChip/public.htm
Summary	Expression profiles of basophils, eosinophils, neutrophils, CD4 cells, CD8 cells, CD14 cells, CD19 cells, platelets, fibroblasts, and mast cells derived from adult peripheral blood progenitors were comparatively examined.
Platforms	Affymetrix GeneChip Human Genome U133 Array Set HG-U133A
Citation	Nakajima T, et al. J Allergy Clin Immunol 2004 (ref. #11)

(continued)

Table 1 (continued)

9.Website	http://www.nch.go.jp/imal/GeneChip/public.htm
Summary	Gene expression profiles of human skin mast cells, lung mast cells, tonsillar mast cells, progenitor-derived mast cells were comparatively examined.
Platforms	Affymetrix GeneChip Human Genome U133 Array Set HG-U133A
Citation	Saito H, et al. Allergol Int 2006 (ref. #12)

Mast Cell-Specific Genes for Drug Targets

When the whole transcripts in a mast cell population are examined by using microarray or some transcriptome database, novel genes that highly expressed by mast cells should be frequently found. By comparing to transcriptomes expressed by other cell types, however, most of those mast cell-expressing genes are not exclusively expressed by mast cells. Crucial adverse reactions of a certain drug should be found on vitally important organs. The safety of anti-inflammatory drugs must be evaluated by comparing its efficacy on inflammatory cells with its toxicity to physiologically important organs. Thus, elucidating the whole information related to the mast cell type-specific functions compared to the other cell types are important especially when you are developing a new drug targeting the mast cell-specific gene.

Mast cells, basophil-, and/or eosinophil-specific genes could be potential therapeutic targets for allergic diseases because these granulocytes play an important role in allergic inflammation [13]. Activation of these cells is generally characterized by an influx of extracellular calcium (Ca^{2+}), which is essential for subsequent release of granule-derived mediators, newly generated lipid mediators, and cytokines [14]. Flow of other ions plays an important role during granulocyte responses because they regulate cell membrane potential and thus influence Ca^{2+} influx [15]. Treatment of mast cells and basophils with pertussis toxin inactivates the Gi-type of G-proteins and abolishes degranulation but not the influx of Ca^{2+} induced by non-immunological ligands such as thrombin and N-formylpeptide [16]. Thus, granulocyte degranulation pathway is sometimes Ca^{2+}-independent and is G protein dependent. Indeed, the thrombin activated receptors and formylpeptide receptors are classified as G protein-coupled receptors (GPCRs), having a seven transmembrane region [17]. As such, ion channels and GPCR both play essential roles in degranulation as well as other cellular function important for granulocytes, and are thought to be good targets of drug development [18]. Receptor genes and ion channel genes are found only in 5 and 1.3% of all genes present in the human genome, respectively [19]. However, receptors and ion channels are, respectively, found in 45 and 5% of the molecular targets of all known drugs [18,20].

Beside their physiological importance, receptors including GPCR and ion channels are considered to be marketable and targeting these molecules should be efficient for pharmaceutical development. In other words, we can concentrate on approximately 2,000 genes as practical drug targets, and can forget about the 30,000 other genes present in the human genome.

Nakajima et al. examined [11] the cell type-selective transcriptome expression of 7 types of leukocytes (basophils, eosinophils, neutrophils, $CD4^+$ cells, $CD8^+$ cells, $CD14^+$ cells, and $CD19^+$ cells), platelets, fibroblasts, and mast cells using high-density oligonucleotide probe arrays. Then, the expression of granulocyte-selective genes for ion channels, GPCR, and other receptors were determined. It was estimated that approximately 50 genes are selectively expressed by mast cells, eosinophils, and basophils among all genes present in the human genome. The representative such "druggable" genes, GPCRs that were selectively expressed by mast cells, basophils, and/or eosinophils were as follows: *HRH4* (histamine H4 receptor), *PTGER3* (prostaglandin E receptor type 3a2), *ADORA3* (adenosine A3 receptor), *P2RY2* (purinergic receptor), *GPR44* (chemoattractant receptor-homologous molecule expressed on Th2 cells, CRTH2), *EMR1* (egf-like module containing, mucin-like, hormone receptor-like sequence 1), *CCR3* (chemokine receptor 3), and *C3AR1* (C3a receptor). As such, analysis of cell type-selective druggable genes from database searches is expected to minimize the efforts required for drug discovery (Fig. 1).

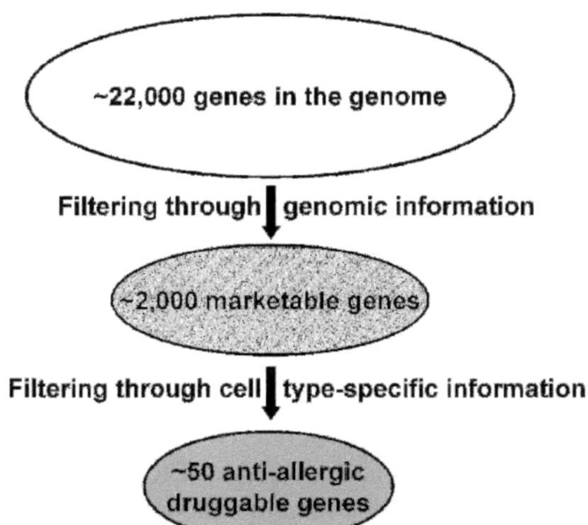

Fig. 1 *Filtering of "druggable" genes through genomic information*. Only 22,000 genes were found to be contained in our genome. Through marketable (easy to obtain the specific antagonist or agonist) merits, 2,000 genes were filtered as drug targets. Using cell-type specific transcriptome database, they were further sub-calcified to be anti-allergic drug targets or other diseases' drug targets. The estimated number of the anti-allergic (mast cell-, basophil-, and eosinophil-specific) drug targets was approximately only 50

Mast Cell Subset-Specific Genes

For genome-wide comprehensive analyses such as transcriptome, it is necessary to obtain a substantial number of mast cells. However, regarding human mast cells, it was not possible to do so for a long time even after establishment of mouse mast cell culture system. We have established the method of generating a substantial number of human mast cells from umbilical cord blood [21] and from adult peripheral blood [22,23]. By the development of microarray technology, it also became possible to examine the levels of whole transcripts even using approximately 10^5 cells. Thus, we can now examine the transcriptome information of subtypes of human mast cells present in various tissues.

Iida et al. comparatively examined the global gene expression in cultured human mast cells derived from umbilical cord blood progenitors and from adult peripheral blood progenitors using microarray [24]. The transcript for Fcε receptor α-chain was found selectively down-regulated in cord blood-derived human mast cells compared to adult counterparts. This down regulation may be controlled by epigenetic mechanisms present in hemopoietic progenitors since the expression level of Fcε receptor α-chain was down-regulated even under the same culture conditions. Indeed, neonatal cord and adult peripheral blood hemopoietic progenitors can produce cell types having somewhat different profiles [25,26].

Kashiwakura et al. reported [8] the transcriptome analysis of human tonsillar mast cells, which locate in the interfollicular areas and may interact with T cells, in comparison with other human mast cells such as lung mast cells. A large fraction of the gene expression profiles of cultured tonsillar mast cells were comparable to other mast cells including cultured lung mast cells. However, macrophage inflammatory protein (MIP)-1α (CCL3, CC-chemokine ligand 3) and MIP-1β (CCL4) were expressed in resting cultured tonsillar mast cells but not in resting cultured lung mast cells. Tumor necrosis factor (TNF)-α expression was also up-regulated in tonsillar mast cells following FcεRI aggregation. It has been reported that CCL3 and CCL4 have the ability to recruit T cells into lymph nodes and mast cells are one of the major source of CCL4 [27], and that both TNF-α concentration and the recruitment of circulating T cells were increased within draining lymph nodes following peripheral mast cell activation [28]. T cells thus may be recruited by tonsillar mast cells. In agreement with the results of chymase expression of tissue mast cells [29], cultured tonsillar mast cells also showed higher intensity of the expression than cultured lung mast cells [8,12]. It is of particular interest that the tissue-specific nature of human mast cells persists after a long period of culture. Kambe et al. have reported a similar observation regarding human skin-derived cultured mast cells [30]. Reactivity toward substance P of the human skin-derived cultured mast cells was not lost even after extensive proliferation of the mast cells under the standard serum-free culture system supplemented with stem cell factor (SCF) [30]. Therefore, it is concluded that cultured mast cells retain some of their characteristics derived from the original tissues, even after proliferation of mast cells under the standard culture condition without specific tissue factors [8,12,30].

Although the microenvironment can change the characterization of mast cells [31], some effects of microenvironment may last long after removal of the environmental factors. These findings may suggest that mast cell progenitors committed to a certain mast cell subtype might be selectively recruited to the tissue. Alternatively, the tissue-specific characters of mast cells may be determined by epigenetic alteration. The mast cells or their progenitors may be epigenetically influenced by environmental factors during their stay in the tissue. Environmental conditions sometimes modify the composition of genomic structure or nucleic acid molecules such as CpG methylation and this modification sometimes last long even beyond generations [32].

Bradding et al. have reported [33] that human skin-derived cultured mast cells express somewhat different types of ion channel profiles in comparison with lung and cord blood-derived mast cells, although the transcriptome profiles of these mast cells were mostly identical. Saito et al. have identified [12] that lung type-cultured mast cells having low levels of chymase transcript and skin type-cultured mast cells having abundant chymase transcript respectively express unique GPCRs. For example, β2 adrenergic receptor transcript is highly expressed by lung mast cells but not by skin mast cells. Indeed, β2 adrenergic agent is not effective for allergic skin diseases. Such observation is particularly important for the future drug discovery for organ-specific allergic diseases.

Mast Cell-Specific Genes in Inflammation

Even before microarray techniques developed, mast cells were known to produce multiple cytokines through transcription of these genes for inducing allergic inflammation, i.e., TNF-α [34], granulocyte-macrophage colony-stimulating factor (GM-CSF) [35], I-309/TCA-3 (CCL1), CCL3, CCL4 [36], monocyte chemotactic peptide (MCP)-1 (CCL2) [37], and interleukin (IL)-3 [38], IL-4 [39], IL-5 [40], IL-6, IL-8 [36], IL-9 [40], IL-10 [41], and IL-13 [42] following IgE-dependent activation. A transcriptome assay for human mast cells seems to be of particular interest as to whether they can produce other unidentified cytokines. According to their microarray data (Table 1) [4–13], the results were not very surprising. Most of the cytokine/chemokine genes expressed by human mast cells after aggregation of FcεRI were identical to the previous reports using non-array methods [34–42].

It was confirmed that Th1 cytokines and CXC-chemokines deriving Th1 cells are not expressed by human mast cells activated through FcεRI aggregation. However, mast cells also express Toll-like receptors (TLRs) which recognize various microbial components [43], and can be activated via challenge with these components. Mouse-cultured mast cells express TLR2, 4, and 6 and produce a variety of cytokines including IL-13 in response to these TLR ligands such as lipopolysaccharide (LPS) [44,45] and release preformed mediators in response to peptideglycan, a TLR2 ligand [46]. Human cord blood-derived cultured mast cells express TLR2 and 6 and produce a variety of cytokines such as GM-CSF [47,48].

On the other hand, adult peripheral blood progenitor-derived cultured mast cells do not significantly respond to TLR stimulation. However, after preincubation with IFN-γ, the expression of TLR4 is up-regulated and that LPS can induce a variety of transcripts in the peripheral blood-derived cultured mast cells. The transcriptome in LPS-stimulated and INF-γ-primed human mast cells are somewhat different from that in anti-IgE-stimulated human mast cells. These LPS-stimulated mast cells produce more TNF-α and RANTES (CXCL5), and produce less IL-5 [49]. Human adult peripheral progenitor-derived mast cells can also produce type I IFNs after exposure to double-stranded RNA via specific interactions with TLR-3, suggesting that mast cells contribute to innate immune responses to viral infection via the production of type I IFNs [50]. Drugs for mast cell-mediated allergic diseases should be targeted for proinflammatory or Th2 inflammation-related molecules without down-regulating innate immunity-related molecules.

Mast Cell-Specific Genes in Airway Tissue Remodeling

Mast cells play an important role not only in immediate hypersensitivity and late phase reactions in the airway but airway remodeling. Bronchial asthma is characterized by airway inflammation, hyperresponsiveness, and remodeling. Airway remodeling is defined as the structural changes in the airways that may affect their functional properties. The structural changes include an increased airway smooth muscle mass, mucus gland hypertrophy, deposition of extracellular matrix components, thickening of the reticular basement membrane, and angiogenesis [51]. Patients with asthma have accelerated loss of lung function over time, and some patients develop progressive fixed airflow obstruction. Although the relationship between remodeling and inflammation has not been fully understood, airway remodeling has been considered to be a consequence of repeated injury and persistent inflammation [51]. However, remodeling processes begin early in the development of asthma and occur in parallel with the establishment of persistent inflammation. Recent reports have demonstrated that persistence of airway hyperresponsiveness is dependent on airway remodeling and not on sustained inflammatory cell recruitment [52–54].

Using microarray technology, Cho and collaborators [55] tried to identify inducible genes in a human mast cell line, HMC-1, activated by phorbol ester and calcium ionophore, finding that expression of the plasminogen activator inhibitor type-1 (PAI-1) was up-regulated. They confirmed by ELISA that activated HMC-1 cells and primary cultured human mast cells secreted PAI-1. PAI-1 inhibits the plasminogen activator converting plasminogen to plasmin, which enhances proteolytic degradation of the extracellular matrix. These results indicated that activated mast cells could play an important role in airway remodeling by secreting PAI-1. Wang et al. [56] and Okumura et al. [57] used oligonucleotide microarrays to examine the up-regulated genes expressed by activated mast cells. These two groups separately identified amphiregulin as a transcript that is markedly increased following aggregation of FcεRI. Amphiregulin induced tissue remodeling, i.e., proliferation of lung fibroblasts and marked induction of MUC5AC transcripts in a human respiratory epithelial cell line. Both groups showed that amphiregulin-positive mast cells were increased in the airways of asthmatics. These investigators employed culture-derived human mast cells for microarray as the first screening and they confirmed the in vivo expression and function of this up-regulated gene. Figure 2 illustrate the typical strategy for identifying a novel steroid-resistant therapeutic target, i.e., amphiregulin in this case, by using microarrays as coincidently employed in the two independent studies [56,57].

Bronchial thermoplasty, which can selectively destroy airway smooth muscles, in subjects with moderate or severe asthma is recently reported to result in an improvement in asthma control [58]. The infiltration of airway smooth muscle by mast cells is associated with the airway hyperresponsiveness in asthma [59]. Tryptase, a highly mast cell-specific molecule is considered to have a potent mitogenic activity [60]. Thus, hypertrophy and hyperplasia of airway smooth muscle cells are now recognized as the most important factors related to airway hyperresponsiveness and the severity of asthma, and that mast cell activation is considered to be involved in the airway smooth muscle cell hypertrophy.

Airway remodeling becomes symptomatic after many years of inflammation and subsequent repairmen and is usually considered to be irreversible. However, most of model experiments that have been reported regarding tissue remodeling are performed at most within a few months and the pathological changes are reversible. In

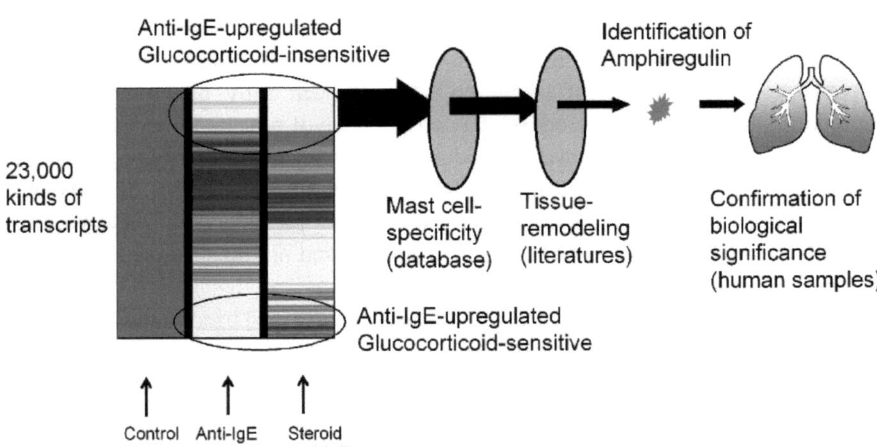

Fig. 2 *The strategy to identify amphiregulin as a glucocorticoid-resistant mast cell-specific molecule.* In [56,57], the authors used GeneChip® (Affymetrix) to find an anti-IgE-upregulated and glucocorticoid-resistant gene cluster. Then, amphiregulin was selected as one of target molecules by filtering with mast cell specificity and descriptions regarding tissue remodeling. Finally, biological significance was confirmed by demonstrating the selected expression in lung mast cells obtained from asthmatics (Adapted from [3])

severe chronic asthma, expression of a gene related to steroid resistance (C/EBPα) in airway smooth muscles is irreversibly and epigenetically down-regulated [61]. Some epigenetic changes such as DNA CpG methylation or histone methylation are considered to be irreversible. An experiment that requires many years does not seem to be practical for the asthma model. Therefore, in the future, it will be required to evaluate whether chromatin remodeling is involve in model experiments related to tissue remodeling.

Conclusions

Regarding mast cell biology and pathogenesis of asthma and allergic diseases, functional genomics such as microarray technology so far provided us the information about comprehensive gene expression profiling and some novel pathogenic mechanisms. This rapidly developing functional genomics soon will provide us the information about the comprehensive role of mast cells in allergic diseases. Someday, we will be able to test a novel drug just by stimulating the personalized mast cells and all other cell types that have an individual genotype and are constructed in silico.

References

1. Saito H, Abe J, Matsumoto K (2005) Allergy-related genes in microarray: an update review. J Allergy Clin Immunol 116:56–59
2. Izuhara K, Saito H (2006) Microarray-based identification of novel biomarkers in asthma. Allergol Int 55:361–367
3. Galli SJ, Nakae S, Tsai M (2005) Mast cells in the development of adaptive immune responses. Nat Immunol 6:135–142
4. Jeffrey KL, Brummer T, Rolph MS, Liu SM, Callejas NA, Grumont RJ, Gillieron C, Mackay F, Grey S, Camps M, Rommel C, Gerondakis SD, Mackay CR (2006) Positive regulation of immune cell function and inflammatory responses by phosphatase PAC-1. Nat Immunol 7:274–283
5. Sayama K, Diehn M, Matsuda K, Lunderius C, Tsai M, Tam SY, Botstein D, Brown PO, Galli SJ (2002) Transcriptional response of human mast cells stimulated via the FcεRI and identification of mast cells as a source of IL-11. BMC Immunol 3:5
6. Jayapal M, Tay HK, Reghunathan R, Zhi L, Chow KK, Rauff M, Melendez AJ (2006) Genome-wide gene expression profiling of human mast cells stimulated by IgE or FceRI-aggregation reveals a complex network of genes involved in inflammatory responses. BMC Genomics 7:210
7. Wiener Z, Kohalmi B, Pocza P, Jeager J, Tolgyesi G, Toth S, Gorbe E, Papp Z, Falus A (2007) TIM-3 is expressed in melanoma cells and is upregulated in TGF-β stimulated mast cells. J Invest Dermatol 127:906–914
8. Kashiwakura J, Yokoi H, Saito H, Okayama Y (2004) T cell proliferation by direct cross-talk between OX40 ligand on human mast cells and OX40 on human T cells: comparison of gene expression profiles between human tonsillar and lung-cultured mast cells. J Immunol 3:5247–5257

9. Nakajima T, Matsumoto K, Suto H, Tanaka K, Ebisawa M, Tomita H, Yuki K, Katsunuma T, Akasawa A, Hashida R, Sugita Y, Ogawa H, Ra C, Saito H (2001) Gene expression screening of human mast cells and eosinophils using high-density oligonucleotide probearrays: abundant expression of major basic protein in mast cells. Blood 98:1127–1134
10. Nakajima T, Inagaki N, Tanaka H, Tanaka A, Yoshikawa M, Tamari M, Hasegawa K, Matsumoto K, Tachimoto H, Ebisawa M, Tsujimoto G, Matsuda H, Nagai H, Saito H (2002) Marked increase in CC chemokine gene expression in both human and mouse mast cell transcriptomes following Fcε receptor I cross-linking: an interspecies comparison. Blood 100:3861–3868
11. Nakajima T, Iikura M, Okayama Y, Matsumoto K, Uchiyama C, Shirakawa T, Yang X, Adra CN, Hirai K, Saito H (2004) Identification of granulocyte subtype-selective receptors and ion channels by using a high-density oligonucleotide probe array. J Allergy Clin Immunol 113:528–535
12. Saito H, Matsumoto K, Okumura S, Kashiwakura JI, Oboki K, Yokoi H, Kambe N, Ohta K, Okayama Y (2006) Gene expression profiling of human mast cell subtypes: an in silico study. Allergol Int 55:173–179
13. Bochner BS (2000) Systemic activation of basophils and eosinophils: markers and consequences. J Allergy Clin Immunol 106:S292–S302
14. Church MK, Pao GJ, Holgate ST (1982) Characterization of histamine secretion from mechanically dispersed human lung mast cells: effects of anti-IgE, calcium ionophore A23187, compound 48/80, and basic polypeptides. J Immunol 129:2116–2121
15. Lin CS, Boltz RC, Blake JT, Nguyen M, Talento A, Fischer PA, Springer MS, Sigal NH, Slaughter RS, Garcia ML (1993) Voltage-gated potassium channels regulate calcium-dependent pathways involved in human T lymphocyte activation. J Exp Med 177:637–645
16. Saito H, Okajima F, Molski TF, Sha'afi RI, Ui M, Ishizaka T (1987) Effects of ADP-ribosylation of GTP-binding protein by pertussis toxin on immunoglobulin E-dependent and -independent histamine release from mast cells and basophils. J Immunol 138:3927–3934
17. Ji TH, Grossmann M, Ji I (1998) G protein-coupled receptors. I. Diversity of receptor-ligand interactions. J Biol Chem 273:17299–17302
18. 8. Zambrowicz BP, Sands AT (2003) Knockouts model the 100 best-selling drugs. Will they model the next 100? Nat Rev Drug Discov 2:38–51
19. Venter JC, Adams MD, Myers EW, Li PW, Mural RJ, Sutton GG, Smith HO, Yandell M, Evans CA, Holt RA, Gocayne JD, Amanatides P, et al. (2001) The sequence of the human genome. Science 291:1304–1351
20. Drews J (2000) Drug discovery: a historical perspective. Science 287:1960–1964
21. Saito H, Ebisawa M, Tachimoto H, Shichijo M, Fukagawa K, Matsumoto K, Iikura Y, Awaji T, Tsujimoto G, Takahashi G, Yanagida M, Uzumaki H, Tsuji K, Nakahata T (1996) Selective growth of human mast cells induced by Steel factor, interleukin 6 and prostaglandin E_2 from cord blood mononuclear cells. J Immunol 157:343–350
22. Ahn K, Takai S, Pawankar R, Kuramasu A, Ohtsu H, Kempuraj D, Tomita H, Matsumoto K, Akasawa A, Miyazaki M, Saito H (2000) Regulation of chymase production in human mast cell progenitors. J Allergy Clin Immunol 106:321–328
23. Saito H, Kato A, Matsumoto K, Okayama Y (2006) Culture of human mast cells from peripheral blood progenitors. Nat Protoc 1:2178–2183
24. Iida M, Matsumoto K, Tomita H, Nakajima T, Akasawa A, Ohtani NY, Yoshida NL, Matsui K, Nakada A, Sugita Y, Shimizu Y, Wakahara S, Nakao T, Fujii Y, Ra C, Saito H (2001) Selective down-regulation of high affinity IgE receptor (FcεRI) α-chain messenger RNA among transcriptome in cord blood-derived versus adult peripheral blood-derived cultured human mast cells. Blood 97:1016–1022
25. Debili N, Robin C, Schiavon V, Letestu R, Pflumio F, Mitjavila-Garcia MT, Coulombel L, Vainchenker W (2001) Different expression of CD41 on human lymphoid and myeloid progenitors from adults and neonates. Blood 97:2023–2030
26. Bracho F, van de Ven C, Areman E, Hughes RM, Davenport V, Bradley MB, Cai JW, Cairo MS (2003) A comparison of ex vivo expanded DCs derived from cord blood and mobilized

adult peripheral blood plastic-adherent mononuclear cells: decreased alloreactivity of cord blood DCs. Cytotherapy 5:349–361
27. Tedla N, Wang HW, McNeil HP, Di Girolamo N, Hampartzoumian T, Wakefield D, Lloyd A (1998) Regulation of T lymphocyte trafficking into lymph nodes during an immune response by the chemokines macrophage inflammatory protein (MIP)-1α and MIP-1β. J Immunol 161:5663–5672
28. McLachlan JB, Hart JP, Pizzo SV, Shelburne CP, Staats HF, Gunn MD, Abraham SN (2003) Mast cell-derived tumor necrosis factor induces hypertrophy of draining lymph nodes during infection. Nat Immunol 4:1199–1205
29. Irani AM, Bradford TR, Kepley CL, Schechter NM, Schwartz LB (1989) Detection of MC_T and MC_{TC} types of human mast cells by immunohistochemistry using new monoclonal anti-tryptase and anti-chymase antibodies. J Histochem Cytochem 37:1509–1515
30. Kambe N, Kambe M, Kochan JP, Schwartz LB (2001) Human skin-derived mast cells can proliferate while retaining their characteristic functional and protease phenotypes. Blood 97:2045–2052
31. Jippo T, Lee YM, Ge Y, Kim DK, Okabe M, Kitamura Y (2001) Tissue-dependent alteration of protease expression phenotype in murine peritoneal mast cells that were genetically labeled with green fluorescent protein. Am J Pathol 158:1695–1701
32. Borish L, Steinke JW (2004) Beyond transcription factor. Allergy Clin Immunol Int 16:2–27
33. Bradding P, Okayama Y, Kambe N, Saito H (2003) Ion channel gene expression in human lung, skin and cord blood-derived mast cells. J Leukoc Biol 73:614–620
34. Gordon JR, Galli SJ (1990) Mast cells as a source of both preformed and immunologically inducible TNF-α/cachectin. Nature 346:274–276
35. Okayama Y, Kobayashi H, Ashman LK, Dobashi K, Nakazawa T, Holgate ST, Church MK, Mori M (1998) Human lung mast cells are enriched in the capacity to produce granulocyte-macrophage colony-stimulating factor in response to IgE-dependent stimulation. Eur J Immunol 28:708–715
36. Burd PR, Rogers HW, Gordon JR, Martin CA, Jayaraman S, Wilson SD, Dvorak AM, Galli SJ, Dorf ME (1989) Interleukin 3-dependent and -independent mast cells stimulated with IgE and antigen express multiple cytokines. J Exp Med 170:245–257
37. Baghestanian M, Hofbauer R, Kiener HP, Bankl HC, Wimazal F, Willheim M, Scheiner O, Fureder W, Muller MR, Bevec D, Lechner K, Valent P (1997) The c-kit ligand stem cell factor and anti-IgE promote expression of monocytes chemoattractant protein-1 in human lung mast cells. Blood 90:4438–4449
38. Lorentz A, Schwengberg S, Sellge G, Manns MP, Bischoff SC (2000) Human intestinal mast cells are capable of producing different cytokine profiles: role of IgE receptor cross-linking and IL-4. J Immunol 164:43–48
39. Bradding P, Feather IH, Wilson S, Bardin PG, Heusser CH, Holgate ST, Howarth PH (1993) Immunolocalization of cytokines in the nasal mucosa of normal and perennial rhinitic subjects. The mast cell as a source of IL-4, IL-5, and IL-6 in human allergic mucosal inflammation. J Immunol 151:3853–3865
40. Jaffe JS, Glaum MC, Raible DG, Post TJ, Dimitry E, Govindarao D, Wang Y, Schulman ES (1995) Human lung mast cell IL-5 gene and protein expression: temporal analysis of upregulation following IgE-mediated activation. Am J Respir Cell Mol Biol 13:665–675
41. Ishizuka T, Okayama Y, Kobayashi H, Mori M (1999) Interleukin-10 is localized to and released by human lung mast cells. Clin Exp Allergy 29:1424–1432
42. Toru H, Pawankar R, Ra C, Yata J, Nakahata T (1998) Human mast cells produce IL-13 by highaffinity IgE receptor cross-linking: enhanced IL-13 production by IL-4-primed human mast cells. J Allergy Clin Immunol 102:491–502
43. Takeda K, Kaisho T, Akira S (2003) Toll-like receptors. Annu Rev Immunol 21:335–376
44. Supajatura V, Ushio H, Nakao A, Okumura K, Ra C, Ogawa H (2001) Protective roles of mast cells against enterobacterial infection are mediated by Toll-like receptor 4. J Immunol 167:2250–2256

45. Masuda A, Yoshikai Y, Aiba K, Matsuguchi T (2002) Th2 cytokine production from mast cells is directly induced by lipopolysaccharide and distinctly regulated by c-Jun N-terminal kinase and p38 pathways. J Immunol 169:3801–3810
46. Supajatura V, Ushio H, Nakao A, Akira S, Okumura K, Ra C, Ogawa H (2002) Differential responses of mast cell Toll-like receptors 2 and 4 in allergy and innate immunity. J Clin Invest 109:1351–1359
47. McCurdy JD, Olynych TJ, Maher LH, Marshall JS (2003) Cutting edge: distinct Toll-like receptor 2 activators selectively induce different classes of mediator production from human mast cells. J Immunol 170:1625–1629
48. Varadaradjalou S, Feger F, Thieblemont N, Hamouda NB, Pleau JM, Dy M, Arock M (2003) Toll-like receptor 2 (TLR2) and TLR4 differentially activate human mast cells. Eur J Immunol 33:899–906
49. Okumura S, Kashiwakura J, Tomita H, Matsumoto K, Nakajima T, Saito H, Okayama Y (2003) Identification of specific gene expression profiles in human mast cells mediated by Toll-like receptor 4 and FcεRI. Blood 102:2547–2554
50. Kulka M, Alexopoulou L, Flavell RA, Metcalfe DD (2004) Activation of mast cells by double-stranded RNA: evidence for activation through Toll-like receptor 3. J Allergy Clin Immunol 114:174–182
51. Busse W, Elias J, Sheppard D, Banks-Schlegel S (1999) Airway remodeling and repair. Am J Respir Crit Care Med 160:1035–1042
52. Holgate ST, Holloway J, Wilson S, Bucchieri F, Puddicombe S, Davies DE (2004) Epithelial-mesenchymal communication in the pathogenesis of chronic asthma. Proc Am Thorac Soc 1:93–98
53. Kariyawasam HH, Aizen M, Barkans J, Robinson DS, Kay AB (2007) Remodeling and airway hyperresponsiveness but not cellular inflammation persist after allergen challenge in asthma. Am J Respir Crit Care Med 175:896–904
54. Southam DS, Ellis R, Wattie J, Inman MD (2007) Components of airway hyperresponsiveness and their associations with inflammation and remodeling in mice. J Allergy Clin Immunol 119:848–854
55. Cho SH, Tam SW, Demissie-Sanders S, Filler SA, Oh CK (2000) Production of plasminogen activator inhibitor-1 by human mast cells and its possible role in asthma. J Immunol 165:3154–3161
56. Wang SW, Oh CK, Cho SH, Hu G, Martin R, Demissie-Sanders S, Li K, Moyle M, Yao Z (2005) Amphiregulin expression in human mast cells and its effect on the primary human lung fibroblasts. J Allergy Clin Immunol 115:287–294
57. Okumura S, Sagara H, Fukuda T, Saito H, Okayama Y (2005) FcεRI-mediated amphiregulin production by human mast cells increases mucin gene expression in epithelial cells. J Allergy Clin Immunol 115:272–279
58. Cox G, Thomson NC, Rubin AS, Niven RM, Corris PA, Siersted HC, Olivenstein R, Pavord ID, McCormack D, Chaudhuri R, Miller JD, Laviolette M, AIR Trial Study Group (2007) Asthma control during the year after bronchial thermoplasty. N Engl J Med 356:1327–1337
59. Brightling CE, Bradding P, Symon FA, Holgate ST, Wardlaw AJ, Pavord ID (2002) Mast-cell infiltration of airway smooth muscle in asthma. N Engl J Med 346:1699–1705
60. Brown JK, Jones CA, Rooney LA, Caughey GH (2001) Mast cell tryptase activates extracellular-regulated kinases (p44/p42) in airway smooth-muscle cells: importance of proteolytic events, time course, and role in mediating mitogenesis. Am J Respir Cell Mol Biol 24:146–154
61. Roth M, Johnson PR, Borger P, Bihl MP, Rudiger JJ, King GG, Ge Q, Hostettler K, Burgess JK, Black JL, Tamm M (2004) Dysfunctional interaction of C/EBPα and the glucocorticoid receptor in asthmatic bronchial smooth-muscle cells. N Engl J Med 351:560–574

Neuropeptide S Receptor 1: an Asthma Susceptibility Gene

Juha Kere

Introduction

Asthma is a complex disorder, and there is no single biochemical or clinical feature that would allow one to set the diagnosis unequivocally. It is also a disease that can have its onset at different ages, and often there is a period of increasing symptoms before the diagnosis is set. Asthma occurs in different degrees of severity, and it may co-occur with other distinct but related atopic disorders. All these disorders are characterized by the body's response to environmental irritants, but they also tend to run in families. Therefore, asthma is naturally viewed as a disorder with both environmental and hereditary determinants. We know more or less about what the external irritants are that the body responds to; but until recently we have been completely ignorant about the specific genes that affect an individual's risk of developing asthma. For some time, however, we have known that the genetic effect on the risk is large, perhaps even stronger than the combined environmental effects [1].

The accumulation of knowledge about human genes, the human genome structure, genetic variation at the population level, and concomitant development of technology to apply this information to studying diseases have recently allowed us to outline a draft picture of the genetics of asthma and other atopic disorders. The picture is by no means complete, and we cannot claim to know all the genes that have a somewhat important role in influencing risk for asthma. New genes are likely to emerge in the coming years, most likely from efforts that are based on genetic association studies on combined, large patient and control cohorts, collected from many countries, that are studied using hundreds of thousands of single-nucleotide polymorphisms (SNPs). There are already strong signs that such studies can identify genes

J. Kere
Department of Biosciences and Nutrition, Karolinska Institutet, Hälsovägen 7, 14157 Huddinge, Sweden;
Clinical Research Centre, Karolinska University Hospital Huddinge, Huddinge, Sweden;
Department of Medical Genetics, Biomedicum, University of Helsinki, Haartmaninkatu 8, 00014 Helsinki, Finland
e-mail: juha.kere@biosci.ki.se

R. Pawankar et al. (eds.), *Allergy Frontiers: Future Perspectives*,
DOI 10.1007/978-4-431-99365-0_12, © Springer 2010

Table 1 Synonymous names for the new G protein-coupled receptor on chromosome 7p. HGNC, Human Gene Nomenclature Committee (www.gene.ucl.ac.uk/nomenclature/)

Name	Explanation	Reference
GPRA	G Protein-coupled Receptor in Asthma	[13]
PGR14	Previously not described GPCR number 14	[15]
VRR1	Vasopressin-Related Receptor 1	[16]
GPR154	G Protein-coupled Receptor, number 154	HGNC
NPSR	Neuropeptide S Receptor	[17]
NPSR1	Neuropeptide S Receptor 1	HGNC

not previously identified by candidate gene studies or genome-wide linkage scans and positional cloning projects [2].

Nevertheless, work completed in the past decade has revealed to us several genes that are likely to essentially contribute to the genetic risk of asthma in a proportion of individuals, and perhaps influence the pathogenesis of asthma even more commonly [3,4]. The purpose of this review is to summarize work that led to the identification of one of these genes, and present further work that has been undertaken to understand the mechanisms and role of this gene in the pathogenesis of asthma. To complicate matters, at least half a dozen of synonymous names have been used for this gene (Table 1). In this review, I will use systematically the currently approved symbol for the gene, neuropeptide S receptor 1 (NPSR1), unless other nomenclature is required by the context.

Genetic Mapping of an Asthma Susceptibility Locus to Chromosome 7p14–p15

The Kainuu Asthma Project started in 1994 by recruitment of individuals with asthma and family members from Kainuu, a rural area of Finland that to geneticists was known as a prototype founder subpopulation. The concept includes a small number of founders, little later immigration, little admixture with neighbors, relatively rapid recent growth, and consequent large effect of a small number of alleles that the founding individuals had brought with them [5,6]. The motivation for starting a study in such a population was the expected simplified genetic architecture of any disease prevalent in the population, hopefully reducing both locus heterogeneity and narrowing the allelic spectrum [7]. Such hopes were supported by previous studies of recessive monogenic disorders in the same geographic region [5,6]. We carefully ascertained the patients using three primary inclusion criteria: (a) asthma had been already verified by a physician, (b) asthma had also been diagnosed in additional family members, and (c) at least the parents had been born in the geographic region (for most families, even the grandparents could be verified to originate from the same region). All diagnoses and family structures were verified from hospital and population registries, respectively [8,9].

Selecting the most informative families for a genetic linkage study (86 pedigrees including 443 individuals), we obtained evidence for a significantly linked locus on chromosome 7p [10]. We replicated the linkage finding in two additional cohorts of families, one ascertained for asthma from the Saguenay-Lac-St-Jean region of Northeastern Quebec, Canada, and another selected on the basis of high serum IgE values from a population based clinical trial conducted in North Karelia, Finland. All three family cohorts showed evidence for linkage that exceeded the genome-wide significance threshold for high serum IgE values in the original Kainuu population sample and nominal significance for both replication sets for either asthma or high serum IgE phenotype. The results suggested an approximately 20 cM genomic region as the likely susceptibility gene position. Linkage to the same region on chromosome 7p had been previously suggested by the first genome-wide linkage scan in asthma [11]. Even though the T cell receptor gamma gene (TCRG) was an attractive positional candidate gene, it failed to show genetic associations to asthma in the mapping cohort [12]

Molecular Cloning of NPSR1

A new gene was identified within a narrow time window by more than one group of investigators. All groups worked on the gene from completely different starting points, and thus only our group was involved in a project of positionally cloning a gene affecting asthma susceptibility. Our approach also implicated that we had no *a priori* idea what kind of a gene we were searching for.

After the initial genetic mapping [10], we genotyped 76 additional microsatellite markers within the peak of 20 cM [13]. We then applied the Haplotype Pattern Mining (HPM) analysis, developed for the purpose of genetic fine-mapping of disease loci under the hypothesis of common founder shared by an excess of patients; the significance of associations was tested by a permutation test [14]. The result suggested that one microsatellite marker and a pattern of markers flanking it were significantly associated with the high IgE phenotype. To exclude or support the identity-by-descent of the pattern-sharing chromosomes, we genotyped additional markers. A repeated HPM analysis suggested that the pattern prevailed and was supported also by newly typed markers, a finding that would be unlikely if the chromosomes were not identical by descent. Moreover, more shared chromosomes with a shorter shared pattern were detected, focusing the interest to a 300 kb segment. Finally, to test for identity-by-descent of a haplotype pattern that occurred in significant excess ($p<0.01$ by permutation, 0.00001 by uncorrected chi-square calculation) among subjects with high IgE values, we selected a patient homozygous for the "risk" haplotype. Sequencing of the nonrepetitive segments over 130 kb revealed no instance of heterozygosity, whereas the sequence differed from the published genomic sequence for altogether 80 SNPs or deletion/insertion polymorphisms (DIPs). More SNPs were discovered by sequencing six additional homozygous DNA samples with different haplotype patterns [13].

We next identified genes within the implicated segment by a combination of ab initio predictions and reverse-transcriptase polymerase chain reaction (RT-PCR) verification of exons. We found one protein-coding gene (GPRA, NPSR1) and one without long ORFs (AAA1); the genomic structure and protein model of NPSR1 are shown in Fig. 1. Variation within the gene included one coding polymorphism, Asn107Ile, in the first extracellular loop of the predicted protein. Subsequent experiments, including Western blot and immunohistochemical analyses with polyclonal rabbit antibodies verified NPSR1 as a protein-coding gene with two main isoforms that we named GPRA-A and GPRA-B (now called NPSR1-A and NPSR1-B, respectively). Further analyses employing the French Canadian and North Karelian Finnish sample sets supported the association of SNPs with asthma or high IgE in all three populations, consistent with the common susceptibility allele hypothesis (the best p-value 0.004 for a single SNP in three populations combined, all contributing) [13].

The NPSR1-A isoform, referred to as PGR14, had also been identified by Vassilatis et al. [15]. They performed a systematic survey of genomic sequences similar to G protein coupled receptors (GPCRs) for endogenous ligands, and identified altogether 367 GPCRs in human, 26 of them new (including PGR14). PGR14 was listed as a new GPCR as an orphan receptor in the class A vasopressin family.

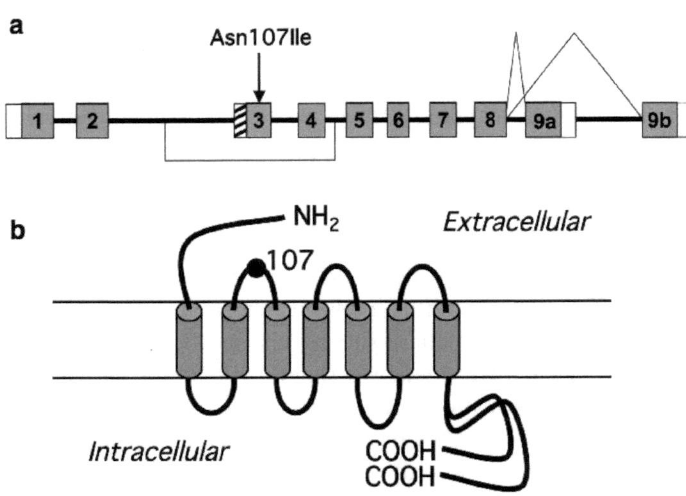

Fig. 1 The genomic structure and a protein threading model of NPSR1. (**a**) The numbered exons of NPSR1 are depicted as gray boxes and untranslated regions are shown as *white boxes*. The position of Asn107Ile polymorphism is indicated, and there are alternative splice sites 5' of exon 3 (*striped box*). The alternative splicing of exons 9a and 9b is shown with thin lines. The approximate position of asthma-associated haplotype block is indicated with a square bracket around exons 3 and 4 (modified from [13]). (**b**) NPSR1 protein is a typical seven-transmembrane segment GPCR. The position of polymorphic amino acid 107 is indicated as a *black dot*. The two isoforms with alternative C-terminal tails are depicted

Gupte et al. [16] identified the same new GPCR, referring to it as vasopressin-related receptor 1 (VRR1). VRR1 was identical to NPSR1-A. According to their results, VRR1 was expressed only in the hypothalamus and retina, and thus there was no suggestion for any role for the new gene in asthma. Gupte et al. further constructed a chimeric receptor by joining the intracellular signaling part of the vasopressin V1a receptor, including all intracellular loops, to the C terminal segment of VRR1. This chimeric receptor was activated by arginine vasopressin, but not by vasopressin or oxytocin. They showed that VRR1 had dual signaling properties and coupled to both Gq and Gs pathways.

Neuropeptide S, a Ligand for NPSR1 with a Role in Brain Functions

Gupte et al. [16] reported a ligand to stimulate the native NPSR1-A. The ligand, a newly identified linear peptide, induced both adenylase cyclase accumulation and intracellular calcium mobilization in a dose-dependent manner [16]. The gene for the polypeptide, translated as a still poorly characterized precursor (not annotated in current MapViewer, www.ncbi.nlm.nih.gov/mapview), maps to human chromosome 10q26 and is conserved in mammals.

The name for Neuropeptide S (NPS) was coined by Xu et al. [17] who referred to the same peptide as Gupte et al. [16]. They also reported the same receptor that was identical to NPSR1-A, named as NPSR in their paper. Xu et al. characterized extensively the expression of both Nps and Npsr1 in 45 types of rat tissues, finding in general highest expression in specific areas of the brain, glandular organs, such as salivary, mammary and thyroid glands, and testis, and low put present in the stomach, duodenum, heart, aorta, thymus, and lungs. They used a radiolabelled NPS and stably NPSR-transfected chinese hamster ovary (CHO) and human embryonic kidney 293 cell lines to measure intracellular Ca^{2+} levels as marker of Gq protein coupling, concluding that NPS-NPSR signaling has high potency and specificity. Injection of NPS in the brain ventricles of mice increased their locomotor activity, and in open-field, light-dark box, elevated plus maze and marble burying tests they exhibited NPS dose-dependent reduction of anxiety as compared to control mice. Electroencephalogram recordings on rats injected with NPS revealed increased wakefulness [17].

Beck et al. [18] expanded the study of NPS effects injected in brains of rats. Injection of 1 ug or 10 ug of NPS in the lateral ventricle caused rats to consume >50% less chow than controls after overnight fasting. Comparison to the effects of corticotropin-releasing hormone or Neuropeptide Y (NPY) and measurements of ghrelin, insulin and leptin suggested that NPS acts independent of these known pathways regulating appetite. The authors suggested NPS agonists as a new treatment for obesity.

Taken together, these results demonstrated that NPS, acting through NPSR1, was a new, potent neuropeptide, with central pharmacological effects inducing locomotion, arousal, anxiety and anorexia in rodents. Expression pattern in rats suggested that brain is a major organ for this new pathway, but many other organs, including glands, might possibly use this pathway as well. In rats, only low expression levels were observed in the lungs, but the resolution did not allow the researchers to comment on epithelial glands present in airways.

Two NPSR1 Isoforms in Human but Not in Rodents

Remarkably, all investigations performed in rodents have failed to detect the alternative exon 9b (Fig. 1) that characterized in human the NPSR1-B isoform, detected by specific antibodies in the bronchial and intestinal epithelia and asthmatic smooth muscle [13]. Vendelin et al. [19] studied alternative transcription in a human bronchoalveolar carcinoma cell line (NCI-H358), and confirmed the presence of both A and B transcripts. The predicted translocation of both A and B isoforms to cell membrane was verified using transient transfections of tagged constructs in COS-1 cells. Using in situ hybridization, Vendelin et al. also verified the presence of low levels of NPS transcripts in bronchial epithelial cells and more abundant expression in the colon in humans. A screening of 30 human tissues by in situ hybridization detected NPSR1 mRNA in many human submucosal or glandular epithelial organs. Immunohistochemical verification of the same tissues suggested preferentially the presence of NPSR1-B, rather than the A isoform in these tissues, although most often both were positive. This observation was also made in several human cell lines. Finally, the signaling effect of NPS through NPSR1-A was confirmed using stably transfected HEK293H cells and GTP binding assays, and the results suggested that NPS stimulation of NPSR1-transfected cells slowed down their growth [19].

Signaling Properties of Neuropeptide S

NPSR1 had been found to have two main isoforms, NPSR1-A and B, and NPSR1-B was differentially expressed in bronchial epithelial cells and smooth muscle cells from asthmatic individuals in comparison to healthy controls [13]. The consistency of this finding in several samples suggested that altered isoform balance might be a common characteristic of asthma, and therefore it was useful to understand their functional differences.

Two groups have characterized in detail the pharmacologic and signaling properties of NPS and NPSR1 protein variants. Reinscheid et al. [20] engineered stable cell lines both for the Asn107 and Ile107 variants as well as both the NPSR1-A and -B isoforms. They found that the Ile107 variant of human NPSR1-A (NPSR1-A*Ile107) had an increased agonist potency compared to the Asn107 variant (as assayed by mobilization of intracellular Ca^{2+}, stimulation of cAMP formation or induction of MAPK phosphorylation), but did not change the binding affinity of

NPS or the constitutive receptor activity. Mouse Npsr1, mimicking in structure human NPSR1-A*Ile107, displayed an intermediate pharmacological profile. The NPSR1-B*Asn107 variant showed a pharmacological profile similar to NPSR1-A*Asn107, whereas our results have suggested differences in the signaling by NPSR1-A and -B [19]. Reinscheid et al. found that the N-terminus of NPS was critical for NPSR1 activation and concluded that the approximately tenfold enhanced signaling potency of the Ile107 isoform of NPSR1 might have physiological significance [20].

The critical residues for NPS activity were mapped by Roth et al. [21]. Their results indicated that the first ten residues of NPS maintained a similar level of agonist potency as the full 20-mer. Amino acids 2–4 (Phe-Arg-Asn) were crucial for biological activity, and residues 8–10 (Thr-Gly-Met) were needed for receptor activation, and positions 6–7 (Val-Gly) acted as a hinge between the two domains. However, for in vitro activity, the C-terminal part of the peptide may influence the stability of NPS or other critical properties, as NPS(1–10) injected to cerebral ventricles in mice did not yield similar effect as the full-length peptide on locomotory stimulation.

Replication of NPSR1 Associations to Asthma and Allergic Disorders

The positional cloning of NPSR1 as an asthma susceptibility gene and the very different route of discovery of NPS as a mood-modifying effector appeared puzzling. Therefore, it has been essential to seek replication of the genetic association in independent cohorts of patients with asthma or allergic symptoms. Presently, five replication studies have been published (Table 2) that confirm a moderate but consistent genetic effect of NPSR1 alleles or haplotypes on asthma and allergic disorders.

The first replication study, performed on a cohort of Korean patients used only one SNP, and failed to detect association [22]. All subsequent studies, however,

Table 2 Published replication studies of NPSR1 associations to asthma and allergic diseases. BHR, bronchial hyperrectivity. In studies where different phenotypes were considered, the number of patients for the largest subcohort is shown (Nr. of cases)

Population, reference	Nr. of cases	Nr. of SNPs	Best OR or p value, phenotype
Korea, adults [22]	439	1	none
5 European countries, children [23]	1087	7	OR = 1.47, allergic asthma
Germany, children [24]	671	6	OR = 3.5, asthma + BHR
China, mixed [25]	715	8	OR = 0.61 (protective haplotype)
Italy, mixed [26]	511	7	p = 0.008, high IgE
European Americans, children	497	26	p = 0.0006, asthma
Puerto Rico, children [27]	439		p = 0.003, asthma

using larger cohorts of patients and controls and 6–8 SNPs to assess haplotype structure within the gene, have detected genetic associations to different asthmatic or atopic subphenotypes. The studies of Melén et al. [23] and Kormann et al. [24] expanded the finding by detecting associations to asthmatic disorders in children. A study of patients of different ages in China used different SNPs than previous studies to assess variation, and found significant protective effect for some NPSR1 variants [25]. It should be emphasized that a genetic effect may be expressed in either direction, and often the convenient direction depends on the frequency of the associating variant in a particular population. In Italian populations, Malerba et al. [26] confirmed linkage of elevated IgE, asthma and atopy to chromosome 7p in 119 families and subsequently verified associations to NPSR1 SNPs and haplotypes. Finally, Hersh et al. [27] studied family-based samples collected from European Americans and another designated Hispanic from Puerto Rico. In both sample sets independently, NPSR1 SNPs associated significantly with asthma. Of interest in both the Malerba and Hersh studies [26,27], the opposite direction of associations in two subsets of families with possibly different environmental exposures suggested that either environmental factors or epistasis with another gene might play a role in modifying the genetic effects of NPSR1.

Recently, we have revisited the PARSIFAL cohort studied earlier by Melén et al. for genetic association of NPSR1 [23]. The PARSIFAL study (Prevention of Allergy Risk factors for Sensitisation In children related to Farming and Anthroposophic Lifestyle) is a cross-sectional study designed to investigate the role of lifestyle and environmental exposures in farm children, children from Steiner schools (who often have an anthroposophic lifestyle) and their reference groups in five European countries [28]. The results suggested that there was an interaction between current regular contact to farm animals and several NPSR1 SNPs, and the effect seemed to depend on the timing of the start of exposure. Bruce et al. also found that monocyte levels of NPSR1-A protein as well as mRNA were upregulated in response to lipopolysaccharide (LPS) exposure in vitro [Bruce S, Nyberg F, Melén E, James A, Pulkkinen V, Orsmark-Pietras C, Bergström A, Dahlén B, Wickman M, von Mutius E, Doekes G, Lauener R, Riedler J, Eder W, van Hage M, Pershagen G, Scheynius A, Kere J, unpublished observations].

These results conform well with epidemiological studies that have found a lower prevalence of IgE-mediated allergic disease among children living on farms [28–31], and with experimental studies on the NPS-NPSR1 pathway and its immune-modifying effects [32]. The protective effects of farm living have been correlated with contact to farm animals and farm milk consumption [33,34], with exposure to endotoxins or moulds as a possible explanation at the molecular level [35,36].

The NPS—NPSR1 Pathway in Immune System Cells

Pulkkinen et al. [32] extended the study of NPSR1 into human immune system cells. Of human blood and sputum cell types, monocyte/macrophages, eosinophils and CD4+ T cells express relatively high levels of NPSR1. Activation of peripheral blood cells with lipopolysaccharide (LPS) resulted in increased NPS and NPSR1 expression in monocytes. Similar increase was not observed if T cells were activated by anti-CD3/CD28 antibodies. NPS treatment of a mouse macrophage cell line stimulated phagocytosis of Escherichia coli in a dose-dependent manner. The results suggested that the NPS—NPSR1 pathway is active in macrophages and that phagocytosis of unopsonized bacteria can be modified by stimulation of the pathway [32].

So far, no studies are available that would consider the possible different effects of different NPSR1 coding variants or haplotype variants directly on such biological functions, and indeed, the possible regulatory effects of intronic SNPs remain uncharted. Such studies require relatively large sample sets in order to identify sufficient numbers of individuals representing different combinations of the putative risk-increasing and protective haplotypes.

Target Genes of NPS—NPSR1 Signaling

The identification of the NPS—NPSR1 pathway and its signaling mechanisms did not suggest any likely downstream targets of the pathway. To identify which genes would be modulated by NPS stimulation of NPSR1, Vendelin et al. [37] engineered HEK-293H cell lines stably overexpressing NPSR1-A*Asn107. By monitoring the expression of 47,000 transcripts on Affymetrix arrays, Vendelin et al. found 104 genes that were significantly upregulated and 42 that were downregulated by NPS—NPSR1 signaling. A Gene Ontology enrichment analysis indicated that the regulated genes most often fell in the categories "cell proliferation", "morphogenesis" and "immune response". Among the upregulated genes, all those tested, namely matrix metalloproteinase 10 (MMP10), activin A (INHBA), interleukin 8 (IL8) and ephrin receptor A2 (EPHA2) displayed a significant NPS dose–response regulatory relationship [37]. Table 3 lists some of the genes regulated by NPS—NPSR1 signaling that are of interest for the pathogenesis of asthma.

These results suggested a first set of NPS—NPSR1 regulated genes. It will be necessary to extend these findings in other cell types, especially neurons that constitutively express high levels of the pathway components and that may have quite a different transcriptional regulatory environment. Interestingly, the list of regulated genes includes many of relevance for neuronal cells (Table 3, [37]). Any such studies will be further facilitated by the availability of specific synthetic agonist and antagonist compounds.

NPSR1 Knockout Mice

At least two distinct knockout strains of mice have been engineered. In a carefully planned and thorough study, Allen et al. [38] failed to detect significant NPSR1/Npsr1 expression in human or mouse lungs (a signal was obtained after 35–36 cycles of PCR). Among many respiratory parameters monitored, Npsr1 deficient

Table 3 A partial list of genes regulated by the NPS–NPSR1 pathway. Listed here are genes subjectively judged to be of interest for asthma pathogenesis. The genes are listed according to the magnitude of the regulatory effect (24-fold for CGA, fourfold for BMP2). Adapted from Vendelin et al. [37]; for a complete list of genes, please refer to the original study

Gene symbol	Systematic name
CGA	Glycoprotein hormones, alpha polypeptide
SV2C	Synaptic vesicle glycoprotein 2C
TFPI2	Tissue factor pathway inhibitor 2
EGR3	Early growth response 3
INHBA	Inhibin, beta A (activin A, activin AB alpha polypeptide)
ARC	Activity-regulated cytoskeleton-associated protein
MMP10	Matrix metalloproteinase 10 (stromelysin 2)
NR4A1	Nuclear receptor subfamily 4, group A, member 1
FOS	v-fos FBJ murine osteosarcoma viral oncogene homolog
EGR2	Early growth response 2 (Krox-20 homolog, Drosophila)
AREG	Amphiregulin (schwannoma-derived growth factor)
CTGF	Connective tissue growth factor
EGR1	Early growth response 1
TAC1	Tachykinin, precursor
SERPINB2	Serine (or cysteine) proteinase inhibitor, clade B, member 2
GLIPR1	GLI pathogenesis-related 1 (glioma)
NR4A3	Nuclear receptor subfamily 4, group A, member 3
FOSL1	FOS-like antigen 1
CYR61	Cysteine-rich, angiogenic inducer, 61
TNC	Tenascin C (hexabrachion)
FOSB	FBJ murine osteosarcoma viral oncogene homolog B
RGC32	Response gene to complement 32
IL6R	Interleukin 6 receptor
DUSP1	Dual specificity phosphatase 1
NR4A2	Nuclear receptor subfamily 4, group A, member 2
SERPINE2	Serine (or cysteine) proteinase inhibitor, clade E (nexin, plasminogen activator inhibitor type 1), member 2
BMP2	Bone morphogenetic protein 2

mice showed as the only consistent effect an attenuated response to thromboxane, a bronchoconstricting agent dependent on the cholinergic receptor. The authors suggested that Npsr1 might contribute to the asthma phenotype by altering the activity of neurally mediated mechanisms or other pathways. They suggest that the high expression of NPSR1 in the nervous system might influence the tone of the airway smooth muscle or the response to external stimuli [38]. Expression of NPSR1 in neural cells in the airways might dramatically impact the pathogenesis of asthma, in particular bronchial hyperreactivity [38].

The laboratory of Dr. Harri Alenius (Institute of Occupational Health, Helsinki, Finland) in collaboration with our group has studied a different strain of Npsr1 knockout mouse. Our results largely support the observation that in mouse, the Nps—Npsr1 pathway components are mostly expressed in the brain (unpublished).

There appear to be important species differences between human and mouse in this respect. Of note, mouse lacks the alternative exon 9b that gives rise to the NPSR1-B isoform in human (Fig. 1), and a possibly highly relevant difference between human and mouse involves the expression of NPSR1/Npsr1 in immune system cells [32]. It has been pointed out that the value of short-term mouse models of asthma may be limited, because such models often do not reproduce many features of human asthma, such as infiltration of epithelia with inflammatory cells, tissue remodeling and sustained bronchial hyperreactivity [39].

Is NPSR1 a Susceptibility Gene for Other Disorders?

Asthma is comorbid not only with a large number of partially overlapping atopic and allergic disorders, but also other, more distinct diseases. For example, in a large study investigating a cohort of over 2,00,000 babies, respiratory distress syndrome (RDS) or transient tachypnoea of the newborn associated with an increased risk of later hospital admission with a diagnosis of asthma with a hazard ratio of 1.7 (95% confidence interval, 95% CI = 1.4–2.2) [40]. Indeed, in a case-control study of 176 preterm babies with RDS, some of the same NPSR1 haplotypes associated with an increased risk (H4/H5) of RDS for babies born at 32–35 weeks of gestation [41]. This results warrants further confirmation.

Inflammatory bowel disease (IBD), comprising Crohn disease and ulcerative colitis, was recently found to increase risk for asthma in a large population-based study of over 8,000 cases of IBD [42]. Both types of IBD patients had a significantly greater frequency of extraintestinal inflammatory diseases than population controls, and asthma was the most common comorbidity increased in Crohn disease patients (prevalence ratio = 1.34, 95% CI = 1.24–1.46). We undertook a study of NPSR1 risk effects in IBD among over 2,400 subjects from Italy, Sweden, and Finland, and found by global analysis of the whole dataset a significant association. Furthermore, the risk-increasing NPSR1 haplotype correlated with higher expression of NPSR1 mRNA in the inflamed gut [43].

On the other hand, even though atopic dermatitis associates with asthma (ratio of proportion, RP = 1.45, 95% CI 1.16–1.80) and allergic rhinoconjunctivitis (RP=2.25, CI 1.77–2.85) [44], NPSR1 SNPs do not appear to associate with atopic dermatitis [45,46].

Asthma and psychiatric disorders such as panic disorder are not infrequently comorbid. In a recent large prospective community-based follow-up study of 591 young adults, asthma and panic disorder were cross-sectionally significantly associated with an odds ratio (OR) of 4.0 (CI = 1.7–9.3). Asthma predicted subsequent panic disorder (OR = 4.5, 95% CI = 1.1–20) and panic disorder predicted asthma (OR = 6.3; 95% CI = 2.8–14) [47]. Another large study of over 3,000 adults [48] indicated that self-reported respiratory disease (asthma, chronic bronchitis, or emphysema) was associated with a significantly increased likelihood of panic attacks (OR = 1.7, 95% CI = 1.2–2.4).

Interestingly, a locus for panic disorder in humans was mapped to the position 57–69 cM on chromosome 7p15 based on 23 large families [49]. A previous study supported mapping of panic disorder to 7p, although the result was not significant [50]. In yet another study, a significant locus for quantitative traits typical of neuroticism was mapped to position 42 cM on chromosome 7p [51]. The peak linkage positions flank NPSR1; the asthma-associated segment is at position 54 cM [12,13]. Taken together, the observation of NPS effects on anxiety in rodents, mapping of a panic disorder or neuroticism gene within a few cM of NPSR1, and the comorbidity of asthma and panic disorder suggest that it will be highly relevant to consider NPSR1 as a candidate gene predisposing to such psychiatric symptoms.

Conclusions and Prospects

In asthma as well as other complex disorders, several robust, multiply replicated genetic association findings have been presented in the past decade (for a critical review of candidate gene studies, see [3]), a few positionally cloned genes are available, and results of genome-wide association studies are forthcoming. These results allow now a systematic molecular mechanistic analysis of asthma pathways in the critical tissues. At the same time, the results also suggest that studies of joint genetic risks ("gene-gene interactions") and genetic modification of environmental risks are required to understand the complexity of asthma pathogenesis. All identified susceptibility genes present such low risk effects (typical OR about 1.5 or eve lower) that significant interactions are likely to exist for some common risk allele combinations. Some of the new genes offer promise of entirely new pharmaceuticals, as natural genetic variation associating with asthma risk also suggests that pharmacological modification of the product of the particular gene might have a desired effect. This may be especially true of NPSR1, because it as a GPCR offers a particularly "druggable" target. Asthma research has entered a new phase of unforeseen excitement.

Acknowledgements The author wishes to thank members of the Karolinska Institutet and University of Helsinki groups and our collaborators for excellent contributions and stimulating discussions. Our research on asthma is supported by Swedish Research Council, Heart and Lung Foundation (Sweden), Academy of Finland, Sigrid Jusélius Foundation, and Päivikki and Sakari Sohlberg Foundation.

References

1. Laitinen T, Räsänen M, Kaprio J, Koskenvuo M, Laitinen LA (1998) Importance of genetic factors in adolescent asthma - A population based twin-family study. Am J Respir Crit Care Med 157:1073-1078
2. The Wellcome Trust Case Control Consortium (2007) Genome-wide association study of 14,000 cases of seven common diseases and 3,000 shared controls. Nature 447:661-678

3. Hoffjan S, Nicolae D, Ober C (2003) Association studies for asthma and atopic diseases: a comprehensive review of the literature. Respiratory Research 4:14
4. Kere J, Laitinen T (2004) Positionally cloned susceptibility genes in allergy and asthma. Curr Opin Immunol 16:689-694
5. de la Chapelle A, Wright FA (1998) Linkage disequilibrium mapping in isolated populations: the example of Finland revisited. Proc Natl Acad Sci U S A 95:12416-12423
6. Kere J (2001) Human population genetics: lessons from Finland. Annu Rev Genomics Hum Genet 2:103-128
7. Lander ES, Schork NJ (1994) Genetic dissection of complex traits. Science 265:2037-2048
8. Laitinen T, Kauppi P, Ignatius J, Ruotsalainen T, Daly MJ, Kääriäinen H, Kruglyak L, Laitinen H, de la Chapelle A, Lander ES, Laitinen LA, Kere J (1997) Genetic control of serum IgE levels and asthma: linkage and linkage disequilibrium studies in an isolated population. Hum Mol Genet 6:2069-2076
9. Kauppi P, Laitinen LA, Laitinen H, Kere J, Laitinen T (1998) Verification of self-reported asthma and allergy in subjects and their family members volunteering for gene mapping studies. Resp Med 92:1281-1288
10. Laitinen T, Daly MJ, Rioux JD, Kauppi P, Laprise C, Petäys T, Green T, Cargill M, Haahtela T, Lander ES, Laitinen LA, Hudson TJ, Kere J (2001) A susceptibility locus for asthma-related traits on chromosome 7 revealed by genome-wide scan in a founder population. Nature Genet 28:87-91
11. Daniels SE, Bhattacharrya S, James A, Leaves NI, Young A, Hill MR, Faux JA, Ryan G, Le Souef P, Lathrop MG, Musk WA, Cookson WOGM (1996) A genome-wide search for quantitative trait loci underlying asthma. Nature 383:247-250
12. Polvi A, Polvi T, Sevon P, Petäys T, Haahtela T, Laitinen LA, Kere J, Laitinen T (2002) Physical map of an asthma susceptibility locus in 7p15-p14 and an association study of TCRG. Eur J Hum Genet 10:658-665
13. Laitinen T, Polvi A, Rydman P, Vendelin J, Pulkkinen V, Salmikangas P, Mäkelä S, Rehn M, Pirskanen A, Rautanen A, Zucchelli M, Gullstén H, Leino M, Alenius H, Petäys T, Haahtela T, Laitinen A, Laprise C, Hudson TJ, Laitinen LA, Kere J (2004) Characterization of a common susceptibility locus for asthma-related traits. Science 304:300-304
14. Toivonen HTT, Onkamo P, Vasko K, Ollikainen V, Sevon P, Mannila H, Herr M, Kere J (2000) Data mining applied to linkage disequilibrium mapping. Am J Hum Genet 67:133-145
15. Vassilatis DK, Hohmann JG, Zeng H, Li F, Ranchalis JE, Mortrud MT, Brown A, Rodriguez SS, Weller JR, Wright AC, Bergmann JE, Gaitanaris GA (2003) The G protein-coupled receptor repertoires of human and mouse. Proc Natl Acad Sci U S A 100:4903-4908
16. Gupte J, Cutler G, Chen JL, Tian H (2004) Elucidation of signaling properties of vasopressin receptor-related receptor 1 by using the chimeric receptor approach. Proc Natl Acad Sci U S A 101:1508-1513
17. Xu Y-L, Reinscheid RK, Huitron-Resendiz S, Clark SD, Wang Z, Lin SH, Brucher FA, Zeng J, Ly NK, Henriksen SJ, de Lecea L, Civelli O (2004) Neuropeptide S: a neuropeptide promoting arousal and anxiolytic-like effects. Neuron 43: 487–497
18. Beck B, Fernette B, Stricker-Krongrad A (2005) Peptide S is a novel potent inhibitor of voluntary and fast-induced food intake in rats. Biochem Biophys Res Comm 332 859–865
19. Vendelin J, Pulkkinen V, Rehn M, Pirskanen A, Räisänen-Sokolowski A, Laitinen A, Laitinen LA, Kere J, Laitinen T (2005) Characterization of GPRA, a novel G protein-coupled receptor related to asthma. Am J Resp Cell Mol Biol 33:262-270
20. Reinscheid RK, Xu Y-L, Okamura N, Zeng J, Chung S, Pai R, Wang Z, Civelli O (2005) Pharmacological characterization of human and murine Neuropeptide S Receptor variants. J Pharmacol Exp Therap 315:1338–1345
21. Roth AL, Marzola E,Rizzi A, Arduin M, Trapella C, Corti C, Vergura R, Martinelli P, Salvadori S, Regoli D, Corsi M, Cavanni P, Calo G, Guerrini R (2006) Structure-activity studies on Neuropeptide S. Identification of the amino acid residues crucial for receptor activation. J Biol Chem 281:20809–20816

22. Shin HD, Park KS, Park C (2004) Lack of association of GPRA (G protein-coupled receptor for asthma susceptibility) haplotypes with high serum IgE or asthma in a Korean population. J Allergy Clin Immunol 5:1226–1227
23. Melén E, Bruce S, Doekes G, Kabesch M, Laitinen T, Lauener R, Lindgren CM, Riedler J, Scheynius A, van Hage-Hamsten M, Kere J, Pershagen G, Wickman M, Nyberg F, the PARSIFAL Genetics study group (2005) Haplotypes of G-protein-coupled receptor 154 are associated with childhood allergy and asthma. Am J Resp Crit Care Med 171:1089-1095
24. Kormann MS, Carr D, Klopp N, Illig T, Leupold W, Fritzsch C, Weiland SK, von Mutius E, Kabesch M (2005) G-Protein-coupled receptor polymorphisms are associated with asthma in a large German population. Am J Respir Crit Care Med 171:1358-1362
25. Feng Y, Hong X, Wang L, Jiang S, Chen C, Wang B, Yang J, Fang Z, Zang T, Xu X, Xu X (2006) G protein-coupled receptor 154 gene polymorphism is associated with airway hyperresponsiveness to methacholine in a Chinese population. J Allergy Clin Immunol; 117:612-617
26. Malerba G, Lindgren CM, Xumerle L, Kiviluoma P, Trabetti E, Laitinen T, Galavotti R, Pescollderungg L, Boner AL, Kere J, Pignatti PF (2007) Chromosome 7p linkage and GPR154 gene association in Italian families with allergic asthma. Clin Exp Allergy 37:83-89
27. Hersh CP, Raby BA, Soto-Quirós ME, Murphy AJ, Avila L, Lasky-Su J, Sylvia JS, Klanderman BJ, Langel C, Weiss ST, Celedón JC (2007) Comprehensive testing of positionally cloned asthma genes in two populations. Am J Resp Crit Care Med doi:10.1164/rccm.200704-592OC
28. Alfven T, Braun-Fahrlander C, Brunekreef B, von Mutius E, Riedler J, Scheynius A, van Hage M, Wickman M, Benz MR, Budde J, Michels KB, Schram D, Ublagger E, Waser M, Pershagen G; PARSIFAL study group (2006) Allergic diseases and atopic sensitization in children related to farming and anthroposophic lifestyle — the PARSIFAL study. Allergy 61:414-421
29. von Ehrenstein OS, von Mutius E, Illi S, Baumann L, Bohm O, von Kries R (2000) Reduced risk of hay fever and asthma among children of farmers. Clin Exp Allergy 30:187-193
30. Riedler J, Eder W, Oberfeld G, Schreuer M (2000) Austrian children living on a farm have less hay fever, asthma and allergic sensitization. Clin Exp Allergy 30:194-200
31. Klintberg B, Berglund N, Lilja G, Wickman M, van Hage-Hamsten M (2001) Fewer allergic respiratory disorders among farmers' children in a closed birth cohort from Sweden. Eur Respir J 17:1151-1157
32. Pulkkinen V, Majuri M-L, Wang G, Holopainen P, Obase Y, Vendelin J, Wolff H, Rytilä P, Laitinen LA, Haahtela T, Laitinen T, Alenius H, Kere J, Rehn M (2006) Neuropeptide S and G protein-coupled receptor 154 modulate macrophage immune responses. Hum Mol Genet 15:1667-1679
33. Riedler J, Braun-Fahrlander C, Eder W, Schreuer M, Waser M, Maisch S, Carr D, Schierl R, Nowak D, von Mutius E; ALEX Study Team (2001) Exposure to farming in early life and development of asthma and allergy: a cross-sectional survey. Lancet 358:1129-1133
34. von Mutius E, Braun-Fahrlander C, Schierl R, Riedler J, Ehlermann S, Maisch S, Waser M, Nowak D (2000) Exposure to endotoxin or other bacterial components might protect against the development of atopy. Clin Exp Allergy 30:1230-1234
35. Braun-Fahrlander C, Riedler J, Herz U, Eder W, Waser M, Grize L, Maisch S, Carr D, Gerlach F, Bufe A, Lauener RP, Schierl R, Renz H, Nowak D, von Mutius E, Allergy and Endotoxin Study Team (2002) Environmental exposure to endotoxin and its relation to asthma in school-age children. N Engl J Med 347:869-877
36. Schram D, Doekes G, Boeve M, Douwes J, Riedler J, Ublagger E, von Mutius E, Budde J, Pershagen G, Nyberg F, Alm J, Braun-Fahrländer C, Waser M, Brunekreef B, PARSIFAL Study Group (2005) Bacterial and fungal components in house dust of farm children, Rudolf Steiner school children and reference children--the PARSIFAL Study. Allergy 60:611-618
37. Vendelin J, Bruce S, Holopainen P, Pulkkinen V, Rytilä P, Pirskanen A, Rehn M, Laitinen T, Laitinen LA, Haahtela T, Saarialho-Kere U, Laitinen A, Kere J (2006) Downstream target genes of the Neuropeptide S—NPSR1 pathway. Hum Mol Genet 15:2923-2935

38. Allen IC, Pace AJ, Jania LA, Ledford JG, Latour AM, Snouwaert JN, Bernier V, Stocco R, Therien AG, Koller BH (2006) Expression and function of NPSR1/GPRA in the lung before and after induction of asthma-like disease. Am J Physiol Lung Cell
39. Fulkerson PC, Rothenberg ME, Hogan SP (2005) Building a better mouse model: experimental models of chronic asthma. Clin Exp Allergy 35:1251–1253
40. Smith GCS, Wood AM, White IR, Pell JP, Cameron AD, Dobbie R (2004) Neonatal respiratory morbidity at term and the risk of childhood asthma. Arch Dis Childr 89:956-960
41. Pulkkinen V, Haataja R, Hannelius U, Helve O, Pitkänen OM, Karikoski R, Rehn M, Marttila R, Lindgren CM, Hästbacka J, Andersson S, Kere J, Hallman M, Laitinen T (2006) G protein-coupled receptor for asthma susceptibility associates with respiratory distress syndrome. Ann Med 38:357-366
42. Bernstein CN, Wajda A, Blanchard JF (2005) The clustering of other chronic inflammatory diseases in inflammatory bowel disease: a population-based study. Gastroenterol 129:827–836
43. D'Amato M, Bruce S, Bressol F, Zucchelli M, Ezer S, Pulkkinen V, Lindgren C, Astegiano M, Rizzetto M, Gionchetti P, Riegler G, Sostegni R, Daperno M, D'Alfonso S, Momigliano-Richiardi P, Torkvist L, Puolakkainen P, Lappalainen M, Paavola-Sakki P, Halme L, Farkkila M, Turunen U, Kontula K, Lofberg R, Pettersson S, Kere J (2007) Neuropeptide S receptor (NPSR1) gene polymorphism is associated with susceptibility to inflammatory bowel disease. Gastroenterol 2007 (in press)
44. Bohme M, Lannero E, Wickman M, Nordvall SL, Wahlgren CF (2002) Atopic dermatitis and concomitant disease patterns in children up to two years of age. Acta Derm Venereol 82:98-103
45. Veal CD, Reynolds NJ, Meggitt SJ, Allen MH, Lindgren CM, Kere J, Trembath RC, Barker JNWN (2005) Absence of association between asthma and high serum Immunoglobulin E associated GPRA haplotypes and adult atopic dermatitis. J Invest Dermatol 125:399-401
46. Söderhäll C, Marenholz I, Nickel R, Grüber C, Kehrt R, Rohde K, Griffioen RW, Meglio P, Tarani L, Gustafsson D, Hoffmann U, Gerstner B, Müller S, Wahn U, Lee Y-A (2005) Lack of association of the G protein–coupled receptor for asthma susceptibility gene with atopic dermatitis. J Allergy Clin Immunol 116:220-221
47. Hasler G, Gergen PJ, Kleinbaum DG, Ajdacic V, Gamma A, Eich D, Rössler W, Angst J (2005) Asthma and panic in young adults. A 20-year prospective community study. Am J Respir Crit Care Med 171:1224–1230
48. Goodwin RD, Pine DS (2002) Respiratory disease and panic attacks among adults in the United States. Chest 122:645–650
49. Crowe RR, Goedken R, Samuelson S, Wilson R, Nelson J, Noyes R Jr (2001) Genomewide survey of panic disorder. Am J Med Genet (Neuropsychiatr Genet) 105:105–109
50. Knowles JA, Fyer AJ, Vieland VJ, Weissman MM, Hodge SE, Heiman GA, Haghighi F, de Jesus GM, Rassnick H, Preud'homme-Rivelli X, Austin T, Cunjak J, Mick S, Fine LD, Woodley KA, Das K, Maier W, Adams PB, Freimer NB, Klein DF, Gilliam TC (1998) Results of a genome-wide genetic screen for panic disorder. American Journal of Medical Genetics (Neuropsychiatr Genet) 81:139–147
51. Fullerton J, Cubin M, Tiwari H, Wang C, Bomhra A, Davidson S, Miller S, Fairburn C, Goodwin G, Neale MC, Fiddy S, Mott R, Allison DB, Flint J (2003) Linkage analysis of extremely discordant and concordant sibling pairs identifies quantitative-trait loci that influence variation in the human personality trait neuroticism. Am J Hum Genet 72:879–890

Probiotics in the Treatment of Asthma and Allergy

Bengt Björkstén and Susan L. Prescott

Introduction

The prevalence of allergies, diabetes, Inflammatory Bowel Disease and other "immunologically mediated diseases of affluence" has increased progressively, particularly over the last 50 years. Over this time there has been growing recognition of the contributing role of declining microbial burden (the "hygiene hypothesis"). There has also been intense interest in the health benefits of dietary supplements (probiotic and prebiotic) that promote favourable colonisation. These two distinct, but rapidly converging, areas of research have emphasised the need to understand, and ultimately to manipulate, our physiological interactions with commensal microbiota.

According to the "hygiene hypothesis", an apparent decline in microbial exposure during early childhood is one of the most plausible causes of the escalating rates of allergic disease. Epidemiological support for this hypothesis has been progressively consolidated by a growing understanding of effects of microbial factors on immune development. While this story began with allergic disorders, autoimmune conditions (such as type I diabetes and inflammatory bowel disease) are now being increasingly included in these models. It is proposed that the underlying concepts of immune regulation by microbes are similar for several immunologically mediated diseases, which have also been considered as "microbial deficiency syndromes" [1].

There is longstanding interest in the relationship between microbial exposure and allergic disease. It is common knowledge among clinicians and patients that respiratory infections can trigger and enhance allergic manifestations, such as an asthma attack in sensitised individuals. It was therefore also assumed for many

B.Björkstén (✉)
Institute of Environmental Medicine, Division of Lung Fysiology, Karolinska Institutet, 171 77 Stockholm, Sweden
e-mail: bengt.bjorksten@cfa.ki.se

S.L. Prescott
School of Paediatrics and Child Health, University of Western Australia, Perth, Australia

R. Pawankar et al. (eds.), *Allergy Frontiers: Future Perspectives*,
DOI 10.1007/978-4-431-99365-0_13, © Springer 2010

years that infections would enhance sensitisation and the development of allergies. Consequently parents were advised to protect their infants from infections. In 1976, the Canadian paediatrician John Gerrard suggested that infections may actually protect against the development of allergies [2]. It was not until 1989, however, when David Strachan suggested that infections early in life might prevent allergic rhinoconjunctivitis in adults, that this notion raised general interest [3]. This formed the basis of the so called "hygiene hypothesis". The term is potentially misleading, as it would appear to question the enormous gains in Public Health caused by improved hygiene and vaccination programmes. It also soon became obvious that a reduction in the number of respiratory infections in certain regions could not explain the global increase in allergic diseases.

Even if altered patterns of respiratory infections cannot explain the rise in allergic disease, changes in exposure to other microbial agents that stimulate the immune system early in life, may potentially do so. Gut flora exert effects beyond the mucosal microenvironments and appear to influence systemic precursor compartments such as bone marrow and thymus. The underlying mechanism(s) are likely to include stimulation of functional maturation of cells within the innate and adaptive immune systems during the early postnatal period. This process may ultimately determine the overall efficiency of immune/tolerance induction during early life, with major flow-on effects into adulthood. A full understanding of the underlying mechanisms may therefore open new venues for the prevention of allergies and other immunologically mediated diseases by modification of the gut microbiota. Thus, not only local disease manifestations, such as food allergies would be modified, but conceivably also diseases with manifestations at distant sites, such as diabetes and respiratory allergies.

This chapter will review the current knowledge of the role of probiotics in the treatment and prevention of asthma and other manifestations of allergy will be discussed. The immunological background and rationale for exploring a potential role for probiotics in allergic disease will be briefly discussed. However, the main focus is on published evidence of the clinical effects of these products.

Immunological Background

It is clear that T-cells responsive to both dietary and inhalant allergens, as measured by lymphoproliferation and cytokine secretion, are present in cord blood from virtually all subjects [4,5]. Additionally, T-cell cloning and subsequent genotyping studies indicate that the responsive cells are of foetal origin and exhibit a Th2-polarised and/or Th0 cytokine profile. Although these may not represent true memory responses [6], the observed correlations with atopic predisposition raise the possibility that the reactive clones could play a role in the development of allergen-specific tolerance.

The early T-cell responses are subject to a variety of regulatory mechanisms postnatally, which are driven by exposure of the infant immune system to environmental antigen. Cross-sectional and prospective studies indicate that in atopic children, consolidation of Th2-polarised immunity against inhalant allergens is initiated in early infancy and may be completed by the end of the preschool years, or even earlier [4] in children who do not develop clinically manifest allergy [7]. However, a number of observations challenge the notion that allergy is the simple result of Th2 polarisation, including stronger Th1 responses to allergens that have also been noted in allergic children [7–9]. The observations suggest that increased inappropriate reactivity to allergens is a result of failure of underlying regulatory pathways. There is also evidence that these pathways may be under environmental influence. For example, prospective studies from Estonia, with a low, and Sweden with a high prevalence of allergy, indicate that the regulatory mechanisms are established more rapidly in Estonia [4].

It is possible that a traditional life style is associated with an early induction of a general regulation of T-cell immunity. This notion is supported by the close correlation globally between the prevalence of "Th2" mediated conditions (asthma and wheezing) and "Th1" mediated conditions (type-1 diabetes) [10]. Thus, modern environments may be promoting immune disease through effects on underlying regulatory immune function, rather than separate (and potentially paradoxical) effects on Th1 or Th2 immunity. This notion has become the unifying link to explain the parallel increase in both Th1-dependent autoimmune disease and Th2-linked atopic allergy. The main consequence of this model has been intense interest in factors (such as microbial exposure) that can influence the development of regulatory function.

Studies investigating the relationship between early childhood infection and atopy risk have been inconsistent or difficult to interpret. The immunological effects of microbial agents differ with the type of infectious agent and the site of infection. For example, only infections in the gastrointestinal tract appear to be protective [11]. Furthermore, non-pathogenic colonising organisms are also likely to play a central role in immune development [12]. A recent large Danish national cohort study including more than 24,000 mother-child pairs found that early infections do not protect from atopic dermatitis [13]. However, they confirmed that other environmental factors, sometimes taken for indirect markers of microbial exposure (such as early daycare attendance, having three or more siblings, farm residence, and pet keeping) were protective. It is possible though, that these protective factors are due to other than microbial exposure. For example, the inverse relationship between number of older siblings and allergy risk may be due to altered maternal immunity as a consequence of repeated pregnancies and exposure to animals could possibly be explained by high zone tolerance induction. Of relevance is also that one of our research groups very recently observed differences in gut microbiota between 4-year old children with and without older siblings [66]. This highlights the emerging concept that overall "microbial burden", rather than specific infections may be more relevant in early life [14]. In this respect, gut microbiota are a more likely source than the considerably less diverse microbial exposure in the respiratory tract.

Microbial Ecology

The intestinal tract performs many different functions. In addition to absorption and digestion, it is also the body's largest organ of host defence. Part of the intestinal mucosal barrier function is formed by a common mucosal immune system, which provides communication between the different mucosal surfaces of the body [15]. The total mucosal surface area of the adult human gastrointestinal tract is up to 300 m^2, making it the largest body area interacting with the environment. It is colonised with over 10^{14} microorganisms, weighing over 1 kg and corresponding to more than ten times the total number of cells in the body.

Our gut microbiota can be pictured as a microbial organ placed within a host organ [16]. It is composed of different cell lineages with a capacity to communicate with one another and the host. The gut microbiome contains >100 times the number of genes in our genome and endows us with functional features that we have not had to evolve ourselves [17].

The gastrointestinal tract of the newborn baby is sterile. Soon after birth, however, it is colonised by numerous types of micro-organisms. Colonisation is complete after approximately 1 week, but the numbers and species of bacteria fluctuate markedly during the first 3 months of life. There is a continuous interaction between the microbial flora and the host, comprising a dynamic eco system that, once established, is surprisingly stable under normal conditions [18]. Environmental changes, e.g. a treatment period with antibiotics, only temporarily change the composition of the microbiota. A study of adult monozygotic twins living apart and their marital partners has emphasised either the potential dominance of host genotype over diet in determining microbial composition of the gut microbiota [19], or alternatively the significance of early life environment.

Microbial colonisation of the gastrointestinal tract, linked with lifestyle and/or geographic factors, may be important determinants of the heterogeneity in disease prevalence throughout the world [20] and ongoing cohort studies are focusing in detail on this complex question. These suggestions are supported by observations that germ free mice do not develop tolerance in the absence of a gut flora [21,22] and by the demonstration of differences in the composition of the gut flora between infants living in countries with a high and a low prevalence of allergy and between healthy and allergic infants (summarised in [20]. The clinical studies on microbial ecology published so far only indicate that there are geographic differences in the composition of gut microbiota and that there have been pronounced changes over the past 40–50 years in affluent countries with a market economy. However, virtually nothing is known about which changes are significant with regard to human health in general and immune regulation in particular. The reason is that until very recently, all ecological studies relied on rather crude, time consuming conventional isolation of bacteria in various media. Recent progress allowing the analysis of bacterial DNA and powerful statistical methods borrowed from analyses of gene expression, will allow a better analysis and understanding of the complex microbial interactions in our gut, as well as of microbe-host interactions.

Gut Microbiota and Immune Regulation

Recent epidemiological studies and experimental research suggest that the microbial environment and exposure to microbial products in infancy modify immune responses and enhance immune regulation and tolerance to ubiquitous antigens. The intestinal microbiota seem to play a particular role in this respect, as they are the major external driving force in the maturation of the immune system after birth.

The gut microbiota are thus the quantitatively most important source of microbial stimulation and may provide a primary signal for driving the postnatal maturation of the immune system and the development of a balanced immunity [15]. Thus, there is mounting evidence that commensal microbes acquired during the early postnatal period are required for the development of tolerance, not only to themselves, but also to other antigens. For example, Th2-mediated immune responses are not susceptible to oral tolerance induction in germ free mice [21]. Oral tolerance was only induced after the introduction of components of normal microbiota. It is also recognised that interaction with microbes, especially the normal microbial flora of the gastrointestinal tract, is the principal environmental signal for postnatal maturation of T-cell function (in particular the Th1 component).

Bacteria are the most powerful immunostimulants in the normal environment, activating the immune system through a range "pattern recognition receptors" system (Toll-like receptors, TLR). It is also recognised that interaction with the normal microbial flora of the gastrointestinal tract is the principal environmental signal for postnatal maturation of T-cell function (in particular the Th1 component) [23]. Although TLR are found principally on cells of the innate immune system (including granulocytes, monocytes, and natural killer cells), they are also present on cells involved in programming and regulating "adaptive" immune responses (such as APC and regulatory T cells). It has been proposed that early microbial activation of both APC and regulatory T cells may promote Th1 maturation and play an important role in reducing the risk of Th2 mediated allergic responses [24]. This is supported by animal studies, demonstrating that bacterial lipopolysacharide (LPS) endotoxin exposure can prevent allergic sensitisation if given before allergic responses are established [25]. These effects may be of greater significance in genetically susceptible individuals who appear to have weaker Th1 responses in the perinatal period [7]. Genetic studies also support a role for the CD14/LPS [26] and TLR [27] pathways in the development of allergic disease.

In animals, bacterial antigens (mycobacteria) have been used successfully to modify allergic inflammation in sensitised animals with evidence that effects are mediated by TGFβ and IL-10 producing regulatory T cells [28]. Supplementation with probiotic bacteria has also been shown to induce regulatory populations [29]. There are also preliminary reports that bacteria may affect regulatory immune function in humans, with an increase in the in vitro production of regulatory cytokines (IL-10) after probiotic ingestion [30]. A potentially significant role of the gut microbiota in the development of immune regulation is suggested by observations that germ free mice when immunised respond with higher production of both Th1 and Th2 cytokines [31]. In support of this, one of our research groups has recently noted significant correlations between colonisation with bifidobacteria species in the first 6 months of life and the level of allergen-associated regulatory activity (detected as FoxP3 expression in response to allergen stimulation) (Martino, Prescott et al. submitted for publication).

Intestinal microbiota are considered to be the most abundant source of early immune stimulation, and contribute significantly to "microbial burden" in early life. A number of studies have suggested differences in colonisation patterns between allergic and non-allergic children (reviewed in [12]). Interestingly, prospective studies have shown that these differences were already apparent at 1 week of age, i.e. well before the infants had developed any allergic manifestations, suggesting that early colonisation can influence subsequent patterns of immune development. Observed differences include higher microbial counts of gramme positive bacteria in neonates who do not develop allergic manifestations, less clostridia and a higher prevalence of bifidobacteria through the first year of life [32]. These differences are present at least during the first 5 years of life [33]. Interestingly, similar differences were noted when comparing the gut microbiota in healthy one-year old infants living in two countries with a low and high prevalence of allergy (Estonia and Sweden) [34]. It was noted that the gut microbiota in Estonia in many respects was similar to that described in Western Europe in the early 1960s, before the emergence of the major difference in allergy prevalence between Eastern and Western Europe [35]. As already mentioned, studies in germfree animals confirm that microbial gut flora are essential for the development of oral tolerance and for the induction of normal immune regulation [21,22]. The controversy regarding the role of gut bacteria in allergy development thus lies in the clinical consequences of these clinical and experimental findings and not as much to what extent they affect the immune system.

Probiotics and Allergy Treatment

Probiotics are live non-pathogenic micro-organisms which, when ingested, exert a positive influence on the health or physiology of the host beyond their nutritional value. The term "prebiotic" is used for eaten compounds that promote microbiota that are beneficial to health. Although used for many years, it is only recently that the mechanisms of action and effects of pre- and probiotics have began to be studied using the same pharmacological approach as for drugs. Probiotic strains with documented clinical efficacy on e.g. infant infectious diarrhoea [36,37] other infections [38] and antibiotic-associated diarrhoea [39] predominantly belong to the *Lactobacillus* and *Bifidobacterium* families. They and other lactic acid-producers are commensal bacteria common to the gut of all mammals, as well as non-mammalian vertebrates.

Several strains of probiotic bacteria have been tried both for treatment of clinical manifestations of allergy (Table 1). The studies are limited to three species of lactobacilli,

Table 1 Summary of placebo-controlled probiotic treatment studies for eczema with and without allergy in infants and young children

Investigators, Country (reference)	Study population	Age, months	*N*=	Treatment duration	Probiotica used	Outcomes and comments
Majamaa and Isolauri. Finland [40]	Infants with mild Eczema+CMA		27	1 month	*Lactobacillus GG*	Improved SCORAD, decreased Fecal TNFα and α1-AT
Isolauri et al. Finland[41]	Breast fed babies with mild eczema	Mean age 4.6 months	27	2 months	*Lactobacillus GG & Bifidobacterium lactis Bb-12*	Improved SCORAD in both probiotics. Reduced serum CD4 and urinary EPX
Rosenfeldt et al. Denmark [44]	Eczema	1–13 years		6 weeks	*Lactobacillus rhamnosus & L.reuteri*	Reduced extent of eczema ($p=0.02$), particularly in sensitised children
Viljanen et al. Finland [42]	AEDS and Suspected CMA		230	4 weeks	*Lactobacillus GG* or Mixture of four strains	Reduced SCORAD by *L.GG* in subgroup of IgE-sensitised infants
Weston et al. Australia [46]	Moderate or severe AEDS	6–18 months	53	8 weeks	*Lactobacillus fermentum*	Reduced SCORAD in treatment group ($p=0.03$) and more common improvement (93% vs. 65%, $p=0.01$)
Brouwer et al. Netherlands [47]	AEDS	<5 months	50	3 months	*Lactobacillus GG* or *Lactobacillus rhamnosus*	No difference as compared with placebo
Sistek et al. New Zealand [45]	AEDS		59	12 weeks	*Lactobacillus GG & Bifidobacterium lactis Bb-12* 2×10^{10}cfu	Reduced SCORAD in subgroup of food sensitive children

i.e. *Lactobacillus rhamnosus, fermentum* and *reuteri* and *Bifidobacterium lactis Bb-12*. The first study was published in 1997 and reported that a one-month treatment with a strain of *Lactobacillus GG* added to an extensively hydrolysed infant formula for 1 month improved eczema in cow's milk allergic infants with mild eczema. The study only included 27 treated infants and although symptoms improved significantly in 13 infants, but not in the 14 babies who only received the hydrolysate, there was no significant difference in symptom scores between the two groups at the end of the study [40]. Of interest is that faecal levels of both TNFα and α1-AT decreased significantly in the infants who were treated with lactobacilli but not in the placebo group, indicating an anti-inflammatory effect on the gut mucosa.

The second study also included 27 breast fed infants with mild eczema and documented a complete resolution in all participants after 6 months, although this occurred more rapidly in the group receiving probiotics (*Lactobacillus GG* ($n=9$) or *Bifidobacterium lactis* ($n=9$)) [41]. The authors also observed reduced soluble CD4 in serum and eosinophil protein X in urine in the treated infants, suggesting a systemic effect. The changes did not correlate with clinical improvement in these small study groups, however.

The two studies were both small and only included infants with mild disease, who are less likely to be atopic and less likely to develop persistent skin disease or new respiratory allergy. More recently, a study of a larger cohort, comprising 230 infants (aged around 6 months) with atopic eczema/dermatitis syndrome (AEDS) and suspected cow's milk allergy were treated with the same probiotic strain (*Lactobacillus GG*), a mixture of four probiotic strains, or placebo for 4 weeks [42]. Beneficial clinical effects of the probiotics were in this study only seen in children with evidence of allergic sensitization and not in children with atopic dermatitis but no sensitization. This suggests that atopic dermatitis is a heterogeneous condition and that the effect of immune modifying agents, such as probiotics will depend on the pattern of disease. Paired pre- and posttreatment plasma samples were analysed for concentrations of IL-2, IL-4, IL-6, IL-10, TNFα, IFNγ, soluble intercellular adhesion molecule 1, soluble E-selectin, TGF-β1, TGF-β2, and C-reactive protein [43]. In infants with IgE-associated AEDS, treatment with LGG induced higher C-reactive protein levels than in the placebo group ($P=0.021$). The IL-6 levels also increased after treatment with LGG ($P=0.023$) and soluble E-selectin levels were higher after probiotic than after placebo treatment in infants with IgE-mediated CMA. Furthermore, faecal levels of α1-AT decreased in infants receiving lactobacilli, thus confirming a previous study with the same micro-organism [40].

Three other studies, including two with other strains of lactobacilli and one with a combination of *Lactobacillus rhamnosus* GG and *Bifidobacterium lactis Bb-12*, have also suggested some favourable effects on atopic dermatitis extent and severity [44–46], while one study was negative [47]. In the Danish study [44], treatment with a combination of *Lactobacillus reuteri* and *L. rhamnosus* was associated with reduced extent of eczema ($p=0.02$), particularly in the subgroup of infants who also had a positive skin prick test. There was also a significant ($p=0.03$) decrease in serum eosinophil cationic protein (ECP), but no significant changes in the production of the cytokines IL-2, IL-4, IL-10, or IFNγ.

In an Australian study, treatment with a strain of *Lactobacillus fermentum* (given at a dose of 10^9 colony forming units, cfu, twice daily) improved infantile eczema as assessed after 16 weeks [46]. This study included infants with more severe eczema than any of the previously cited studies. The reduction in the SCORAD index was significant in the probiotic ($p=0.03$) but not placebo group. Furthermore, significantly more children receiving probiotics had a SCORAD (SCORing index Atopic Dermatitis) that was better than baseline at week 16 (93% vs. 63% in the placebo group, $p=0.01$). Interestingly, probiotic administration was associated with increased polyclonal Th1 IFNγ responses in the infants and the improvement in atopic dermatitis was directly proportional to the increase in IFNγ responses to Staphylococcus enterotoxin B. ($r=0.445$, $P=0.026$) [48]. Increased IFNγ responses by probiotics have also recently been observed in infants treated for cow's milk allergy [49].

In a study from New Zealand, the effect of two probiotics (*Lactobacillus rhamnosus* and *Bifidobacterium lactis*) given at a high dose (2×10^{10}) was studied in 59 children with established AEDS [45]. Although there was no significant difference between the probiotic and placebo groups after 12 weeks, a significant improvement was noted in the subgroup of food allergic children receiving probiotics.

A recent Dutch study could not document any beneficial effects of probiotics on infant eczema [47]. After 4–6 weeks of baseline and double-blind, placebo-controlled challenges for diagnosis of cow's milk allergy (CMA), infants less than 5 months old with AD received a hydrolysed whey-based formula as placebo ($n=17$), or supplemented with either *Lactobacillus rhamnosus* ($n=17$) or *Lactobacillus GG* ($n=16$) for 3 months. Before, during and after intervention, the clinical severity of AD was evaluated using SCORAD. Allergic sensitization was evaluated by measurement of total IgE and a panel of food-specific IgEs as well as skin prick testing for cow's milk. Inflammatory parameters were blood eosinophils, eosinophil protein X in urine, faecal alpha-1-antitrypsin and production of IL-4, IL-5 and IFNγ by peripheral blood mononuclear cells after polyclonal stimulation. There was no statistically significant effect of probiotic supplementation on SCORAD, sensitization, inflammatory parameters or cytokine production between groups. Only four infants were diagnosed with CMA, however, in this rather small study.

Thus, of the seven studies in which probiotics were assessed for the treatment of eczema in infants, six showed some beneficial effects, at least in subgroups of infants with documented allergy. The treatment was only associated with a small or modest reduction in symptoms. Most of the studies were small, however, and mostly included only infants with mild eczema. In three of the studies there were also recorded effects on laboratory parameters, e.g. increased polyclonal IFNγ responses [46] or faecal chemokines [40,50], lower serum ECP levels [44], lower urinary eosinophil protein X and serum CD4 [41] and stabilised mucosal barrier function [51].

There are also studies comprising older children and adults, in which probiotics have been tried as treatment of respiratory allergies. In one study, 36 teenagers and young adults with pollen allergy were randomised to a 5.5-month treatment with *Lactobacillus rhamnosus* or placebo [52]. The treatment had no effect on seasonal symptoms, or on the outcome of provocations. In contrast, in a study of 80 adults with perennial rhinitis a strain of *Lactobacillus paracasei* for 30 days was reported to slightly although significantly reduce frequency and severity of symptoms [53].

A strain of *Bifidobacterium longum* has been tried as treatment of Japanese Cedar pollinosis (JCP). In one randomised, double-blind trial, 44 patients received probiotic bacteria or placebo for 13 weeks during the pollen season [54]. The treatment was associated with decreases in rhinorrhea, nasal blockage and composite scores. The same authors also tried the same strain given in yoghurt for 14 weeks to patients with JCP [55]. Slightly less eye symptoms were reported in the treatment as compared to the placebo group, but most differences did not reach statistical significance. The same group very recently reported similar results on ocular symptoms in a placebo-controlled study with cross-over design [56].

Probiotics and Allergy Prevention

It is logical from an immunological standpoint to explore the benefits of probiotics very early in life when immune responses are still developing, and there are now a number of studies addressing the role or probiotics in primary allergy prevention (Table 2). The first study to assess the role of probiotics in this context administered *Lactobacillus rhamnosus* to mothers (starting 2–4 weeks before delivery) and to infants in the first 6 months of life. This was reported to reduce the incidence of eczema at 2 years by around 50% [57]. Although the cumulative effect on eczema was still evident at 4 years, there was no reduction in respiratory allergy, IgE levels or allergic sensitisation [58]. This was confirmed by a follow-up at 7 years [59]. Effects on underlying immune response were not reported and a number of methodological concerns have been raised about the study [60]. A major concern was that many of the children (28 out of 64) included in the probiotic supplement group did not receive probiotics directly, as the supplement was given to the mother if babies were breastfed. These issues have made the results difficult to interpret.

There are three other recently published studies, in which the potential to prevent the development of allergic disease by probiotics has been tested (Table 2). In addition, there are numerous similar ongoing studies in Australia, Germany, The Netherlands, New Zealand, Singapore and United Kingdom with three strains of lactobacilli and four strains of bifidobacteria in doses ranging from 10^8 to 10^9 cfu daily. The results of these studies are awaited with interest. The second of the so far published studies (using a *Lactobacillus acidophilus*) failed to show any reduction in allergic disease despite changes in colonisation [61]. Rather, there was a worrying increase in sensitization and in IgE-associated atopic eczema. In this study, the treatment was started after birth, while in the study by Kalliomäki et al and the two studies summarised below, the pregnant women were given the probiotic during the last month of gestation.

The second study showed a reduction in atopic eczema but no effects on sensitization or other allergic disease [62]. A mixture of four probiotic bacteria were

Table 2 Summary of primary prevention studies in infants using strains of *Lactobacillus, Bifidobacterium* and/or *Proprionibacterium*

	Study protocol				Outcomes				
Investigators, country (reference)	Population characteristics	organism(s) and dosage	Prenatal treatment	Postnatal (duration)	Less eczema	Less sensitisation	Reduction in other AD	Effect on colonisation	Comment
Kalliomaki et al. Finland [57–59]	First degree relative with allergy $n=132/159$ completed	*L. rhamnosus GG*, 1×10^{10} cfu daily	2–4 weeks	6 months Only to mother if breast-feeding	Yes at 2, 4, 7 years	No	No	Yes	
Taylor et al. Australia [61]	Mother SPT+ and allergic $n=189/230$ completed	*L. acidophillus* (3×10^8 cfu daily)	No	6 months	No	No	No	Yes	More often sensitised in probiotic group
Kukkonen et al. Finland [62]	Parent(s) with allergic disease $n=925/1223$ completed	*L. rhamnosus GG & LC705& B. breve & Proprionibact. freudenreichii* ($2–5\times10^9$ cfu twice daily)	2–4 weeks	6 months	YES (at 2 years)	No	No	Yes	Probiotic group also received prebiotics (galacto-oligosaccharides
Abrahamsson et al. Sweden [63]	First degree relative with allergy $n=188/232$ completed	*L. reuteri* (1×10^8 cfu daily)	2–4 weeks	12 months	Less eczema with IgE second year	Only in subgroup with atopic mothers	Only in subgroup with atopic mothers	Yes	
Kopp et al. Germany [67]	First degree relative with allergy $n=94/102$ completed	*L. rhamnosus GG*, 1×10^{10} cfu daily	4–6 weeks	6 months (first 3 months only to mother if breast feeding	No	No	No		No

given to the mothers during the last 2–4 weeks of pregnancy and then to the babies for 6 months. The statistical power is high in the study, since over 900 infants participated in the follow-up at 2 years. Probiotic treatment compared with placebo showed no effect on the cumulative incidence of allergic diseases but tended to reduce IgE-associated (atopic) diseases (odds ratio [OR], 0.71; 95% CI, 0.50–1.00; $P=0.052$). The treatment also reduced eczema (OR, 0.74; 95% CI, 0.55–0.98; $P=0.035$) and atopic eczema (OR, 0.66; 95% CI, 0.46–0.95; $P=0.025$). Thus, the treatment significantly prevented eczema and especially atopic eczema. Of note, this study used a combination of strains and prebiotic galacto-oligosaccharides.

In the fourth published study, *Lactobacillus reuteri* was given to pregnant mothers during the last 4 weeks and then daily to the infants for 1 year [63]. The incidence of eczema and other potentially allergic manifestations was similar in the treatment and placebo groups. However, subgroup analyses showed that the probiotic treatment was associated with less IgE-associated atopic eczema during the second year of life. Furthermore, in the infants with atopic mothers there was a reduction not only in IgE associated eczema, but also in the prevalence of allergen-specific IgE antibodies. In contrast, there was no effect of the treatment in infants who only had paternal allergy. This observation is interesting as the levels of IL-10 were higher and TGFβ lower in colostrum of mothers who had eaten probiotics during the last month of pregnancy [64]. Prospective analysis of these populations is necessary to assess long-term outcomes, particularly any possible effects on respiratory allergy.

Despite all of the immunomodulatory effects described in experimental models, so far none of these studies has shown any clear effect preventive sensitization on any allergic disease other than eczema. Possible explanations for the varied results in the treatment and prevention studies include differences in the bacterial strains used, host factors that could influence microbial responsiveness and allergic propensity, and other environmental factors that could influence colonisation or immune development. *Firstly*, there are significant variations in the strains claimed to be probiotic. It is also of note that the three studies suggesting at least some preventive effects started supplementation in pregnancy, whereas the study that showed increased sensitisation [61] did not. This may indicate that the supplementation to the mothers in late pregnancy is of a crucial importance. In light of this, it is of interest to note that in one study the levels of IL-10 were higher and TGFβ lower in colostrum of mothers receiving a probiotic as compared to placebo treated mothers [64]. *Secondly*, there are differences in host susceptibility to microbial influence and to colonisation with a particular strain of bacteria. Functional genetic polymorphisms in microbial recognition pathways are well described (including TLR), and it is likely that this could result in individual variation in the effects of probiotics. Similarly there is some heterogeneity in the level of allergic risk in the study groups. *Thirdly*, there are likely to be many environmental factors that influence both colonisation (such as maternal microbiota and other sources of microbial exposure, delivery method, antibiotics, and prebiotics in the diet and general microbial burden) and immune development. It is quite conceivable that administration of a certain strain may affect microbial ecology in one environment, but not in another.

For example, in the Swedish study of allergy prevention [63], the probiotic *Lactobacillus reuteri* was isolated at least once in 12% of the mothers and the infants belonging to the placebo group. Thus the strain, which was originally isolated from breast milk, is a transient component of the gut microbiota, at least in Scandinavia. All of these factors are likely to make robust meta-analyses problematic to perform as more studies are completed.

Prebiotics

Although some studies have reported benefits in the treatment and prevention of atopic eczema, none has had any effects on the development of Th2 mediated allergic responses. It appears unlikely that supplementation with a single probiotic strain would be sufficient to have a major influence on the very diverse intestinal microbiota and the complex interaction between the gut bacteria and the host. This has lead to an interest in dietary substrates that could have a more global effect on gut microbiota, namely prebiotics (non-digestible, fermentable oligosaccharides which stimulate the growth of *Bifidobacterium* and *Lactobacillus* species). Altering the intake of foods containing these products can directly influence the composition and activity of intestinal microbiota. This could explain some of the protective effects of grains and cereals that have been seen in epidemiologic studies. To date there is only one controlled study in which the effects of probiotics has been studied without simultaneous administration of probiotic bacteria. A mixture of neutral short-chain oligosaccharides and long-chain fructooligosacharides added to a hypoallergenic infant formula given for the first six months of life to infants with a family history of allergy was associated with a reduction in the incidence of atopic dermatitis, recurrent wheezing and allergic urticaria [68]. The treatment was also associated with a slight reduction in the plasma levels of IgE, IgG2 and IgG3, but not IgG4 [69].

Concluding Comments

While there is a sound theoretical basis for anticipating benefits of probiotic supplementation in allergic disease, there is currently insufficient data to recommend this as a part of standard therapy in allergic conditions in general, or for prevention. Although there has been promise in atopic dermatitis, it is generally accepted that more studies are needed to confirm this, and that any benefits are likely to be modest. However, faced with the stress and severe discomfort that can be associated with atopic dermatitis, many families are choosing to try probiotics in conjunction with their prescribed products. Although probiotics are part of normal gut microbiota and not associated with any serious adverse effects, further studies are needed to determine the significance of the increased rates of sensitisation associated with the use of probiotics in some prevention studies.

Although the potential role of the gut microbiota for human health was pointed out a century ago [65], a detailed study of microbial ecology has only recently become possible, thanks to novel technology. Studies on the potential use of probiotic bacteria are still complicated by our lack of understanding of the interaction between the various components of the human “microbiome”. Usually clinical trials are executed with a reductionistic approach, in which ideally the effect of one molecule or compound is tested against a single well-defined disease. It may be necessary to apply a much more holistic approach to fully understand how and under what conditions certain bacteria will interact with each other and with the host. At this stage there is still very little data to directly confirm the immunological or therapeutic effects of prebiotic supplements, but a number of studies are underway.

References

1. Rook GA, Stanford JL (1998) Give us this day our daily germs. Immunol Today 19:113–116.
2. Gerrard J, Geddes C, Reggin P, Gerrard C, Horne S (1976) Serum IgE levels in white and metis communities in Saskatchewan. Ann Allergy 37:91–100.
3. Strachan D (1989) Hay fever, hygiene and household size. Brit Med J 299:1259–1256.
4. Böttcher MF, Jenmalm MC, Voor T, Julge K, Holt PG, Björkstén B (2006) Cytokine responses to allergens during the first 2 years of life in Estonian and Swedish children. Clin Exp Allergy 36:619–628.
5. Holt PG, Macaubas C (1997) Development of long term tolerance versus sensitisation to environmental allergens during the perinatal period. Curr Opin Immunol 9:782–787.
6. Thornton CA, Upham JW, Wikstrom ME, Holt BJ, White GP, Sharp MJ, Sly PD, Holt PG (2004) Functional maturation of CD4+CD25+CTLA4+CD45RA+ T regulatory cells in human neonatal T cell responses to environmental antigens/allergens. J Immunol 173:3084–3092.
7. Prescott SL, Macaubas C, Smallacombe T, Holt BJ, Sly PD, Holt PG (1999) Development of allergen-specific T-cell memory in atopic and normal children. Lancet 353:196–200.
8. Ng T, Holt P, Prescott S (2002) Cellular immune responses to ovalbumin and house dust mite in egg-allergic children. Allergy 57:207–214.
9. Smart J, Kemp A (2002) Increased Th1 and Th2 allergen-induced cytokine responses in children with atopic disease. Clin Exp Allergy 32:796–802.
10. Stene LC, Nafstad P (2001) Relation between occurrence of type 1 diabetes and asthma. Lancet 257:607–608.
11. Matricardi PM, Rosmini F, Panetta V, Ferrigno L, Bonini S (2002) Hay fever and asthma in relation to markers of infection in the United States. J Allergy Clin Immunol 110:381–387.
12. Björkstén B (2004) Effects of intestinal microflora and the environment on the development of asthma and allergy. Springer Semin Immunopathol 25:257–270.
13. Benn CS, Melbye M, Wohlfahrt J, Bjorksten B, Aaby P (2004) Cohort study of sibling effect, infectious diseases, and risk of atopic dermatitis during first 18 months of life. BMJ 328:1223–1230.
14. Martinez FD (2001) The coming-of-age of the hygiene hypothesis. Respir Res 2:129–132.
15. Hooper L, Gordon J (2001) Commensal host-bacterial relationships in the gut. Science 292:1115–1118.
16. Bäckhed F, Ley R, Sonnenburg J, Peterson D, Gordon J (2007) Host-bacterial mutualism in the human intestine. Science 307:1915–1920.
17. Gill SR, Pop M, Deboy RT, Eckburg PB, Turnbaugh PJ, Samuel BS, Gordon JI, Relman DA, Fraser-Liggett CM, Nelson KE (2006) Metagenomic analysis of the human distal gut microbiome. Science 312:1355–1359.

18. Zoetendal EG, Akkermans AD, De Vos WM (1998) Temperature gradient gel electrophoresis analysis of 16S rRNA from human fecal samples reveals stable and host-specific communities of active bacteria. Appl Environ Microbiol 64:3854–3859.
19. Zoetendal EG, Ben-Amor K, Akkermans AD, Abee T, de Vos WM (2001) DNA isolation protocols affect the detection limit of PCR approaches of bacteria in samples from the human gastrointestinal tract. Syst Appl Microbiol 24:405–410.
20. Björkstén B (2005) Genetic and environmental risk factors for the development of food allergy. Curr Opin Allergy Clin Immunol 5:249–253.
21. Moreau MC, Coste M, Gaboriau V, Dubuquoy C (1995) Oral tolerance to ovalbumin in mice: effect of some paramters on the induction and persistence of the suppression of systemic IgE and IgG antibody responses. Adv Exp Med Biol 371B:1229–1234.
22. Sudo N, Sawamura S-A, Tanaka K, Aiba Y, Kubo C, Koga Y (1997) The requirement of intestinal bacterial flora for the development of an IgE production system fully susceptible to oral tolerance induction. J Immunol 159:1739–1745.
23. Demengeot J, Zelenay S, Moraes-Fontes MF, Caramalho I, Coutinho A (2006) Regulatory T cells in microbial infection. Springer Semin Immunopathol 28:41–50.
24. Wills-Karp M, Santeliz J, Karp CL (2001) The germless theory of allergic disease: revisiting the hygiene hypothesis. Nat Rev Immunol 1:69–75.
25. Blumer N, Herz U, Wegmann M, Renz H (2005) Prenatal lipopolysaccharide-exposure prevents allergic sensitisation and airway inflammation, but not airway responsiveness in a murine model of experimental asthma. Clin Exp Allergy 35:397–402.
26. Baldini M, Lohman IC, Halonen M, Erickson RP, Holt PG, Martinez FD (1999) A polymorphism in the 5′-flanking region of the CD14 gene is associated with circulating soluble CD14 levels with total serum IgE. Am J Respir Cell Mol Biol 20:976–983.
27. Eder W, Klimecki W, Yu L, von Mutius E, Riedler J, Braun-Fahrlander C, Nowak D, Martinez FD (2004) Toll-like receptor 2 as a major gene for asthma in children of European farmers. J Allergy Clin Immunol 113:482–488.
28. Zuany-Amorim C, Sawicka E, Manlius C, Le Moine A, Brunet LR, Kemeny DM, Bowen G, Rook G, Walker C (2002) Suppression of airway eosinophilia by killed *Mycobacterium vaccae*-induced allergen-specific regulatory T-cells. Nat Med 8:625–629.
29. Di Giacinto C, Marinaro M, Sanchez M, Strober W, Boirivant M (2005) Probiotics ameliorate recurrent Th1-mediated murine colitis by inducing IL-10 and IL-10-dependent TGF-beta-bearing regulatory cells. J Immunol 174:3237–3246.
30. Lammers KM, Brigidi P, Vitali B, Gionchetti P, Rizzello F, Caramelli E, Matteuzzi D, Campieri M (2003) Immunomodulatory effects of probiotic bacteria DNA: IL-1 and IL-10 response in human peripheral blood mononuclear cells. FEMS Immunol Med Microbiol 38:165–172.
31. Bowman L, Holt P, Björkstén. Immune regulation of the newborn using germ-free and conventional dendritic cells. In: World Immunology Congress 2001; abs 541, Stockholm, 2001.
32. Björkstén B, Sepp E, Julge K, Voor T, Mikelsaar M (2001) Allergy development and the intestinal microflora during the first year of life. J Allergy Clin Immunol 108:516–520.
33. Sepp E, Julge K, Mikelsaar M, Björkstén B (2005) Intestinal microbiota and immunoglobulin E responses in 5-year-old Estonian children. Clin Exp Allergy 35:1141–1146.
34. Sepp E, Julge K, Vasar M, Naaber P, Björkstén B, Mikelsaar M (1997) Intestinal microflora of Estonian and Swedish infants. Acta Paediatr 86:956–961.
35. Nicolai T, Bellach B, Mutius EV, Thefeld W, Hoffmeister H (1997) Increased prevalence of sensitization against aeroallergens in adults in West compared with East Germany. Clin Exp Allergy 27:886–892.
36. Allen S, Okoko B, Martinez E, Gregorio G, Dans L (2004) Probiotics for treating infectious diarrhoea. Cochrane Database Syst Rev 2:CD003048.
37. D'Souza AL, Rajkumar C, Cooke J, Bulpitt CJ (2002) Probiotics in prevention of antibiotic associated diarrhoea: meta-analysis. Brit Med J 324:1361–1364.
38. Weizman Z, Asli G, Alsheikh A (2005) Effect of a probiotic infant formula on infections in child care centers: comparison of two probiotic agents. Pediatrics 115:5–9.

39. Johnston B, Supina A, Vohtra S (2006) Probiotics for pediatric antibiotic-associated diarrhea: a meta-analysis of randomized placebo-controlled trials. Can Med Assoc J 175:377–383.
40. Majamaa H, Isolauri E (1997) Probiotics: a novel approach in the management of food allergy. J Allergy Clin Immunol 99:179–185.
41. Isolauri E, Arvola T, Sutas Y, Moilanen E, Salminen S (2000) Probiotics in the management of atopic eczema. Clin Exp Allergy 30:1604–1610.
42. Viljanen M, Savilahti E, Haahtela T, Juntunen-Backman K, Korpela R, Poussa T, Tuure T, Kuitunen M (2005) Probiotics in the treatment of atopic eczema/dermatitis syndrome in infants: a double-blind placebo-controlled trial. Allergy 60:494–500.
43. Viljanen M, Kuitunen M, Haahtela T, Juntunen-Backman K, Korpela R, Savilahti E (2005) Probiotic effects on faecal inflammatory markers and on faecal IgA in food allergic atopic eczema/dermatitis syndrome infants. Pediatr Allergy Immunol 16:65–71.
44. Rosenfeldt V, Benfeldt E, Nielsen SD, Michaelsen KF, Jeppesen DL, Valerius NH, Paerregaard A (2003) Effect of probiotic *Lactobacillus* strains in children with atopic dermatitis. J Allergy Clin Immunol 111:389–395.
45. Sistek D, Kelly R, Wickens K, Stanley T, Fitzharris P, Crane J (2006) Is the effect of probiotics on atopic dermatitis confined to food sensitized children? Clin Exp Allergy 36:629–633.
46. Weston S, Halbert A, Richmond P, Prescott SL (2005) Effects of probiotics on atopic dermatitis: a randomised controlled trial. Arch Dis Child 90:892–897.
47. Brouwer ML, Wolt-Plompen SA, Dubois AE, van der Heide S, Jansen DF, Hoijer MA, Kauffman HF, Duiverman EJ (2006) No effects of probiotics on atopic dermatitis in infancy: a randomized placebo-controlled trial. Clin Exp Allergy 36:899–906.
48. Prescott SL, Dunstan JA, Hale J, Breckler L, Lehmann H, Weston S, Richmond P (2005) Clinical effects of probiotics are associated with increased interferon-gamma responses in very young children with atopic dermatitis. Clin Exp Allergy 35:1557–1564.
49. Pohjavuori E, Viljanen M, Korpela R, Kuitunen M, Tiittanen M, Vaarala O, Savilahti E (2004) *Lactobacillus GG* effect in increasing IFN-gamma production in infants with cow's milk allergy. J Allergy Clin Immunol 114:131–136.
50. Viljanen M, Pohjavuori E, Haahtela T, Korpela R, Kuitunen M, Sarnesto A, Vaarala O, Savilahti E (2005) Induction of inflammation as a possible mechanism of probiotic effect in atopic eczema-dermatitis syndrome. J Allergy Clin Immunol 115:1254–1259.
51. Rosenfeldt V, Benfeldt E, Valerius NH, Paerregaard A, Michaelsen KF (2004) Effect of probiotics on gastrointestinal symptoms and small intestinal permeability in children with atopic dermatitis. J Pediatr 145:612–616.
52. Helin T, Haahtela S, Haahtela T (2002) No effect of oral treatment with an intestinal bacterial strain, *Lactobacillus rhamnosus* (ATCC 53103), on birch-pollen allergy: a placebo-controlled double-blind study. Allergy 57:243–246.
53. Wang MF, Lin HC, Wang YY, Hsu CH (2004) Treatment of perennial allergic rhinitis with lactic acid bacteria. Pediatr Allergy Immunol 15:152–158.
54. Xiao JZ, Kondo S, Yanagisawa N, Takahashi N, Odamaki T, Iwabuchi N, Miyaji K, Iwatsuki K, Togashi H, Enomoto K, Enomoto T (2006) Probiotics in the treatment of Japanese cedar pollinosis: a double-blind placebo-controlled trial. Clin Exp Allergy 36:1425–1435.
55. Xiao JZ, Kondo S, Yanagisawa N, Takahashi N, Odamaki T, Iwabuchi N, Iwatsuki K, Kokubo S, Togashi H, Enomoto K, Enomoto T (2006) Effect of probiotic *Bifidobacterium longum* BB536 in relieving clinical symptoms and modulating plasma cytokine levels of Japanese cedar pollinosis during the pollen season. A randomized double-blind, placebo-controlled trial. J Investig Allergol Clin Immunol 16:86–93.
56. Xiao JZ, Kondo S, Yanagisawa N, Miyaji K, Enomoto K, Sakoda T, Iwatsuki K, Enomoto T (2007) Clinical efficacy of probiotic *Bifidobacterium longum* for the treatment of symptoms of Japanese cedar pollen allergy in subjects evaluated in an environmental exposure unit. Allergol Int 56:67–75.
57. Kalliomäki M, Salminen S, Arvilommi H, Kero P, Koskinen P, Isolauri E (2001) Probiotics in primary prevention of atopic disease: a randomised placebo-controlled trial. Lancet 357: 1076–1079.

58. Kalliomäki M, Salminen S, Poussa T, Arvilommi H, Isolauri E (2003) Probiotics and prevention of atopic disease: 4-year follow-up of a randomised placebo-controlled trial. Lancet 361:1869–1871.
59. Kalliomäki M, Salminen S, Poussa T, Isolauri E (2007) Probiotics during the first 7 years of life: a cumulative risk reduction of eczema in a randomized, placebo-controlled trial. J Allergy Clin Immunol 119:1019–1021.
60. Matricardi P, Björkstén B, Bonini S, Bousquet J, Djukanovic R, Dreborg S, Gereda J, Malling H, Popov T, Raz E, Renz H, Wold A (2003) Microbial products in allergy prevention and therapy. Allergy 58:461–471.
61. Taylor AL, Dunstan JA, Prescott SL (2007) Probiotic supplementation for the first 6 months of life fails to reduce the risk of atopic dermatitis and increases the risk of allergen sensitization in high-risk children: a randomized controlled trial. J Allergy Clin Immunol 119:184–191.
62. Kukkonen K, Savilahti E, Haahtela T, Juntunen-Backman K, Korpela R, Poussa T, Tuure T, Kuitunen M (2007) Probiotics and prebiotic galacto-oligosaccharides in the prevention of allergic diseases: a randomized, double-blind, placebo-controlled trial. J Allergy Clin Immunol 119:192–198.
63. Abrahamsson TR, Jakobsson T, Böttcher MF, Fredrikson M, Jenmalm MC, Björkstén B, Oldaeus G (2007) Probiotics in prevention of IgE-associated eczema: a double-blind, randomized, placebo-controlled trial. J Allergy Clin Immunol 119:1174–1180.
64. Böttcher M, Abrahamsson T, Fredriksson M, Jakobsson T, Björkstén B (2008) Low breast milk TGF-b2 is induced by *Lactobacillur reuteri* supplemenation and associates with reduced risk of sensitisation during infancy. Pediatr Allergy Immunol 19:497–504
65. Metchnikoff E. The prolongation of life. London: William Heinemann; 1907.
66. Sjögren YM, Jemalm MC, Böttcher MF, Björkstén B, Sverremark-Ekström E (2009) Altered early infant gut microbiota in children developing allergy up to 5 years of age. Clinical and Experimental allergy 39:518–526.
67. Kopp MV, Hennemuth I, Heinzmann A, Urbanek R (2008) Randomized double-blind, placebo-controlled trial of probiotics for primary prevention: no clinical effects of lactobacillus GG supplementation. Pediatrics 121:850–856
68. Arsanoglu S, Moro G, Schmitt J, Tandoi L, Rizzardi S, Boehm G (2008) Early dietary intervention with a mixture of prebiotic oligosacharides reduces the incidence of allergic manifestations and infections during the first two years of life. J Nutr 138:1091–1095
69. van Hoffen E, Ruiter B, FaberJ, M´Rabet L, Knol EF, Stahl B, Arsanoglu S, Moro G, Boehm G, Garssen J (2009) A specific mixture of short-chain galoco-oligosacharides and long-chain fructooligosacharides induces a beneficial immunoglobulin profile in infants at high risk for allergy. Allergy 64:484–487

Hypersensitivity Reactions to Nanomedicines: Causative Factors and Optimization of Design Parameters

S. Moein Moghimi and Islam Hamad

Introduction

Advances in nanomedicine are beginning to transform the detection/diagnosis and treatment of diseases, and are turning promising molecular discoveries into benefits for patients. Examples of nanomedicines (ranging in size from a few to hundreds of nanometres) that have been administered into the body include liposomes, polymeric nanospheres, micelles, late-generation dendrimers, protein cages, vault nanocapsules, composite nanoshells, iron oxide nanocrystals and carbon nanotubes [1,2]. Some of these entities (e.g. liposomes and polymeric nanospheres, Fig. 1) can efficiently encapsulate or incorporate drug molecules, thus following administration affording protection against drug degradation or inactivation en-route to the target site. This may even result in a reduction of the amount of active agent needed to obtain a beneficial effect, and may effectively reduce drug-induced toxicity and other side effects [1].

Encapsulation capacity, drug release profiles (over a period of days or even weeks), and biological performance of nanomedicines vary with parameters such as chemical make-up, morphology and size [1]. These parameters can be tailored in relation to the type, developmental stage and location of a given disease. For instance, intravenously injected polymeric nanoparticles and liposomes are rapidly intercepted by the hepatic and splenic macrophages [1,3]. This propensity of macrophages for the phagocytic/endocytic clearance of foreign entities provides a rational approach to macrophage-specific delivery of drugs, toxins, antigens and diagnostic agents, Fig. 1e [1]. Indeed, liposome-mediated macrophage suicide (i.e. delivery of macrophage toxins) has proved to be a powerful approach in removing

S.M. Moghimi (✉)
Department of Pharmaceutics and Analytical Chemistry, Faculty of Pharmaceutical Sciences, University of Copenhagen, Universitestparken 2, DK2100, Copenhagen Ø, Denmark
e-mail: momo@farma.ku.dk

I. Hamad
Molecular Targeting and Polymer Toxicology Group, School of Pharmacy, University of Brighton, Brighton BN2 4GJ, UK

R. Pawankar et al. (eds.), *Allergy Frontiers: Future Perspectives*,
DOI 10.1007/978-4-431-99365-0_14, © Springer 2010

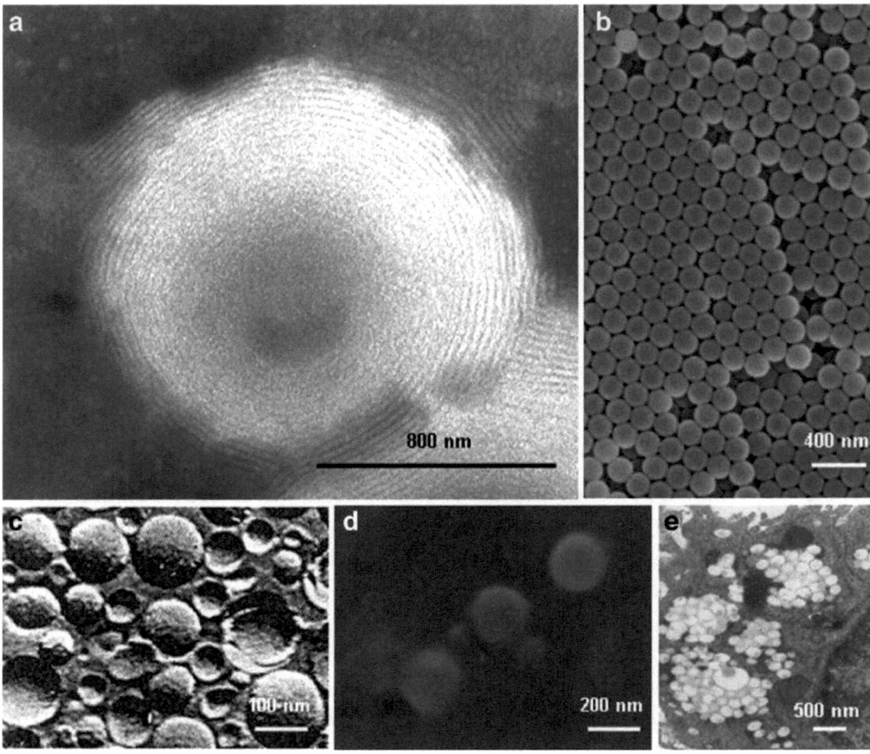

Fig. 1 Electron micrograph representation of liposomes and polymeric nanospheres. (**a**) Transmission electron micrograph of a multilamellar vesicle. (**b**) Scanning electron micrograph of polystyrene nanospheres. (**c**) Freeze fracture electron micrograph of small unilamellar vesicles. (**d**) Scanning electron micrograph of poly(lactideco-glycolide) nanospheres. (**e**) Accumulation of intravenously injected polystyrene nanospheres in lysosomes of a rat Kupffer cell

unwanted macrophages during gene therapy, or in autoimmune blood disorders or spinal cord injury [3]. Furthermore, nanomedicines can be engineered to be pH-sensitive or fusion-competent; these properties aid the release of their entrapped cargo from the endo-lysosomal compartment into the cytosol within minutes of internalization [4,5]. This is a useful strategy for channelling antigens into highly polymorphic MHC class-I molecules of macrophages and dendritic cells for subsequent presentation to $CD8^+$ T-lymphocytes. Alternatively, pharmacokinetic profiles of nanoparticles can be altered by tailoring their size, shape and surface properties (e.g. by polymer grafting), thus providing opportunities for targeting non-macrophage sites [6]. For example, 'macrophage-evading' drug carriers of ≤150 nm size exhibit prolonged circulation times in the blood and may escape from the vasculature at sites where the capillaries have open fenestrations or when the integrity of the endothelial barrier is perturbed by inflammatory processes or tumour growth. Indeed, there are many reported cases of successful delivery of drugs and contrast agents with different long-circulating entities to the underlying parenchyma of solid tumours and injured arteries [1,6].

The biggest commercial opportunities in the nanomedicine sector are envisaged to arise from the development of multifunctional entities capable of simultaneously detecting and treating diseases, as well as for follow-up monitoring of a particular pathology. Here, advances in the development of composite metal nanoshells, iron oxide nanocrystals and carbon nantotubes have been of paramount importance [2]. As a result of their nanosize (and hence different atomic arrangements), these materials exhibit a wide spectrum of unique physical and chemical properties [1,2]. Composite metal nanoshells, for example, consist of a spherical dielectric core of 20–80 nm (e.g. made from silica) surrounded by a thin metal shell of 5–20 nm (e.g. made from gold). In such entities, incident light can couple to the plasmon excitation of the metal; a process that involves the light-induced motion of all valence electrons. Consequently, the type of plasmon that exists on the surface of a metallic nanoparticle is directly related to the shape and curvature of the nanoparticle. Hence, by controlling the relative thickness of the core and shell layers, the plasmon resonance and resultant optical absorption properties can be adjusted from near-UV to mid-infrared [7]. Drugs can be incorporated within the nanoshell core, and the surface of a nanoshell is further amenable for decoration with biological ligands and polymers for site-specific targeting. The plasmon resonance property of near-infrared-responsive gold nanoshells has been exploited for irreversible photothermal ablation of cancer cells in vivo under magnetic resonance guidance [8], and is currently undergoing phase II testing for treatment of glioblastoma and astrocytoma. Here, the temperature change is induced only in nanoshell-associated cells with an external infrared light, which is transmitted through tissue at depths of a few cm with relatively little attenuation and no local damage. Such interventions are more precise than chemotherapy (being targeted) and exert fewer side effects; they are also potentially less expensive and therefore more affordable to poorer countries.

However, as a consequence of their small size, composition and altered pharmacokinetics, nanomedicines may induce inflammatory reactions and adverse immune toxicity [1]. For instance, acute allergic reactions with symptoms that fit in Coombs and Gell's Type I category (but, which are not initiated or mediated by pre-existing IgE antibodies) have been reported to occur following administration of clinically available nanomedicines (e.g. liposomes, micelles and polymeric nanospheres) [9–16]. An understanding of the causative and molecular basis of these reactions is of great importance, and could lead to better material design and nanoengineering strategies for preventing hypersensitivity to future nanomedicines. These concepts are discussed in this article.

Hypersensitivity to Liposomes

Liposomes are vesicular structures that form on hydration of dry phospholipids above their phase transition temperature, and that are classified on the basis of their size and number of bilayers [1]. Drug molecules can be either entrapped in the aqueous space or intercalated into the lipid bilayer of liposomes, depending on the physicochemical characteristics of the drug. Cholesterol may also be incorporated into the liposomal bilayer to control membrane fluidity and hence influence vesicular stability. Clinical formulations of liposomes include Ambisome®, which is used for treatment of visceral leishmaniasis or confirmed infections caused by special fungal species, and DuanoXome®, a danuorubicin-encapsulated vesicle of 45 nm in size for HIV-related Kaposi's sarcoma [1].

Acute allergic reactions have been reported to occur in some patients within 5–10 min of liposome infusion [9–13]; the frequency of these reactions to liposomes shows large variation of between 3 and 45% [17]. Some of the observed symptoms are similar to those of IgE-mediated Type I allergy. These include symptoms of cardiopulmonary distress such as dyspnea, tachypnea, hypertension/hypotension and chest and back pain. However, unlike Type I allergy, the response to liposomes arises at the first exposure without prior sensitization, and the symptoms may lessen or disappear on later treatments. Liposome-induced haemodynamic changes are highly reproducible in the porcine model following intravenous injection of minute amounts (5–10 mg total lipid) and include a massive rise in pulmonary arterial pressure, and a decline in systemic arterial pressure, cardiac output and left ventricular end-diastolic pressure [17,18]. In pigs, these haemodynamic changes are associated with massive but transient ECG alterations including tachycardia, bradycardia, ST-segment depression and T-wave changes, ventricular fibrillation or cardiac arrest [18].

Pseudoallergic reactions to liposomes are strongly correlated with complement activation, which leads to rapid production of anaphylatoxins C3a and C5a and subsequent release of thromboxane A2 and other anaphylatoxin-derived mediators [17,18]. Indeed, inhibitors of complement activation such as soluble complement receptor Type 1 (sCR1) and anti-C5a monoclonal antibody can dramatically suppress liposome-induced cardiopulmonary changes in the porcine model [18]. Complement activation by liposomes depends on vesicular lipid composition, bilayer packing, surface characteristics, morphology and size [19–21]. Liposomal activation of the classical pathway occurs when natural antibodies to phospholipids and cholesterol bind to the vesicles. Liposomes also activate complement through non-antibody-mediated mechanisms via the classical pathway (e.g. following direct C1q binding to vesicles bearing anionic phospholipids in their bilayer), as well as via the alternative pathway (e.g. following direct C3 adsorption and conformational changes, leading to exposure of neo-antigenic epitopes capable of forming an initiating C3 convertase, or even following antibody binding). For vesicles composed of zwitterionic phospholipids, complement activation seems to proceed only after prolonged exposure to serum/plasma, presumably via the C-reactive protein-binding pathway.

Surface camouflaging of liposomes by methoxypoly(ethyleneglycol), mPEG, has been shown to suppress protein adsorption and limit the opsonization processes (including complement activation and fixation) [6,22]. Such engineered vesicles (PEGylated liposomes) display prolonged circulation times in the blood due to poor macrophage capture and as a result have been formulated for delivery of therapeutic agents to solid tumours [6]. For example, Doxil® is a 100 nm PEGylated liposome with encapsulated doxorubicin approved for HIV-related Kaposi's sarcoma and refractory ovarian carcinoma [1,6]. Interestingly, infusion of Doxil® and other PEGylated liposomes has also induced cardiopulmonary distress in a substantial percentage of human subjects [13,17,23]. A recent investigation has reported acute allergic reactions to Doxil® infusion in 13 out of 29 cancer patients [23]. In spite of the general view that surface modification with mPEG would dramatically suppress complement activation [22], Doxil®, however, induced complement activation in 21 out of those 29 patients (72%), as reflected by significant elevation of SC5b-9 (the terminal complex activation marker) levels in plasma within 10–30 min of infusion [23]. Remarkably, among the 13 sensitive patients, 12 (92%) had elevated plasma SC5b-9 levels, whereas within the 16 non-responding individuals significant rises in plasma SC5b-9 level occurred in 9 (56%). Similarly, in a study involving radio-labelled PEGylated liposomes for scintigraphic detection of bowel inflammation, pseudoallergy was observed in three out of nine patients, and in the case of one sensitive patient the plasma levels of C3, C4 and factor B decreased substantially [24]. Collectively, these observations indicate that PEGylated liposome-induced cardiopulmonary distress may be a manifestation of complement activation-related pseudoallergy. In this context, it is worth mentioning that complement has been known to be involved in the effector arm of antibody-mediated Type II and Type III allergic reactions. However, the elevated plasma SC5b-9 levels in non-responders (as in the Doxil® study [23]) suggest that complement activation per se cannot solely account for liposome-induced pseudoallergy and that other contributing factors therefore must be considered. The differences between sensitive and non-responding individuals, for instance, may depend on the extent of activation of other plasma cascades such as the kallikrein-kinin system that results in generation of a co-stimulus for mast cell activation. Alternatively, the mast cells and basophils of sensitive individuals may have a lower than normal threshold for degranulation following the binding of anaphylatoxins to their G-protein coupled receptors. It is also plausible that the risk of complement activation-related pseudoallergic cardiopulmonary reactions may be highest in a complement-responder with atopic constitution.

But why do PEGylated liposomes activate complement? Our recent studies [25] have indicated the importance of a spatial relationship between the headgroup of zwitterionic phospholipids in the liposomal bilayer and the net anionic charge on the phosphate moiety of phospholipid-mPEG conjugate in controlling antibody binding and its orientation into a complement activating posture (Fig. 2). In addition, a direct role for C1q binding to PEGylated vesicles and subsequent complement activation was speculated [25], where C1q may interact with the ether oxygen groups of the projected mPEG chains via hydrophobic interactions and/or hydrogen bonding as well as with the anionic phosphate oxygen of the phospholipid-mPEG through the top of its basic head. If complement activation is a pre-condition to liposome-mediated hypersensitivity, then it is highly desirable to engineer liposomes and related structures that circumvent complement activation; this is despite the fact that slow intravenous liposome infusion together with high-dose steroid and antihistamine premedication substantially reduces the risk of hypersensitivity. Some progress has now been made towards design of non-complement activating

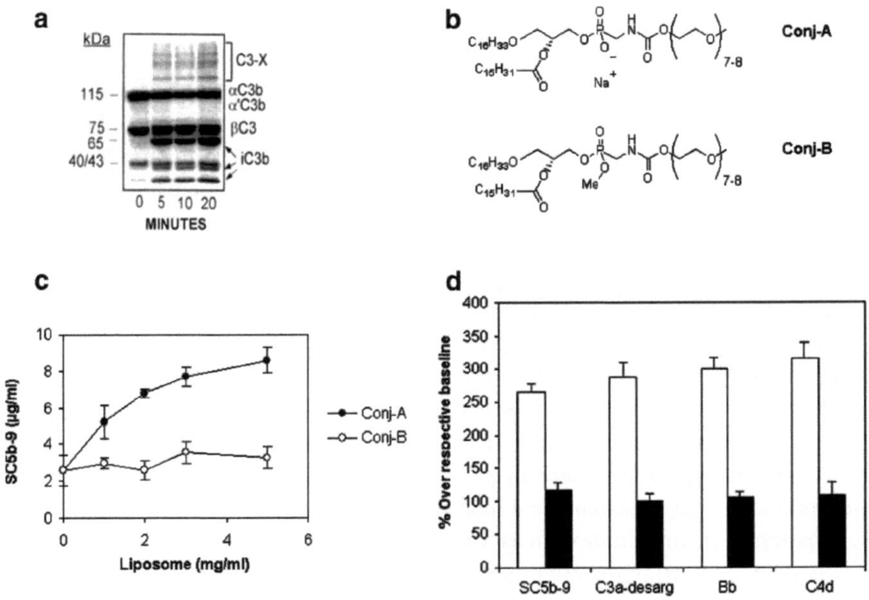

Fig. 2 Complement activation by PEGylated liposomes. (**a**) SDS–PAGE analysis of Doxil®-mediated complement activation in human serum supplemented with ^{125}I-labelled C3 for the given times. (**b**) Structure of mPEG-lipid conjugates with and without (methylated) the presence of the negative charge on the phosphate oxygen (see [25] for details). (**c**) The effect of PEGylated liposome (70–110 nm) concentration on generation of SC5b-9 in a healthy human serum. Liposomes were composed of dipalmitoylphosphatidylcholine (DPPC) and mPEG-lipid in a mole ratio of 95:5 and incubated in serum for 30 min prior to SC5b-9 analysis. (**d**) The effect of the mPEG-lipid conjugate incorporation (5 mol%) on DPPC liposome-mediated generation of SC5b-9 and complement split product (C3a-desarg, Bb and C4d) in a healthy human serum. Liposome concentration was 3 mg lipid/ml serum. Open columns refer to Conj-A and black columns refer to Conj-B incorporated vesicles, respectively

PEGylated liposomes; these include zwitterionic vesicles with incorporated non-ionic lipid-mPEG conjugates (Fig. 2b–d) [25] or other related lipopolymers in their bilayer [26].

Hypersensitivity to Cremophor EL

Cremophor EL (CrEL) is a non-ionic solubilizer and emulsifier obtained by reacting ethylene oxide with castor oil. The main component of CrEL is glycerol-PEG-ricinoleate, which together with fatty acid esters of PEG represents the hydrophobic components of the product. The hydrophilic components of CrEL include free

PEG chains and ethoxylated glycerol. In aqueous solution, and at a concentration above 60 μg/ml, CrEL can form micelles of 8–25 nm in size thus allowing solubilization of hydrophobic/amphipathic drugs such as paclitaxel, teniposide and cyclosporine [27]. CrEL-based formulations may contain ethanol as a co-solvent to further aid drug solubilization and micelle formation.

The occurrence of hypersensitivity reactions to CrEL-based pharmaceuticals is common and is extensively documented in the case of Taxol-® (paclitaxel solubilized in CrEL/ethanol) [15,28]. Reactions to Taxol-® infusion occur in about 2–7% of cancer patients despite premedication with high-dose dexamethasone, antihistamines and H2-receptor antagonists, and are severe and life-threatening in some 2% of the recipients [17,28,29]. Hypersensitivity to Taxol-® has been referred to in some studies as a Type I allergic reaction, primarily on the basis of its clinical course and symptoms, but conclusive evidence for a role of IgE in Taxol-®-mediated hypersensitivity has never been established. In addition, a direct effect of paclitaxel on basophils and/or mast cells has never been proven. Most reactions to Taxol-® occur during the first or second treatment cycle. However, the reactions may spontaneously disappear on slowing the infusion rate and may be associated with transient pulmonary infiltration, hypertension and major cardiac arrhythmia [17]. These symptoms are consistent with complement-activation related pseudoallergy. Indeed, recent in vitro studies have shown that at clinically relevant concentrations both Taxol-® and its vehicle (CrEL/ethanol micelles) can equally induce complement activation in human sera (based on the generated levels of SC5b-9), thus suggesting that the vehicle, and not paclitaxel, is a complement activating agent [30]. It also appears that the complement system of most humans is susceptible to activation by Taxol-® or its vehicle [30]. Nevertheless, in vivo studies are still necessary to establish whether complement activation is a causal factor to CrEL-mediated hypersensitivity reactions.

Taxol-® or CrEL/ethanol-mediated complement activation in human serum occurs via both calcium-sensitive and alternative pathways, and can be inhibited by sCR1 and human intravenous immunoglobulin [27,30]. The exact mechanisms of complement activation by CrEL components or CrEL/ethanol micelles remain unknown. It is plausible that in human serum ethanol may cause an increase in C3 conversion through inhibition of factor I. On the contrary, ethanol was shown to be ineffective in elevating levels of SC5b-9 and Bb (the alternative pathway marker) in human serum [30]. Alternatively, it has been shown that in serum CrEL can substantially decrease the electrophoretic mobility of both HDL and LDL, resulting in de novo formation of larger molecular size complexes with no evidence of lipoprotein dissociation into smaller fragments [27,31]. These alterations were speculated to arise from incorporation of some of the hydrophobic components of CrEL into lipoproteins [27]. The components of CrEL that did not associate with lipoproteins were suggested to form large droplets (100–300 nm) capable of assembling C3 convertases, presumably as a result of direct C3 binding to the surface exposed hydroxyl and ethylene oxide residues [27].

Complement Activation by Poloxamers and the Risk of Hypersensitivity

Poloxamers are a family of non-ionic surfactants composed of a central polypropylene oxide chain flanked at either side by a polyethylene oxide segment, thus forming an ABA block co-polymer structure [32]. Among the members of the poloxamer family, poloxamer 188 and 407 have found many applications in experimental and therapeutic medicine. For example, poloxamer 188 has been used in the development of fluorocarbon-based artificial blood substitutes (e.g. Fluosol-DA) [33]. Poloxamer 407 at a concentration of 250 mg/ml can form a thermoreversible gel; the polymer is in aqueous solution at temperatures below 5°C, but will gel at higher temperatures due to micellization and micelle entanglements [34]. As a result of its thermo-gelation properties, poloxamer 407 was recently used for reversible occlusions during percutaneous endovascular procedures [35]. Adverse cardiorespiratory reactions to poloxamers have also been noted, which again may be linked to complement activation. For example, infusion of Fluosol-DA into rabbits and dogs has been associated with a transient, profound haemodynamic collapse accompanied by leukopenia and thrombocytopenia [33,36], and the effects were reproducible following administration of relevant quantities of poloxamer 188 [33]. In addition, poloxamer 188 was capable of activating complement in rabbit plasma via the alternative pathway [33]. In a clinical study, symptoms of complement activation related pseudoallergy were also reported in up to 30% of patients receiving Fluosol-DA as an adjunct to radiation treatment for advanced squamous tumours of the head and neck [37].

Recently, we demonstrated that both poloxamer 188 (at sub-micellar concentrations) and 407 (in micellar form) can activate human complement system via calcium-sensitive as well as alternative pathways [25,38]. Poloxamer-mediated complement activation, however, is an intrinsic property of the polymer, and is independent of the degree of sample polydispersity or the presence of trace organic volatiles [38]. The mechanisms of poloxamer-mediated complement activation are still poorly understood, but activation of the alternative pathway may be related to inhibition of factors H and I. However, direct interaction between poloxamer and C3 or C4, which could lead to generation of products resembling activated C3 and C4 is unlikely, since complement activation by poloxamer is totally abolished in the presence of the sCR1, an inhibitor of C3/C5 convertases [38]. Furthermore, our recent studies have strongly indicated a role for the involvement of the lectin pathway in poloxamer-mediated complement activation (Hamad and Moghimi 2009, unpublished observations).

Quasi-elastic light scattering studies have recently confirmed that poloxamers favourably interact with both HDL and LDL [38]. For example, poloxamer 188 caused a slight but significant increase in the hydrodynamic size of human HDL particles. Remarkably, the presence of poloxamer 188 generated two distinct populations of particles from LDL; one population of particles of 10–20 nm in size and a second population with particles in the range of 30–50 nm [38]. It is not clear whether these structures can activate complement, but elevation of serum HDL and

LDL levels (corresponding to increased cholesterol levels of 30 and 100% above normal, respectively) significantly reduced poloxamer 188-mediated rises of SC5b-9 [38]. These observations are in line with the reported low incidence of poloxamer-mediated hypersensitivity reactions in subjects with abnormal or elevated lipid profiles [33,39]. The protective role of HDL against poloxamer-mediated rises of SC5b-9 levels may be due to the inhibitory effect of apolipoproteins A-I and A-II on C9 polymerization [40], thus minimizing the capacity of C5b-9 complex to elicit non-lytic stimulatory responses on vascular endothelial cells. On the basis of these studies it is imperative to examine possible regulatory and modulatory roles of lipoproteins and apolipoproteins on complement system during health and in chronic inflammatory conditions.

Polymeric Nanoparticles and Acute Hypersensitivity Reactions: Optimization of Design Parameters

Polymeric nanoparticles are colloidal systems of <1,000 nm in size that are assembled either directly from a variety of preformed synthetic polymers of different architecture or by polymerization of monomers. In addition, polymers of natural origin (e.g. albumin, dextran or chitosan) and pseudosynthetic polymers such as poly(amino acids) have also been used in nanoparticle construction [41]. Some poly(amino acids) such as poly(lysine)s and poly(histidine)s, as well as synthetic polycations like poly(ethylenemine)s, can condense DNA and RNA into nanoparticulate-like structures (polyplexes) for transfection [41]. Generally, polymeric nanoparticles and polyplexes are capable of activating complement via all the three known pathways [22,41,42]; this again could lead to complement activation-related pseudoallergy in susceptible individuals. Indeed, complement-related acute hypersensitivity reactions were noted in patients receiving intravenous doses of doxorubicin encapsulated poly(isohexylcyanoacrylate) nanoparticles [16]. However, complement activation by polymeric nanoparticles and nanospheres can be reduced dramatically by coating their surface with non-ionic polymers to include poloxamers and related structures (e.g. poloxamine 908, a tetrafunctional polyethylene oxide/polypropylene oxide ethylenediamine block copolymer, Fig. 3a). Here, the extent of complement activation is related to the surface density and conformation of the attached polymers, Fig. 3b and c [42,43].

Intriguing progress is being made in cancer drug delivery with the development of Abraxane™. This is an albumin nanoparticle-based paclitaxel formulation of 130 nm in size; the only regulatory approved (FDA, USA) solvent-free polymeric nanoparticle formulation for use in cancer patients. Abraxane™ has been reported to cause considerably fewer hypersensitivity reactions compared with Taxol®, despite the fact that it was given to patients without steroid and antihistamine premedication, at a 50% higher dose and with a shorter infusion time [44]. Rapid disassembly of Abraxane™ into albumin molecules in the systemic circulation may account for poor complement activation.

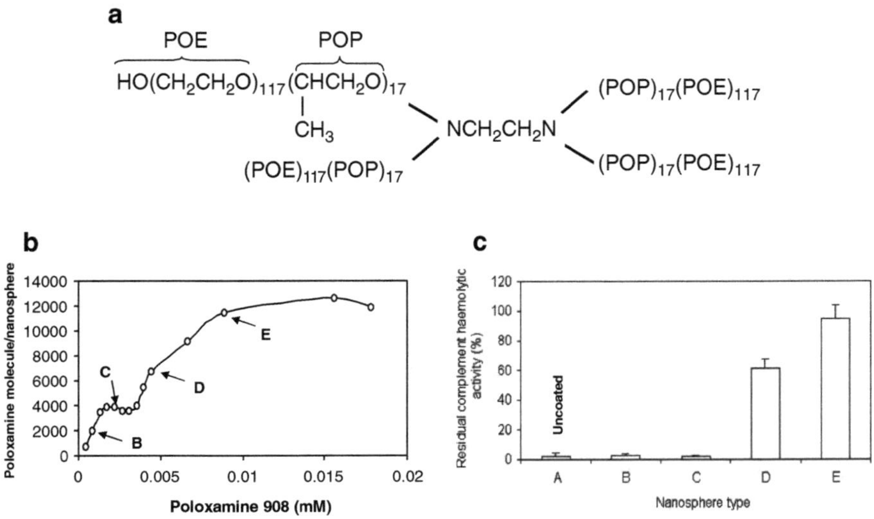

Fig. 3 Complement activation by poloxamine 908-coated polystyrene nanospheres. (**a**) Structure of poloxamine 908. (**b**) Adsorption characteristics of poloxamine 908 on the surface of 232 nm polystyrene nanospheres. (**c**) Consumption of human complement by uncoated and poloxamine 908-coated polystyrene nanospheres. The uncoated nanospheres are referred to as Type A and poloxamine 908-coated nanospheres (Types B–E) refer to selected points on the adsorption characteristic panel

Concluding Remarks

The information delineated above strongly suggests that complement activation may be a contributing, but not a rate limiting factor in eliciting hypersensitivity reactions to nanomedicines in sensitive individuals. The molecular basis of complement activation by nanomedicines is complex and depends on nanomedicine dose and structure. Nevertheless, there are efforts to circumvent nanomedicine-mediated complement activation by optimizing design parameters (as in the case of liposomes and nanospheres). Parallel efforts may include tagging of nanomedicines with complement regulatory proteins or specific complement inhibitors. Several novel complement inhibitors and chimeric or modified human complement regulatory proteins are available for pursuing such studies. Lipoproteins also seem to play an unexpected role in regulating the complement system, and recent studies have further indicated that elevation of serum lipoprotein levels can dramatically suppress liposome- and poloxamer-mediated complement activation. These findings may have important bearings on the future design and development of nanomedicines, as well as in patient selection. On the other hand, complement activation and fixation may be beneficial in scenarios where nanocarriers have been employed for antigen delivery [45]. Indeed, complement activation products such as C3b, C4b, iC3b and C3d act as adjuvants and could aid particle interaction with complement receptors (e.g. CR2) on antigen presenting cells as well as B lymphocytes.

References

1. Moghimi SM, Hunter AC, Murray JC (2005) Nanomedicine: current progress and future prospects. FASEB J 19: 311–330.
2. Moghimi SM, Kissel T (2006) Particulate nanomedicines. Adv Drug Deliv Rev 58: 1451–1455.
3. Moghimi SM (2003) Exploitation of macrophage clearance functions in vivo. In: Gordon S (ed) Handbook of Experimental Pharmacology, Volume 158: The Macrophage as Therapeutic Target. Springer, Berlin, pp 41–54.
4. Drummond DC, Zignani M, Leroux JC (2000) Current status of pH-sensitive liposomes in drug delivery. Prog Lipid Res 39: 409–460.
5. Panyam J, Zhou WZ, Prabha S, Sahoo SK, Labhasetwar V (2002) Rapid endo-lysosomal escape of poly(DL-lactide-co-glycolide) nanoparticles: implications for drug and gene delivery. FASEB J 16: 1217–1226.
6. Moghimi SM, Hunter AC, Murray JC (2001) Long-circulating and target-specific nanoparticles: theory to practice. Pharmacol Rev 53: 283–318.
7. Hirsch LR, Gobin AM, Lowery AR, Tam F, Drezek RA, Halas NJ, West JL (2006) Metal nanoshells. Ann Biomed Engineering 34: 15–22.
8. Hirsch LR, Stafford RJ, Bankson JA, Sershen SR, Rivera B, Price RE, Hazle JD, Halas NJ, West JL (2003) Nanoshell-mediated near-infrared thermal therapy of tumors under magnetic resonance guidance. Proc Natl Acad Sci USA 100: 13549–13554.
9. Sculier JP, Coune A, Brassinne C, Laduron C, Atassi G, Ruysschaert JM, Fruhling J (1986) Intravenous-infusion of high-doses of liposomes containing NSC-251635, a water-insoluble cytostatic agent–A pilot-study with pharmacokinetic data. J Clin Oncol 4: 789–797.
10. Laing RBS, Milne LJR, Leen CLS, Malcolm GP, Steers AJW (1994) Anaphylactic reactions to liposomal amphotericin. Lancet 344:682.
11. Levine SJ, Walsh TJ, Martinez A, Eichacker PQ, Lopez-Berstein G, Ntanson C (1991) Cardiopulmonary toxicity after liposomal amphotericin B infusion. Ann Internal Med 114: 664–666.
12. Richardson DS, Kelsey SM, Johnson SA, Tighe M, Cavenagh JD, Newland AC (1997) Early evaluation of liposomal danuorubicin (DaunoXome, Nexstar) in the treatment of relapsed and refractory lymphoma. Invest New Drugs 15: 247–253.
13. Uziely B, Jeffers S, Isacson R, Kutsch K, Wei-Tsao D, Yehoshua Z, Libson E, Muggia FM, Gabizon A (1995) Liposomal doxorubicin: antitumor activity and unique toxicities during two complementary phase I studies. J Clin Oncol 13: 1777–1785.
14. Kris MG, O'Connell JP, Gralla RJ (1986) A phase I trial of Taxol given as 3-hour infusions every 21 days. Cancer Treat Rep 70: 605–607.
15. Grosen E, Siitari E, Larrison E, Tiggelaar C, Roecker E (2000) Paclitaxel hypersensitivity reactions related to bee-sting allergy. Lancet 355: 288–289.
16. Kattan J, Droz JP, Couvreur P, Marino JP, Boutanlaroze A, Rougier P, Brault P, Vranckx H, Grognet JM, Morge X, Sanchogarnier H (1992) Phase-I clinical-trial and pharmacokinetic evaluation of doxorubicin carried by polyisohexylcyanoacrylate nanoparticles. Invest New Drugs 10: 191–199.
17. Szebeni J (2005) Complement activation-related pseudoallergy: a new class of drug-induced acute immune toxicity. Toxicology 216: 106–121.
18. Szebeni J, Fontana JL, Wassef NM, Mongan PD, Morse DS, Dobbins DE, Stahl GL, Bünger R, Alving CR (1999) Hemodynamic changes induced by liposomes and liposome-encapsulated hemoglobin in pigs. A model for pseudoallergic cardiopulmonary reactions to liposomes: role of complement and inhibition by soluble CR1 and anti-C5a antibody. Circulation 99: 2302–2309.
19. Moghimi SM, Hunter AC (2001) Recognition by macrophages and liver cells of opsonised phospholipid vesicles and phospholipid headgroups. Pharm Res 18: 1–8.
20. Chonn A, Cullis PR, Devine DV (1992) The role of surface charge in the activation of the classical and alternative pathways of complement by liposomes. J Immunol 146: 4234–4241.

21. Bradley AJ, Brooks DE, Norris-Jones R, Devine DV (1999) C1q binding to liposomes is surface charge dependent and is inhibited by peptides consisting of residues 14–26 of the human C1qA chain in asequence independent manner. Biochim Biophys Acta 1418: 19–30.
22. Moghimi SM, Szebeni J (2003) Stealth liposomes and long circulating nanoparticles: critical issues in pharmacokinetics, opsonization and protein-binding properties. Prog Lipid Res 42: 463–478.
23. Chanan-Khan A, Szebeni J, Savay S, Liebes L, Rafique NM, Alving CR, Muggia FM (2003) Complement activation following first exposure to pegylated liposomal doxorubicin (Doxil): possible role in hypersensitivity reactions. Ann Oncol 14: 1430–1437.
24. Dams ET, Oyen WJ, Boerman OC, Storm G, Laverman P, Kok PJ, Buijs WC, Bakker H, van der Meer JW, Corstens FH (2000) ^{99m}Tc-PEG liposomes for the scintigraphic detection of infection and inflammation: clinical evaluation. J Nucl Med 41: 622–630.
25. Moghimi SM, Hamad I, Andresen TL, Jørgensen K, Szebeni J (2006) Methylation of the phosphate oxygen moiety of phospholipid-methoxy(polyethylene glycol) conjugate prevents PEGylated liposome-mediated complement activation and anaphylatoxin production. FASEB J 20: 2592–2593 (E2057–E2067).
26. Zalipsky S, Barenholz Y (2004) Liposome composition for reduction of liposome-induced complement activation. PCT Patent Application W/O 2004/078121.
27. Szebeni J, Alving CR, Savay S, Barenholz Y, Priev A, Danino D, Talmon Y (2001) Formation of complement-activating particles in aqueous solutions of Taxol: possible role in hypersensitivity reactions. Int Immunopharmacol 1: 721–735.
28. Rowinsky EK, Eisenhauer EA, Chaudhry V, Arbuck SG, Donehower RC (1993) Clinical toxicities encountered with paclitaxel (Taxol). Semin Oncol 20: 1–15.
29. Guchelaar HJ, ten Napel CH, de Vries EG, Mulder NH (1994) Clinical, toxicological and pharmaceutical aspects of antineoplastic drug taxol: a review. Clin Oncol 6: 40–48.
30. Szebeni J, Muggia FM, Alving CR (1998) Complement activation by Cremophor EL as a possible contributor to hypersensitivity to paclitaxel: an in vitro study. J Natl Cancer Inst 90: 300–306.
31. Kessel D, Woodburn K, Kecker D, Sykes E (1995) Fractionation of Cremophor EL delineates components responsible for plasma lipoprotein alterations and multidrug resistance reversal. Oncol Res 7: 207–212.
32. Moghimi SM, Hunter AC (2000) Poloxamers and poloxamines in nanoparticle engineering and experimental medicine. Trend Biotechnol 18: 412–420.
33. Vercellotti GM, Hammerschmidt DE, Craddock PR, Jacob HS (1982) Activation of plasma complement by perfluorocarbon artificial blood: probable mechanism of adverse pulmonary reactions in treated patients and rationale for corticosteroid prophylaxis. Blood 59: 1299–1304.
34. Cabana A, Aït-Kadi A, Juhász J (1997) Study of the gelation process of polyethylene oxide$_a$-polypropylene oxide$_b$-polyethylene oxide$_a$ copolymer (poloxamer 407) aqueous solutions. J Colloid Interface Sci 190: 307–312.
35. Raymond J, Metcalfe A, Salazkin I, Schwarz A (2004) Temporary vascular occlusion with poloxamer 407. Biomaterials 25: 3983–3989.
36. Faithfull NS, Cain SM (1988) Cardiorespiratory consequences of fluorocarbon reactions in dogs. Biomaterial Artif Cells Artif Organs 16: 463–472.
37. Lustig R, McIntosh-Lowe N, Rose C, Haas J, Krasnow S, Spaulding M, Prosnitz L (1989) Phase I/II study of Fluosol-DA and 100% oxygen as an adjuvant to radiation in the treatment of advanced squamous cell tumours of the head and neck. Int J Radiat Oncol Biol Phys 16: 1587–1593.
38. Moghimi SM, Hunter AC, Dadswell CM, Savay S, Alving CR, Szebeni J (2004) Causative factors behind poloxamer 188 (Pluronic F68, Flocor™)-induced complement activation in human sera. Protective role against poloxamer-mediated complement activation by elevated serum lipoprotein levels. Biochim Biophys Acta 1689: 103–113.
39. Kent KM, Cleman MW, Cowley MJ, Forman MB, Jaffe CC, Kaplan M, King SB, Krucoff MW, Lassar T, Mcauley B, Smith R, Wisdom C, Wohlgelernter D (1990) Reduction of myocardial

ischemia during percutaneous coronary angioplasty with oxygenated Fluosol. Am J Cardiol 66: 279–284.
40. Hamilton KK, Zhao J, Sims PJ (1993) Interaction between apolipoproteins A-I and A-II and the membrane attack complex of complement. Affinity of the apoproteins for polymeric C9. J Biol Chem 268: 3632–3638.
41. Moghimi SM (2006) Recent development in polymeric nanoparticle engineering and their applications in experimental and clinical oncology. Anti-Cancer Agents Med Chem 6: 553–561.
42. Gbadamosi JK, Hunter AC, Moghimi SM (2002) PEGylation of microspheres generates a heterogeneous population of particles with differential surface characteristics and biological performance. FEBS Lett 532: 338–344.
43. Al-Hanbali O, Rutt KJ, Sarker DK, Hunter AC, Moghimi SM (2006) Concentration dependent structural ordering of poloxamine 908 on polystyrene nanoparticles and their modulatory role on complement consumption. J Nanosci Nanotechnol 6: 3126–3133.
44. Sparreboom A, Scripture CD, Trieu V, Williams PJ, De T, Yang A, Beals B, Figg WD, Hawkins M, Desai N (2005) Comparative preclinical and clinical pharmacokinetics of a Cremophor-free, nanoparticle albumin-bound paclitaxel (ABI-007) and paclitaxel formulated in Cremophor (Taxol). Clin Cancer Res 11: 4136–4143.
45. Singh M, O'Hagan D (1999) Advances in vaccine adjuvants. Nat Biotechnol 17: 1075–1081.

An Environmental Systems Biology Approach to the Study of Asthma

William A. Toscano, Kristen P. Oehlke, and Ramzi Kafoury

The number of people with asthma is estimated at 300 million worldwide. Although asthma is the leading cause of hospitalization in children and is considered the most prevalent chronic childhood disease, the causes of asthma remain unknown [1]. Although causes of asthma are unknown, much is known regarding triggers of asthma. Many factors including genetic makeup, environmental conditions, socio-economic status (SES) and education level of parents, dietary factors, and occupation are thought to play a role in both the cause and exacerbation of asthma in children and adults [2]. One of the reasons for our not knowing much about the mechanism of the cause of asthma is that we lack the in-depth knowledge of which genes are involved and what role the environment plays in the development of asthma. It is recognized that asthma is a disease, which is heterogeneous in presentation and course. Although the causes of asthma are not well understood, many studies suggest its familial nature and others provide evidence for environmental factors, such as dust mite antigens, cockroach antigens, pet antigens, and passive tobacco smoking, involved in triggering asthma-related symptoms, but not as the cause of the disease. Rather than a single condition, the term asthma probably comprises a group of conditions that have similar presentations, but may result from perturbations of more than one physiological pathway or be triggered by a combination of environmental factors [3].

The sequencing of the human genome gave much promise for understanding the underlying causes of chronic conditions such as asthma. Almost immediately after announcement of the genomic sequence it was recognized that simply understanding

W.A. Toscano (✉) and K.P. Oehlke
Division of Environmental Health Sciences, University of Minnesota School of Public Health, Mayo Building, Suite 1260, MMC 807, 420 Delaware St. SE, Minneapolis, MN 55455, USA
e-mail: tosca001@umn.edu

K.P. Oehlke
Minnesota Department of Health, St. Paul, MN 55410, USA

R. Kafoury
Department of Biology, Jackson State University, 1400 Lynch St, Jackson, MS 39217, USA

R. Pawankar et al. (eds.), *Allergy Frontiers: Future Perspectives*,
DOI 10.1007/978-4-431-99365-0_15, © Springer 2010

the sequence of the human genome is not enough to yield causal information on disease development. Many genes have been implicated in asthma, but the reductionist approach of individual gene discovery has not yielded the answer to the question of what causes asthma.

Most studies of genetic influence in asthma have focused on single genes. Those studies however have not yielded general reproducible information on the cause of asthma. A recent paper recognized this approach to find the genetic causes of asthma; this approach needs to be re-thought of, as "....gene variants for asthma are polymorphisms that *exert their influence on the network system controlling biological responses* to asthma-related exposures" [4].

Systems biology offers an integrative approach to understanding causes of complex chronic conditions involving many genes and phenotypic perturbation. In its most basic form, systems biology seeks to understand the complex interactions of molecules in cells. Much of the focus of systems biology has been on understanding gene–gene interactions, and it soon branched off to understanding many other molecular interactions and cellular communication systems. By its nature, systems biology, or in silico biology, involves computer modeling and bioinformatics. A number of excellent books reviewing systems biology with various levels of mathematical sophistication have been published [5–10].

We recently suggested that systems biology approaches are required to understand environmentally caused disease in humans, because the reductionist approaches usually employed are not leading to definitive answers in the exposure-gene-disease continuum [11]. To understand environmentally caused disease it is important to recognize that a perturbation may occur in one part of the system, but because of the complex interaction of the entire –ome of a cell, it may cause a domino-like effect in the cellular system. Thus a minor perturbation of gene expression will yield synergistic changes in protein, metabolite, and signaling paradigms of the cell, resulting in clinical disease. If you change one thing in the balanced-tightly controlled physiological system, you change everything.

Family history of disease is an important public health tool that can be used in a systems approach to elucidate, or at least point to important genomic and gene–environment interactions to design appropriate studies to elucidate, the cause of asthma, and lead to systematic intervention strategies.

Having a family history of asthma is an independent risk factor for the disease. Studies of families and twins consistently show asthma clusters in families [12]. A first degree relative with asthma (mother, father, or sibling) is associated with odds ratios of 1.5–9.7, depending on the population, the family members included in the study, the case definition for asthma, and the population studied. The studies were inconsistent for determining which first degree relative with asthma was associated with the greatest odds ratio for childhood asthma in the study populations. However, in spite of this, most studies identified an odds ratio between 2 and 4 for childhood asthma, when a first degree relative was affected with asthma or an asthma-related phenotype [12]. A positive predictive value for a family history of asthma is less than 50%, although a consistent association between a family history of asthma in first-degree relatives and childhood asthma is often observed. Although a family history of asthma is a strong risk factor for childhood asthma, it does not necessarily involve the majority of children on a population level.

A family history of asthma may also reflect environmental factors that increase risk. In a recent prospective study of Dutch children with a positive family history of physician-diagnosed asthma in a first degree relative, and associated with exposure to environmental tobacco smoke or the house mite antigen *Der p 1*, increased risk for asthma-associated phenotypes was found in the first 2 years of life. Odds ratios in the exposed population were between 3.4- and 6-folds compared to the risk associated with a positive family history alone. Infants with a positive family history of asthma in a first degree relative, and exposure to the same environmental agents had a risk for asthma-associated phenotypes 18-fold greater than that for those with a positive family history without these environmental exposures [13].

Studies of twins have been used to estimate the relative contributions of genetic, shared environmental, and non-shared environmental factors to asthma and related phenotypes such as atopy and bronchial hyper-responsiveness. Interpretation of the data in these studies is on the basis of classic twin theory. Monozygotic twins share 100% of their genes with each other, while dizygotic twins share 50% of their genes, on average. The theory also assumes that the degree to which environmental factors are shared is the same for both monozygotic and dizygotic twins. Consequently, any observed differences in phenotype between monozygotic and dizygotic twins are interpreted to be due to genetic similarities in the case of monozygotic twins [14].

Shared environmental factors are often not observed to be significant while non-shared environmental factors contribute only moderately to asthma and related phenotypes [14–16]. However the design of those studies could not adequately distinguish genetic factors from gene environment interactions. In other words, it is possible that a significant proportion of the factors contributing to causation or pathogenesis of asthma and related phenotypes and to the risk of disease may be related to gene–environment interactions that are not detectable using current study designs [4,14,17].

Studying families with two or more family members affected with asthma have provided opportunities to identify genes and genomic regions that are associated with development of asthma. Strategies for identifying genomic elements that may contribute to asthma risk or pathophysiology include linkage analysis, positional cloning, and whole genome association approaches [18].

In *The Collaborative Study on the Genetics of Asthma*, a genome-wide search of 140 families was conducted. Six novel regions associated with asthma were identified. The genomic regions identified included 5p15 ($p=0.00080$ and 17p11.1-q11.2 ($p=0.0015$) in African Americans; 11p15 ($p=0.0089$) and 19q13 ($p=0.0013$) in Caucasians; and 2q33 ($p=0.0005$) and 21q21 ($p=0.0040$) in Hispanics. The study confirmed linkages to regions of the genome that had been observed by others, including 5q23-31, 6p21.3-23, 12q14-24.2, 13q21.3-qter, and 14q11.2-13 in Caucasians and 12q14-24.2 in Hispanics [19].

Another collaborative study on the genetics of asthma, which included 266 families in the United States from three populations, found linkage to several regions of the genome. The strongest linkage was found at 6p21 in European Americans; at 11q21 in the African Americans; and a region at 1p32 in Hispanic population. Other regions of the genome that showed evidence for linkage included 5q31, 8p23, 12q22, and 15q13 as determined using the conditional analysis and the affected sib pair 2-locus analysis. Several of these regions have been identified as being associated with asthma [20].

In a study seeking connections between a family history of atopic disease and the risk for pediatric atopic-related phenotypes in children aged 0–7 years from 476 families involved in the *Childhood Allergy Study* in Detroit, Michigan, significant associations were found between the asthma and atopy history of the father, especially when the condition presented in childhood. Whether the condition had resolved or was persistent into adulthood did not significantly affect the association. Interestingly, mother's history of asthma or atopy was not strongly predictive for related phenotypes in the offspring. This leads to the conclusion that atopy and related conditions are complex and that a thorough family history of atopy across the lifespan is critical for identifying risk and classifying disease phenotypes [21].

A recent search of the National Center for Biotechnology human genome database (http://www.ncbi.nlm.nih.gov/sites/entrez?db=Genome; visited in July 2007) indicated 170 genes where an association was referenced among susceptibility, pathogenesis, treatment response, or asthma severity. Review of the specific references that documented these associations showed that many of the associations were only reported once in the peer-reviewed literature cited and most of the genes identified were associated with more than one medically relevant phenotype or condition. This was especially true for genes that were associated with pathogenesis or pathophysiology of asthma or closely related phenotypes such as bronchial hyper-responsiveness. It is clear that there is a problem of reproducibility among studies to identify genes related to asthma susceptibility and pathogenesis. Why this is occurring is currently unknown. Reasons for a lack of reproducibility include the following: (1) Asthma is a group of diseases; (2) Different populations have different causative genetic and environmental factors; (3) Different phenotypes are studied, which may not be comparable across populations; and (4) History of asthma is often dependant on patient or parent reports and is not the documented diagnosis of a health care provider. In addition, the designs of studies differ, including the factors that are controlled or considered as confounders, and the appropriateness of the controls also varies. All of these factors could contribute to the lack of reproducibility among many studies.

Asthma is characterized by multiple pathogenetic mechanisms [22]. Extrinsic factors, including airway infections (bacterial and viral), increased levels of air pollution (for example, ozone, nitrogen dioxide, particulate matter, various hydrocarbon emissions, and others), and intrinsic factors, including altered immunity and gene gene interactions contribute to the pathogenesis of atopic (allergic) and non-atopic asthma. Allergic asthma (atopic asthma) is reported to account for nearly 90% of asthma cases in population groups 30 years of age or less. Therefore, it is important to consider cytokine networks when carrying out a systems analysis of asthma. There is increasing evidence of the role of T helper type 2 (Th2) lymphocytes and their released cytokine network, which includes interleukins IL-4, IL-5, IL-9, IL-13, and IL-17 in the pathogenesis of atopic (allergic) and non-atopic asthma [23]. These Th2-derived cytokines initiate and promote complex cascades of allergic and inflammatory responses, including mobilization of eosinophils, activation of mast cells, propagation of Th2 phenotype, activation of alveolar macrophages, and in some instances recruitment of neutrophils [24,25]. In addition to the Th2-derived cytokines, effector inflammatory cells, such as, airway epithelial cells and resident alveolar macrophages respond to allergic and inflammatory stimuli by releasing a diverse array of pro-inflammatory mediators, including leukotrienes (LTs), prostaglandins (PGs), platelet-activating factor (PAF), chemokines (CXC, CC, C, and CX3C), and inflammatory cytokines, including IL-1β, IL-6, IL-8, granulocyte macrophage-colony stimulating factor (GM-CSF), tumor necrosis factor-α (TNF-α), and transforming growth factor-β (β1, β2, and β3). The orchestrated interplay between the immuno-regulatory and inflammatory cells and their products, from the diverse cytokines and chemokines to pro-inflammatory mediators, results in structural changes in the airway wall and remodeling with subsequent narrowing, obstruction, and decreased pulmonary function, which characterize asthma.

T lymphocytes respond to exogenous aeroallergens by releasing an array of cytokines. Mobilization, activation, and trafficking of effector cells to the airways, eosinophils, basophils, and in some instances neutrophils are regulated by a network of T helper type 2 cells (Th2)-specific cytokines. Secretion of a Th2 profile of cytokines occurs after a cognate stimulation of naïve Th2 cells by antigen-presenting cells (APC), mainly dendritic cells and macrophages. Th2 cells produce IL-4, IL-5, IL-9, and IL-13 and are involved in humoral immunity and the allergic response to antigens. In contrast, Th1 cells produce IL-10, INF-γ, and IL-2 and inhibit Th2 cells, as well as provide protection against intracellular pathogens. Genetic mapping has linked asthma to chromosome 5q31–33, which includes the cytokine gene cluster, including IL-4, IL-5, IL-9, and IL-13 [26–28].

Recent studies indicate that innate immune responses are initiated and regulated by an array of pattern recognition receptors (PRRs). Toll-like receptors (TLRs) are members of a family of PRRs [29,30]. TLR proteins initiate pathogen recognition through the innate immune system. Many TLR proteins have been identified in humans (10 TLRs) and animals (13 TLRs), including TLR2, TLR3, TLR4, TLR5, TLR6, TLR7, TLR8, TLR9, TLR10, and TLR11 [4,31,32]. Although the mechanisms underlying the signaling of some of these TLRs remain unknown, it is thought that TLR-mediated signaling pathways regulate pathogen detection and recognition. Unlike macrophage opsonised-phagocytic receptors (Fc and complement factors) that recognize antibodies and particles [33], TLRs are non-phagocytic [32]. TLRs recognize conserved patterns unique to pathogen surfaces [34]. Some reports indicate that TLRs are capable of directly recognizing invading pathogens, others suggest that most TLR-mediated immune responses and induction of pro-inflammatory cytokines are dependent on adapter proteins, especially the myeloid differentiation factor 88 (MyD88) [35]. The cytoplasmic domain of TLRs contains a conserved region known as the Toll/IL-1 receptor (TIR) homology domain [30].

TLR3 and TLR4 have unique signaling pathways that involve both, MyD88-dependent and MyD88-independent pathways in inducing the expression of IFN-β genes. TLRs, 3, 7, 8, and 9 orchestrate the innate response to viruses and modulate the induction of anti-viral cytokines, namely, type I interferons INFα and (INFβ) [36,37]. TLR3 recognizes double-stranded RNA produced during viral replication [38]. TLRs 7 and 8 recognize single-stranded RNA derived from influenza viruses, while TLR9 recognizes bacterial and viral DNA (CpG DNA) [39]. Human influenza A viruses have been reported to induce the induction of the inflammatory cytokines, IL-6, IL-8, and the regulated on activation-normal T cell expressed and secreted (RANTES) chemokine in normal [40] and transformed airway epithelial cells [41]. In addition to the effect of IL-5, RANTES modulates the infiltration of eosinophils, attracts monocytes, and plays a regulatory role in the activation and differentiation of T cells.

TLRs play an important role in the clearance of the respiratory syncytial virus (RSV) [42] in infected lower respiratory airways. TLR4 activates NF-κB binding in alveolar macrophages and modulates their response to RSV [43]. Moreover, exacerbation of asthma in response to ozone and particulate matter (PM_{10-2}) has been linked to TLR2- and TLR4-regulated signaling pathways in murine lung and airway epithelial cells, respectively [44].

Cytokines appear to play a critical role in mediating the inflammatory response in the airways. LPS at high levels can inhibit IL-5 and eotaxin-2 in peripheral blood monocytes (PBMC) [45]. Inhibition of IL-5 and eotaxin subfamily members is attributed to IL-10 and its anti-allergic and anti-inflammatory effect. TLR4-mediated signaling and increased expression of TNF-α evidently are responsible for LPS activation of mast cells [46]. TLR4 is expressed on dendritic cells, macrophages, and B cells [47]. A constitutively active mutant TLR4 that activates NF-κB and induces the expression of the pro-inflammatory genes, IL-1, IL-6, and IL-8 in transfected human cell lines has been reported [30]. TLR2 may also recognize LPS. TLR2 in association with TLR1 or TLR6 recognizes Gram-positive bacteria and other bacterial components, including mycoplasma lipopeptide [48,49].

The intracellular domain of the Toll protein is homologous to that of the IL-1 receptor (IL-1R) suggesting that these receptors share common signaling pathways in regulating the innate response and cytokine induction. The transmembrane and cytoplasmic Toll/IL-1 receptor (TIR) domains are pivotal in all TLR signaling pathways (Fig. 1). TLR-mediated intracellular signaling cascades are propagated by TIR-domain-associated adapter protein MyD88, and downstream members of the IL-R-associated kinase (IRAK; IRAK1, IRAK2, IRAK4, and IRAK-M). IRAK1 and IRAK4 possess serine and threonine kinase activity, but IRAK2 and IRAK-M lack the kinase activity and are suggested to negatively regulate TLR-mediated signaling [37]. Studies in IRAK4-deficient mice support the role of IRAK4 in TLR-mediated signaling downstream from MyD88, IRAK1, and IRAK4, in response to various stimuli to undergo phosphorylation and subsequent activation of tumor necrosis factor-associated factor 6 (TRAF6) [50]. TRAF6 forms complexes with Ubc13 and Uev1A (members of the E3 ubiquitin ligase family),

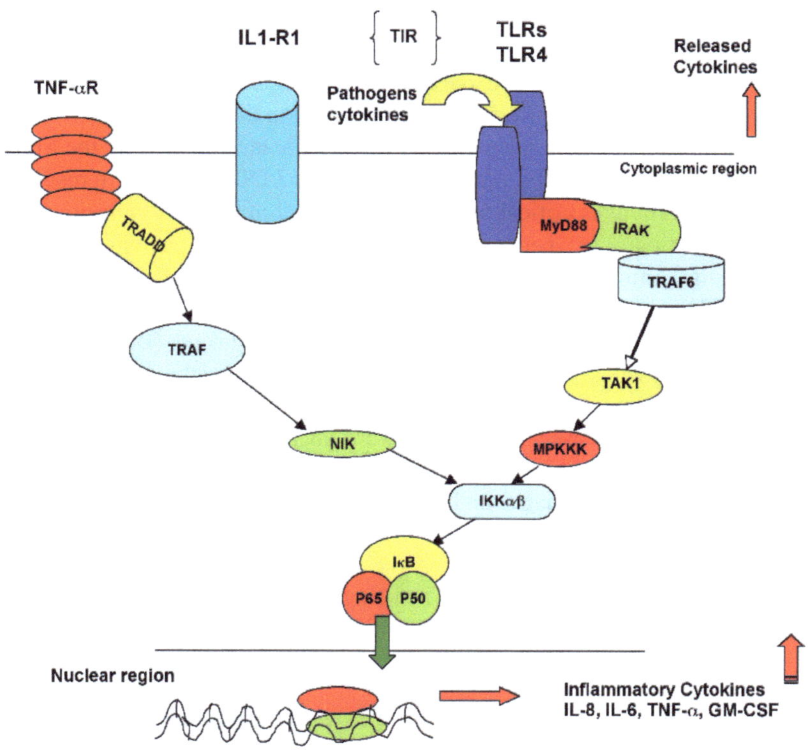

Fig. 1 A schematic diagram illustrating the signaling pathways initiated by binding of pathogens, allergens, and other ligands to TLRs, TNFRs, or IL-1R and subsequent activation of signaling elements, ultimately leading to the activation of NF-κB

promote the synthesis of lysine 63 polyubiquitin chains [40], and activates a member of the MAP kinase kinase kinase (MAPKKK) family, transforming growth factor-β protein kinase 1(TAK1) [40]. TAK1, in turn, activates the inhibitory kinase kinase (IKK) complex resulting in degradation of the inhibitory unit IκB (IκBα, IκBβ), translocation of the NFκB subunits (mainly P65/P50) into the nucleus, and activation of transcription of inflammatory genes [35,40].

Over-expression of pro-inflammatory genes in the lung is regulated at the transcription level [51]. Many pro-inflammatory genes, IL-1β, IL-8, IL-6, TNF-α, and GM-CSF have κB sites in their 5′-flanking regions. Activation of NF-κB results in the expression of many of these inflammatory genes [52,53]. Increased activation of NF-κB has been observed in airways of asthmatics and in sputum macrophages [54]. Moreover, Glucocorticoids that inhibit NF-κB activation have been shown to reduce the survival of eosinophils, a characteristic in immuno-inflammatory asthma [54].

Although TLR signaling pathways are MyD88-dependent, TLR3 and TLR4 are unique because they can signal through MyD88-independent pathways. LPS can induce the expression of the IFNβ in macrophages and DCs through a MyD88-independent mechanism that requires TIR-containing adapter-inducing INFβ protein and TRIF, and is capable of activating NF-κB[55,56]. In contrast, MyD88-mediated pathways are incapable of activation the INFβ promoter [56,57]. Studies using TRIF-deficient mice support the significance of TRIF in the MyD88-independent pathway and INFβ induction [56]. Type I INF produced in response to viral or LPS infections is critical in inducing antiviral immune responses.

Inflammatory cytokine networks play a pivotal role in asthma pathogenesis (Fig. 2). Pro-inflammatory cytokines, particularly TNF-α and IL-1β, play a major role in amplifying the inflammatory response in asthma [34]. This is supported by the observation of TNFα and IL-1β in bronchial alveolar lavage (BAL) fluids from symptomatic asthmatics [58]. TNF-α has been linked to asthma and its severity [34]. Increased expression of membrane-bound TNF-α, TNF-α receptor 1 (TNFR1), and TNF-α converting enzyme by PBMC has been reported [59]. TNF-α levels are significantly increased in induced sputum of asthmatics. TNF-α is produced primarily by macrophages and monocytes following activation by LPS [60]. Over-expression of TNF-α is observed in patients with pneumonia [61]. TNF-α stimulates the generation of reactive oxygen species (ROS) in neutrophils, airway epithelial cells, and endothelial cells and depletes the anti-oxidant, glutathione. Increased levels of TNF-α have been linked to vasoconstriction and hyperplasia of

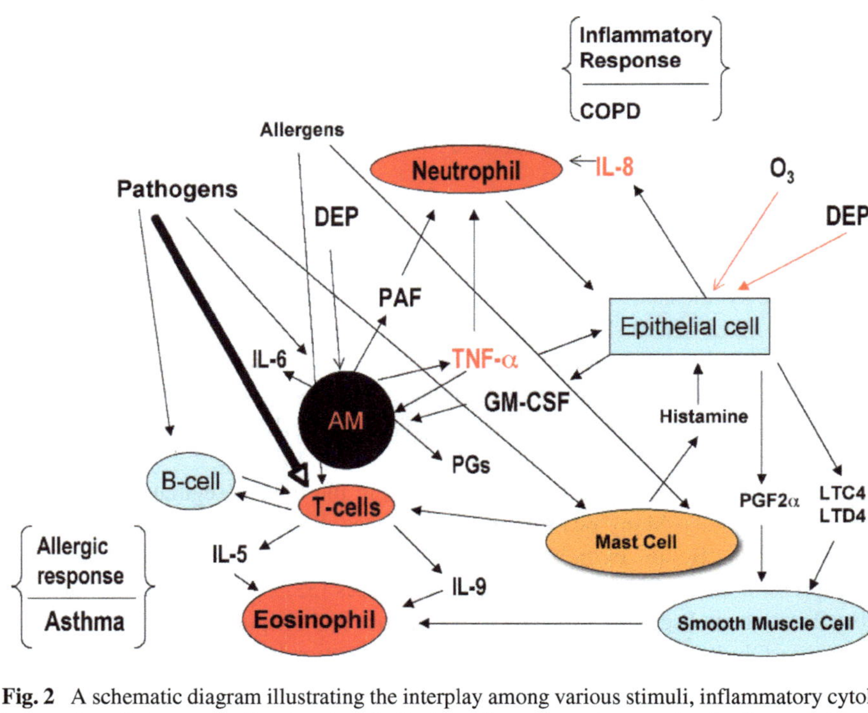

Fig. 2 A schematic diagram illustrating the interplay among various stimuli, inflammatory cytokines, and mediators, as well as target and effector cells, in the pathogenesis of asthma or chronic obstructive pulmonary disease (COPD)

bronchial smooth muscle cells, as well as airway hyper-reactivity and airway epithelium remodeling [62]. Other reports suggest the action of TNF-α on eotaxin (eotaxin-1 and eotaxin-2) induction in airway smooth muscle cells [63]. TNF-α also up-regulates the expression of neurotrophins, nerve growth factors (NGFs) that are linked to prolonged survival of eosinophils [64]. Up-regulation of cell surface expression of intercellular adhesion molecules (ICAMs) and vascular adhesion molecules (VCAMs) on bronchial epithelial cells and leukocyte function-associated antigen (LFA-1) is associated with TNF-α [65]. Bronchial allergic asthma is characterized by eosinophil infiltration of the airways and vasoconstriction. The action of TNF-α on asthma pathogenesis also is linked to increased mucin production by airway epithelial cells. TNF-α also up-regulates the expression of mucin genes, particularly, *MUC5AC* [66,67]. Sequence analysis of the *MUC2* and *MUC5AC* has revealed the presence of NF-κB binding sequences [68]. TNF-α-induced expression of *MUC5AC* is mediated by the P38/MAPK in airway epithelium, which leads to NF-κB activation [40].

TNF-α initiates its action through binding to one of its receptors, p55 (TNFR1) or p75 (TNFR2) [69]. These receptors are expressed on surfaces of most cells, including airway epithelial cells, endothelial cells, macrophages, and airway smooth muscle cells. In response to infection, inflammation, or tissue injury, TNF-α binds to TNF1 or TNF2 and activates signaling elements, members of mitogen-activated protein kinases (MAPKs), and ERK1/2, p42/p44 MAPK, p38/MAPK, or c-Jun NH2-terminal kinase. These serine/threonine phosphorylating kinases play a key role in cellular responses, including inflammation, cell proliferation, and cell cycle progression. TNF-α-activated MAPKs activate downstream signaling elements, in particular, nuclear factor inhibitory kinase (IKK) complex (IKKα, IKKβ, and NEMO) and result in subsequent phosphorylation and degradation of the NF-κB inhibitory subunit IκB and translocation of the NF-κB complex to the nucleus [70]. Therefore, coupling of allergens, pathogens, environmental agents, and inflammatory cytokines to TLRs, TNFRs, or IL-1R initiates signaling cascades that ultimately activate NF-κB and induce the transcription of inflammatory genes that amplify the inflammatory response in the lung.

Besides TNF-α, transforming growth factor-α (TGF-α) also induces MUC5AC expression in airway epithelial cells through epidermal growth factor receptor (EGFR)-mediated tyrosine phosphorylation [71]. Over-expression of EGFR on surfaces of airway epithelial cells and smooth muscle cells has been observed in asthmatic airways [72]. TGF-α plays a role in amplifying the inflammatory response in the lung through mucin overexpression. TGF-β1 has been correlated with smooth muscle cell hypertrophy and basement membrane thickening [73]. TGF-β1, which can be produced by a variety of cells, including macrophages, eosinophils, mast cells, activated lymphocytes, epithelial cells, and smooth muscle cells, has been detected in significant amounts in BAL fluid of asthmatics [74].

In addition to inflammatory cytokines, the role of diverse lipid mediators is well established in asthmatics with lung inflammation as evidenced by increases in BAL fluid of several pro-inflammatory mediators, including prostaglandins (PGs, mainly PGE_2), leukotrienes (LTs, mainly LTB4, LTC4) [75], IL-8, and IL-6 [76]. PLA_2 is a critical enzyme in the liberation of AA, a substrate for and therefore, a rate-limiting step in prostanoid and leukotriene synthesis, including PGE_2 [76,77]. Prostaglandin-H-synthases1/2 (PGHS-1/2) also known as cyclooxygenase1/2 (COX1/2) and lipoxygenase (LO) enzymes are responsible for the generation of prostanoids and leukotrienes from free arachidonic acid (AA) [75], released as a result of preferential PLA_2 cleavage of AA-containing phospholipids in various airway cells, including epithelial cells and macrophages, and from smooth muscle cells [76,77]. Bronchoconstriction of airway smooth muscle cells can be induced in response to cytokine-induced thromboxane B_2 (TXB2) and PGF2α [78]. In contrast, PGE2 serves as a bronchodilator; however, at high levels it can lead to bronchoconstriction by signaling through the TX receptor [79]. Cysteinyl leukotrienes (LTC4, LTD4, and LTE4) can modulate Th2-derived cytokines, for example, IL-4 [4,80] and IL-5 [81]. Furthermore, cysteinyl leukotrienes have been shown to enhance TNF-α production in mast cells [81].

The environmental systems biology approach takes into consideration interacting cellular signaling networks as well as other variables not generally used in systems biology studies of disease. As complex as the pathways are for genes and signals involved in pathophysiology of asthma, it is also important to distinguish complex exposure pathways that could be involved in the onset of asthma. No single environmental exposure evokes asthmatic onset. It may be as varied as diesel exhaust, ozone, dust mites, animal dander, environmental tobacco or passive smoking, and cockroach chitin. In order to dissect the causes of asthma, a systematic understanding of biological systems, and exposure factors is needed. To date, focus has been on genetic aspects of asthma in humans, and while we understand much about complex interacting pathways, we do not have conclusive causal relations yet. It is possible that we should also develop an epigenetic systems biology approach to closely understand environmental control of gene expression networks in addition to susceptibility networks within the genome.

References

1. Gold, D. R., and Wright, R. Population Disparities in Asthma. Annu. Rev. Public Health, *26:* 89–113, 2005.
2. Maddox, L., and Schwartz, D. A. The Pathophysiology of Asthma. Annu. Rev. Med., *53:* 477–498, 2002.
3. Bosse, Y., and Hudson, T. J. Toward a Comprehensive Set of Asthma Susceptibility Genes. Annu. Rev. Med., *58:* 171–184, 2007.
4. Guerra, S., and Martinez, F. D. Asthma Genetics: From Linear to Multifactorial Approaches. Annu. Rev. Med., *59:* 327–348, 2007.
5. Al-Rubeai, M., and Fussinger, M. Systems Biology. Cell Engineering. Amsterdam, Netherlands: Springer, 2007.
6. Kitano, H. Foundations of Systems Biology. Cambridge, MA: MIT Press, 2001.
7. Klipp, E., Herwig, R., Kowald, A., Wierling, C., and Lehrach, H. Systems Biology in Practice. Weinheim, Germany: Wiley-VCH, 2005.
8. Kriete, A., and Eils, R. Computational Systems Biology. Burlington, MA: Elsevier-Academic Press, 2006

9. Palsson, B. Ø. Systems Biology: Properties of Reconstructed Networks. New York: Cambridge University Press, 2006.
10. ZSzallasi, Z., Stelling, J., and Periwal, V. System Modeling in Cellular Biology: From Concepts to Nuts and Bolts. Cambridge, MA: MIT Press, 2006.
11. Toscano, W. A., and Oehlke, K.-P. Systems Biology: New Approaches to Old Environmental Health Problems. Int. J. Environ. Res. Public Health, *2:* 4–9, 2005.
12. Burke, W., Fesinmeyer, M., Reed, K., Hampson, L., and Caristen, C. Family History as a Predictor of Asthma Risk. Am. J. Prev. Med., *24:* 160–169, 2003.
13. Kuiper, S., Muris, J. W., Dompeling, E., Kester, A. D., Wesseling, G., Knottnerus, J. A., and van Schayck, C. P. Interactive Effect of Family History and Environmental Factors on Respiratory Tract-related Morbidity in Infancy. J. Allergy Clin. Immunol., *120:* 388–395, 2007.
14. Koeppen-Schomerus, G., Stevenson, J., and Plomin, R. Genes and Environment in Asthma: A Study of 4 Year Old Twins. Arch. Dis. Child., *85:* 398–400, 2001.
15. Harris, J. R., Magnus, P., Samuelsen, S. O., and Tambs, K. No Evidence for Effects of Family Environment on Asthma. A Retrospective Study of Norwegian Twins. Am. J. Respir. Crit. Care Med., *156:* 43–49, 1997.
16. van Beijsterveldt, C., and Boomsma, D. I. Genetics of Parentally Reported Asthma, Eczema and Rhinitis in 5-yr-Old Twins. Eur. Respir. J., *29:* 516–521, 2007.
17. Martinez, F. D. Gene-environment Interactions in Asthma and Allergies: A New Paradigm to Understand Disease Causation. Immunol. Allergy Clin. North Am., *25:* 709–721, 2005.
18. Smith, A. K., and Meyers, D. A. Family Studies and Positional Cloning of Genes for Asthma and Related Phenotypes. Immunol. Allergy Clin. North Am., *25:* 641–654, 2005.
19. Xu, J., Meyers, D. A., Ober, C., Blumenthal, M. N., Mellen, B., Barnes, K. C., King, R. A., Lester, L. A., Howard, T. D., Solway, J., Langefeld, C. D., Beaty, T. H., Rich, S. S., Bleecker, E. R., Cox, N. J., and Collaborative Study on the Genetics of Asthma. Genomewide Screen and Identification of Gene-gene Interactions for Asthma Susceptibility Loci in Three U. S. Populations: Collaborative Study on the Genetics of Asthma. Am. J. Hum. Genet., *68:* 1437–1446, 2001.
20. Xu, J., Fang, Z., Wang, B., Chen, C., Guang, W., Jin, Y., Yang, J., Lewitzky, S., Aelony, A., Parker, A., Meyer, J., Weiss, S. T., and Xu, X. A. Genomewide Search for Quantitative-trait Loci Underlying Asthma. Am. J. Hum. Genet., *69:* 1271–1277, 2001.
21. Alford, S. H., Zoratti, E., Peterson, E. L., Maliarik, M., Ownby, D. R., and Johnson, C. C. Parental History of Atopic Disease: Disease Pattern and Risk of Pediatric Atopy in Offspring. Allergy Clin. Immunol., *114:* 1046–1050, 2004.
22. Barnes, P. J., and Woolcock, A. J. Difficult Asthma. Eur. Respir. J., *12:* 1209–1218, 1998.
23. Temann, U. A., Laouar, Y., Eynon, E. E., Homer, R., and Flavell, R. A. IL9 Leads to Airway Inflammation by Inducing IL13 Expression in Airway Epithelial Cells. Int. Immunol., *19:* 1–10, 2006.
24. Renauld, J. C. New Insights into the Role of Cytokines in Asthma. J. Clin. Pathol., *54:* 577–589, 2001.
25. Strieter, R. M., Belperio, J. A., and Keane, M. P. Cytokines in Innate Host Defense in the Lung. J. Clin. Invest., *109:* 699–705, 2002.
26. Marsh, D. G., Neely, J. D., Breazeale, D. R., Ghosh, B., Freidhoff, L. R., Ehrlich-Kautzky, E., Schou, C., Krishnaswamy, G., and Beaty, T. H. Linkage Analysis of IL4 and Other Chromosome 5q31.1 Markers and Total Serum Immunoglobulin E Concentrations. Science, *264:* 1152–1156, 1994.
27. Postma, D. S., Bleecker, E. R., Amelung, P. J., Holroyd, K. J., Xu, J., Panhuysen, C. L., Meyers, D. A., and Levitt, R. C. Genetic Susceptibility to Asthma-Bronchial Hyperresponsiveness Coinherited with a Major Gene for Atopy. N. Engl. J. Med., *333:* 894–900, 1995.
28. Rosenwasser, L. J., and Borish, L. Genetics of Atopy and Asthma: The Rationale Behind Promoter-based Candidate Gene Studies (IL-4 and IL-10) Am. J. Respir. Crit. Care Med., *156:* S152–S155, 1997.
29. Janeway, C. A. J., and Medzhitov, R. Innate Immune Recognition. Annu. Rev. Immunol., *20:* 197–216, 2002.

30. Medzhitov, R., and Janeway, C. J. Innate Immunity. N. Engl. J. Med., *343:* 338–344, 2000.
31. Akira, S., Takeda, K., and Kaisho, T. Toll-like Receptors: Critical Proteins Linking Innate and Acquired Immunity. Nat. Immunol., *2:* 675–680, 2001.
32. Basu, S., and Fenton, M. J. Toll-like Receptors: Function and Roles in Lung Disease. Am. J. Physiol., *286:* L887–L892, 2004.
33. Peiser, L., Mukhopadhyay, S., and Gordon, S. Scavenger Receptors in Innate Immunity. Curr. Opin. Immunol., *14:* 123–128, 2002.
34. Mukhopadhyay, S., Hoidal, J. R., and Mukherjee, T. K. Role of TNFα in Pulmonary Pathophysiology. Respir. Res., *7:* 125–133, 2006.
35. Sato, S., Sanjo, H., Takeda, K., Ninomiya-Tsuji, J., Yamamoto, M., Kawai, T., Matsumoto, K., Takeuchi, O., and Akira, S. Essential Function for the Kinase TAK1 in Innate and Adaptive Immune Responses. Nat. Immunol., *6:* 1087–1095, 2005.
36. Akira, S., and Takeda, K. Toll-Like Receptor Signaling. Nat. Rev. Immunol., *4:* 499–511, 2004.
37. Kawai, T., and Akira, S. Innate Immune Recognition of Viral Infection. Nat. Immunol., *7:* 131–137, 2006.
38. Alexopoulou, L., Holt, A. C., Medzhitov, R., and Flavell, R. A. Recognition of Double-stranded RNA and Activation of NF-κB by Toll-Like Receptor 3. Nature, *413:* 732–738, 2001.
39. Krug, A., French, A. R., Barchet, W., Fischer, J. A., Dzionek, A., Pingel, J. T., Orihuela, M. M., Akira, S., Yokoyama, W. M., and Colonna, M. TLR9-dependent Recognition of MCMV by IPC and DC Generates Coordinated Cytokine Responses That Activate Antiviral NK Cell Function Immunity *21:* 107–119, 2004.
40. Chen, Z. J. Ubiquitin Signaling in the NF-kappaB Pathway. Nat. Cell Biol., *7:* 758–765, 2005.
41. Adachi, M., Matsukura, S., Tokunaga, H., and Kokubu, F. Expression of Cytokines on Human Bronchial Epithelial Cells Induced by Influenza Virus A. Int. Arch. Allergy Immunol., *113:* 307–311, 1997.
42. Kurt-Jones, E. A., Popova, L., Kwinn, L., Haynes, L. M., Jones, L. P., Tripp, R. A., Walsh, E. E., Freeman, M. W., Golenbock, D. T., Anderson, L. J., and Finberg, R. W. Pattern Recognition Receptors TLR4 and CD14 Mediate Response to Respiratory Syncytial Virus. Nat. Immunol., *1:* 398–401, 2000.
43. Haeberle, H. A., Takizawa, R., Casola, A., Braiser, A. R., Dieterich, H. J., van Rooijen, N., Gatalica, Z., and Garofalo, R. P. Respiratory Syncytial Virus-Induced Activation of Nuclear Factor-κB in the Lung Involves Alveolar Macrophages and Toll-Like Receptor 4-Dependent Pathways. J. Infect. Dis., *186:* 1199–1206, 2002.
44. Becker, S., Fenton, M. J., and Soukup, J. M. Involvement of Microbial Components and Toll-like Receptors 2 and 4 in Cytokine Responses to Air Pollution Particles. Am. J. Respir. Cell Mol. Biol., *27:* 611–618, 2002.
45. Min, J. W., Park, S. M., Rhim, T. Y., Park, S. W., Jang, A. S., Uh, S. T., Park, C. S., and Chung, I. Y. Effect and Mechanism of Lipopolysaccharide on Allergen-Induced Interleukin-5 and Eotaxins Production by Whole Blood Cultures of Atopic Asthmatics. Clin. Exp. Immunol., *147:* 440–448, 2007.
46. Supajatura, V., Ushio, H., Nakao, A., Akira, S., Okumura, K., Ra, C., and Ogawa, H. Differential Responses of Mast Cell Toll-Like Receptors 2 and 4 in Allergy and Innate Immunity. J. Clin. Invest., *109:* 1351–1359, 2002.
47. Hoshino, K., Takeuchi, O., Kawai, T., Sanjo, H., Ogawa, T., Takeda, Y., Takeda, K., and Akira, S. Toll-like Receptor 4 (TLR4)-deficient Mice are Hyperesponsive to Lipopolysaccharide: Evidence for TLR4 as the LPS Gene Product. J. Immunol., *162:* 3749–3752, 1999.
48. Ozinsky, A., Underhill, D. M., Fontenot, J. D., Hajjar, A. M., Smith, K. D., Wilson, C. B., Schroeder, L., and Aderem, A. The Repertoire for Pattern Recognition of Pathogens by the Innate Immune System Is Defined by Cooperation Between Toll-Like Receptors. Proc. Natl. Acad. Sci. U.S.A., *97:* 13766–13771, 2000.

49. Takeuchi, O., Hoshino, K., Kawai, T., Sanjo, H., Takada, H., Ogawa, T., Takeda, K., and Akira, S. Differential Roles of TLR2 and TLR4 in Recognition of Gram-Negative and Gram-Positive Bacterial Cell Wall Components. Immunity, *11:* 443–451, 1999.
50. Suzuki, N., Suzuki, S., Duncan, G. S., Millar, D. G., Wada, T., Mirtsos, C., Takada, H., Wakeham, A., Itie, A., Li, S., Penninger, J. M., Wesche, H., Ohashi, P. S., Mak, T. W., and Yeh, W. C. Severe Impairment of Interleukin-1 and Toll-Like Receptor Signaling in Mice Lacking IRAK 4. Nature, *416:* 750–756, 2002.
51. Baldwin, A. S. J. Series Introduction: The Transcription Factor NF-κB and Human Disease. J. Clin. Invest., *107:* 3–6, 2001.
52. Christman, J. W., Sadikot, R. T., and Blackwell, T. S. The Role of Nuclear Factor-κβ in Pulmonary Disease. Chest, *117:* 1482–1487, 2000.
53. Kafoury, R. M., Hernandez, J. M., Lasky, J. A., Toscano, W. A. J., and Friedman, M. Activation of Transcription Factor IL-6 (NF-IL-6) and Nuclear Factor-kappaB (NF-kappaB) by Lipid Ozonation Products Is Crucial to Interleukin-8 Gene Expression in Human Airway Epithelial Cells. Environ. Toxicol., *22:* 159–168, 2007.
54. Graziano, F. M., Cook, E. B., and Stahl, J. L. Cytokines, Chemokines, RANTES, and Eotaxin. Allergy Asthma Proc., *20:* 141–146, 1999.
55. Hoebe, K., Du, X., George, P., Janssen, E., Tabeta, K., Kim, S. O., Goode, J., Lin, P., Mann, N., Mudd, S., Crozat, K., Sovath, S., Han, J., and Beutler, B. Identification of Lps2 as a Key Transducer of MyD88-Independent TIR Signaling. Nature, *424:* 743–748, 2003.
56. Yamamoto, M., Sato, S., Hemmi, H., Hoshino, K., Kaisho, T., Sanjo, H., Takeuchi, O., Sugiyama, M., Okabe, M., Takeda, K., and Akira, S. Role of Adapter TRIF in MyD88-Independent Toll-Like Receptor Signaling Pathway. Science *301:* 640–643, 2003.
57. Oshiumi, H., Matsumoto, M., Funami, K., Akazawa, T., and Seya, T. TICAM-1 and Adapter Molecule That Participates in Toll-Like Receptor 3-Mediated Interferon-Beta Induction. Nat. Immunol., *4:* 161–167, 2003.
58. Broide, D. H., Lotz, M., Cuomo, A. J., Coburn, D. A., Federman, E. C., and Wasserman, S. I. Cytokines in Symptomatic Asthma Airways. J. Allergy Clin. Immunol., *89:* 958–967, 1992.
59. Chaplin, D. D. Cell Cooperation in Development of Eosinophil-predominant Inflammation in Airways. Immunol. Res., *26:* 55–62, 2002.
60. Pfeffer, K. Biological Functions of Tumor Necrosis Factor Cytokines and Their Receptors. Cytokine Growth Factor Rev., *14:* 185–191, 2003.
61. Laichalk, L. L., Kunkel, S. L., Strieter, R. M., Danforth, J. M., Bailie, M. B., and Standiford, T. J. Tumor Necrosis Factor Mediates Lung Antibacterial Host Defense in Murine Klebsiella Pneumonia. Infect. Immun., *64:* 5211–5218, 1996.
62. Vignola, A. M., Chanez, P., Bonsignore, G., Godard, P., and Bousquet, J. Structural Consequences of Airway Inflammation in Asthma. J. Allergy Clin. Immunol., *105:* S514–S517, 2000.
63. Ghaffar, O., Hamid, Q., Renzi, P. M., Allakhverdi, Z., Molet, S., Hogg, J. C., Shore, S. A., Luster, A. D., and Lamkhioued, B. Constitutive and Cytokine-Stimulated Expression of Eotaxin by Human Airway Smooth Muscle Cells. Am. J. Respir. Crit. Care Med., *159:* 1933–1942, 1999.
64. Hahn, C., Islamian, A. P., Renz, H., and Nockher, W. A. Airway Epithelial Cells Produce Neurotrophins and Promote the Survival of Eosinophils During Allergic Airway Inflammation. J. Allergy Clin. Immunol., *117:* 787–794, 2006.
65. Wong, C. K., Wang, C. B., Li, M. L., Ip, W. K., Tian, Y. P., and Lam, C. W. Induction of Adhesion Molecules Upon the Interaction Between Eosinophils and Bronchial Epithelial Cells: Involvement of p38 MAPK and NF-kappaB. Int. Immunopharmacol., *6:* 1859–1871, 2006.
66. Amrani, Y., Ammit, A. J., and Panettieri, R. A. J. Tumor Necrosis Factor Receptor (TNFR) 1 but Not TNFR2 Mediates Tumor Necrosis Factor-α-Induced Interleukin-6 and RANTES in Human Smooth Muscle Cells: Role of p38 and p42/44 Mitogen-Activated Protein Kinases. Mol. Pharmacol., *60:* 646–655, 2001.

67. Lora, J. M., Zhang, D. M., Liao, S. M., Burwell, T., King, A. M., Barker, P. A., Singh, L., Keaveney, M., Morgenstern, J., Gutierrez-Ramos, J. C., Coyle, A. J., and Frase, C. C. Tumor Necrosis Factor-α Triggers Mucus Production in Airway Epithelium Through IκB Kinase β-Dependent Mechanism. J. Biol. Chem., *280:* 36510–36517, 2005.
68. Escande, F., Aubert, J. P., Porchet, N., and Buisine, M. P. Human Mucin Gene MUC5AC: Organization of Its 5'-Region and Central Repetitive Region. Biochem. J., *358:* 763–772, 2001.
69. Tartaglia, L. A., Goeddel, D. V., Reynolds, C., Figari, I. S., Weber, R. F., Fendly, B. M., and Palladino, M. A. J. Stimulation of Human T-Cell Proliferation by Specific Activation of the 75-kDa Tumor Necrosis Factor Receptor. J. Immunol., *151:* 4637–4641, 1993.
70. Kafoury, R. M., and Madden, M. C. Diesel Exhaust Particles Induce Over-expression of Tumor Necrosis Factor-α (TNF-α) Gene in Alveolar Macrophages and Failed to Induce Apoptosis Through Activation of Nuclear Factor-κB (NF-κB). Int. J. Environ. Res. Public Health, *2:* 107–113, 2005.
71. Takeyama, K., Dabbagh, K., Lee, H. M., Agusti, C., Lausier, J. A., Ueki, I. F., Grattan, K. M., and Nadel, J. A. Epidermal Growth Factor System Regulates Mucin Production in Airways. Proc. Natl. Acad. Sci. U.S.A., *96:* 3081–3086, 1999.
72. Amishima, M., Munakata, M., Nasuhara, Y., Sato, A., Takahashi, T., Homma, Y., and Kawakami, Y. Expression of Epidermal Growth Factor and Epidermal Growth Factor Receptor Immunoreactivity in the Asthmatic Human Airway. Am. J. Respir. Crit. Care Med., *157:* 1907–1912, 1998.
73. Cohen, M. D., Ciocca, V., and Panettieri, R. A. J. TGF-Beta 1 Modulates Human Airway Smooth Muscle Cell Proliferation Induced by Mitogens. Am. J. Respir. Cell Mol. Biol., *16:* 85–90, 1997.
74. Bradding, P., Redington, A. E., and Holgate, S. T. Airway Wall Remodeling in the Pathogenesis of Asthma: Cytokine Expression in the Airways. *In:* A. G. Stewart (ed.), Airway Wall Remodeling in Asthma: Pharmacology & Toxicology: Basic and Clinical Aspects, pp. 29–63. Boca Raton, FL: CRC Press, 1997.
75. Tilley, S. L., Coffman, T. M., and Koller, B. H. Mixed Messages: Modulation of Inflammation and Immune Responses by Prostaglandins and Thromboxanes. J. Clin. Invest., *108:* 15–23, 2001.
76. Kafoury, R. M., Pryor, W. A., Squadrito, G. L., Salgo, M. G., Zou, X., and Friedman, M. Induction of Inflammatory Mediators in Human Airway Epithelial Cells by Lipid Ozonation Products. Am. J. Respir. Crit. Care Med., *160:* 1934–1942, 1999.
77. Kafoury, R. M., Pryor, W. A., Squadrito, G. L., Salgo, M. G., Zou, X., and Friedman, M. Lipid Ozonation Products Activate Phospholipases A2, C, and D. Toxicol. Appl. Pharmacol., *150:* 338–349, 1998.
78. Pang, L., and Knox, A. J. Effect of Interleukin-1 Beta, Tumor Necrosis Factor-Alpha and Interferon-Gamma on the Induction of Cyclooxygenase-2 in Cultured Human Airway Smooth Muscle Cells. Br. J. Pharmacol., *121:* 579–587, 1997.
79. Jongejan, R. C., de Jongste, J. C., Raatgeep, H. C., Stijnen, T., Bonta, I. L., and Kerrebijn, K. F. Effects of Inflammatory Mediators on the Responsiveness of Isolated Human Airways to Methacholine. Am. Rev. Respir. Dis., *142:* 1129–1132, 1990.
80. Bandeira-Melo, C., Hall, J. C., Penrose, J. F., and Weller, P. F. Cysteinyl Leukotrienes Induce IL-4 Release from Cord Blood-derived Human Eosinophils. J. Allergy Clin. Immunol., *109:* 975–979, 2002.
81. Mellor, E. A., Austen, K. F., and Boyce, J. A. Cysteinyl Leukotrienes and Uridine Diphosphate Induce Cytokine Generation by Human Mast Cells Through an Interleukin-4-Regulated Pathway That Is Inhibited by Leukotriene Receptor Antagonists. J. Exp. Med., *195:* 583–592, 2002.

Targeting Chemokine Receptors in Allergy

Cory M. Hogaboam

Introduction

Asthma is a disease of increasing in frequency in the developed world, and the magnitude of this clinical problem is putting strains on the health care system. For example, in 2002, there were over 15 million self-reported adult cases of asthma in the USA and asthma ranked eighth in terms of visits, with 17 million such visits for clinical care [1]. Without a clear understanding of the etiopathogenesis of asthma, a number of hypotheses have emerged to explain this alarming change in public health. The hygiene hypothesis is among the most heavily cited and draws upon the interesting connection that exists between the innate and acquired immune system [2]. Essentially, as this hypothesis outlines, the increase in asthma reflects the increase in hygiene within the developed world. While this development has all but eliminated many infectious illnesses such as cholera, the lack of pathogen exposure in early childhood appears to predispose to Th2-type immune responses, namely allergy and asthma later in life. No official list of "protective" pathogens has been formulated but according to the hygiene hypothesis any organism that evokes a strong type-1 cytokine response might prevent the development of asthma later in life [3]. Clearly, the lack of appropriate environmental pathogen exposure cannot entirely explain the rise in allergy and asthma, nor does this hypothesis explain the rise of Th1-type autoimmune diseases and the anti-allergic effect of strong Th2-cytokine mediated parasitic infections. At present, it is appreciated that several environmental pathogens and/or their byproducts contribute to allergic exacerbation of asthmatic responses. These environmental factors include viruses, bacteria, animal danders, pollens, house dust mite, cockroach waste products, and mold. In this review, we address the putative role of the mold *Aspergillus fumigatus* in the asthma epidemic and propose that many of the allergic features associated with this mold can be effectively targeted with specific chemokine receptor antagonist approaches.

C.M. Hogaboam
Immunology Program, Department of Pathology, University of Michigan Medical School, Rm 4057 BSRB, 109 Zina Pitcher Place, Ann Arbor, MI 48109-2200, USA
e-mail: Hogaboam@med.umich.edu

R. Pawankar et al. (eds.), *Allergy Frontiers: Future Perspectives*,
DOI 10.1007/978-4-431-99365-0_16, © Springer 2010

Role of *A. fumigatus* in the Asthma Epidemic

Although other fungal genera including *Bipolaris*, *Curvularia*, *Cladosporium*, *Penicillium*, and *Alternaria* are also suspected culprits in the growing epidemic of allergy and asthma [4–6], the airborne fungal pathogens that have received the greatest research attention are found in the genera *Aspergillus*. On the basis of worldwide sampling of indoor and outdoor ambient air, *Aspergillus* is among the most prevalent of airborne fungal spores. *Aspergillus* poses a significant problem in hospital and home environments where it readily infects patients with various forms of immunodeficiency. Englehart and colleagues [7] detected mean indoor and outdoor of *A. fumigatus* counts of 8.1 and 9.4 cfu/m^3, respectively. Alarmingly, their study also showed that portable air filtration units only reduced indoor airborne *Aspergillus* spore counts by approximately 30% meaning that even filtered air poses a major threat to immunocompromised patients.

Aspergillus also affects individuals with an intact immune system. For example, the intrapulmonary growth and persistence of *A. fumigatus* elicit a chronic hypersensitivity reaction in the lung that is commonly referred to as allergic bronchopulmonary aspergillosis (ABPA). Several features of ABPA mirror those of asthma including severe airway hyperactivity, remodeling (i.e. mucus hypersecretion in the airway and subepithelial fibrosis), and inflammation characterized by increased type-2 cytokine levels, eosinophilia, and CD4+ T cell activation. ABPA is typically present in approximately 1–2% of chronic asthmatics, a finding that may be related to the fact that colonization of the lung by *Aspergillus* is rarely observed in immunocompetent individuals.

The lack of *Aspergillus* colonization in the asthmatic lung does not rule out a major exacerbating role for this fungus in the vast majority of other asthmatics that do not present with clinically defined ABPA. Indeed, growing evidence indicates that allergy particularly to mold is related to asthma severity. In patients with persistent asthma requiring physician referral, 20–25% have skin test reactivity to *Aspergillus* or other fungi [8–10]. Mold sensitivity has been associated with increased asthma severity and death, hospital admission and intensive care admissions in adults, and with increased bronchial reactivity in children [11,12]. These alarming clinical data provide an interesting basis for the exploration of the impact of *Aspergillus* on the asthmatic lung. One important consequence of the introduction of Aspergillus into the immunocompetent lung is the elaboration of a number of pro-inflammatory protein factors including chemokines [13].

Chemokines

Chemokines are a group of chemotactic cytokines that attract leukocytes through their corresponding G-protein coupled chemokine receptors to sites of inflammation or infection. Chemokines are primarily divided into two main subfamilies that are referred to as CC ligands (CCLs) and CXCLs. Chemokine nomenclature is based upon the sequence homology and position of the first two cysteines at the amino terminus of these small (8–14 kDa) proteins. In vitro studies suggest that several chemokines exhibit promiscuity for a number of receptors raising the specter that these factors are redundant in their proinflammatory roles. Nevertheless, in vivo studies demonstrate that chemokine synthesis is regulated in several tissues leading to what appears to be a coordinated involvement of distinct chemokines at various stages of disease. Similarly, chemokine receptor expression is regulated in a temporal and spatial manner during allergic disease. The responses induced by the CC chemokines are initiated via specific G protein–coupled receptors, referred to as CCRs, which are abundantly expressed on the cell surface of immune and non-immune cells. While it is not surprising that leukocytes produce significant quantities of chemokines during asthmatic responses, it was unanticipated that structural cells in the lung such as airway epithelial cells and fibroblasts also produce significant amounts of chemokines during the same responses.

Chemokines function at multiple levels during the development and maintenance of asthma. First, chemokines mediate the recruitment of effector leukocytes such as neutrophils, T cells, and eosinophils [14–16]. Second, chemokines influence the outcome of the immune response by altering the activation state of the effector cells such as mast cells that are present in abundance at the peribronchial site [17]. Finally, chemokines appear to regulate the activation of cells resident in the lung including airway epithelial cells and fibroblasts. Given the array of chemokines and receptors present during clinical and experimental asthmatic or allergic airway disease, it could be argued that targeting a single chemokine or chemokine receptor might not eliminate asthma or even provide significant relief from the symptoms asthma [18]. Nevertheless, data arising from studies of allergic airway responses in mice lacking specific chemokines or chemokine receptors suggest that the targeting of specific chemokines and/or their receptors may provide greater benefit than first expected [19]. Thus, the overall theme of this review is that the investigation of the roles of individual chemokines and their receptors in the development and maintenance of allergic airway disease should provide therapeutically relevant information.

Animal Modeling of Chronic Fungal Asthma and Allergy

Acute, Aspergillus Soluble Antigen Driven Model

A murine model of acute Aspergillus antigen driven allergic airway disease has provided substantial evidence that chemokines are important initiators and orchestrators of airway disease. In this model, gene expression profiling revealed that a number of cytokine- and chemokine-related genes including CCR4, CCR5, and

CCL27 were increased in *A. fumigatus*-sensitized mice compared to control mice [20]. Lung concentrations of the CC chemokines CCL3, CCL2, CCL5, CCL6, CCL11, CCL17, CCL22, and the CXC chemokine CXCL1 were increased during acute fungal asthma. Specifically, immunoneutralization of either CCL6 (also known as C10) [21] or CCL11 [22] revealed a role for CCL6 and CCL11 in eosinophilic airway inflammation. Following challenge with *A. fumigatus* antigen, CCL6 blockade significantly reduced airway hyperresponsiveness (AHR), eosinophil and lymphocyte infiltration, and levels of CCL11, CCL2, IL-13, and IL-10 in the BAL, while numbers of BAL macrophages were increased [21]. These data suggest that CCL6 appears to have a prominent role in recruitment of inflammatory cells and development of AHR via the manipulation of the cytokine response. Blockade of CCL11 had a less dramatic effect by reducing eosinophil recruitment and AHR without an effect on lymphocyte recruitment or pulmonary inflammation [22]. Thus, results from these acute models of Aspergillus-induced allergic airway disease clearly show that chemokines have a major role in the recruitment of immune cell types that contribute to changes in airway physiology.

Chronic, Aspergillus Conidia-Driven Model of Fungal Asthma

While studies with acute models of allergic airway disease have provided insight into the potential role of chemokines in leukocyte recruitment during acute allergic aspergillosis, we have focussed most of our research attention on the role of chemokines using a chronic model of *A. fumigatus*-induced allergic lung disease. This model of chronic fungal asthma is characterized by an elaborate interplay between the innate immune responses directed against *A. fumigatus* conidia and Th2-mediated events that modulate peribronchial inflammation, AHR, and airway remodeling. To date, our findings strongly suggest that the persistence of fungal material in the lungs of allergic mice promotes the chronicity of eosinophilic and T-cell driven inflammation, thereby promoting allergic airway hyper-reactivity (Fig. 1) and airway remodeling (Fig. 2). Importantly, the elimination of this fungal material from these mice reverses these major features [23]. Chemokines affect almost every type of immune cell and are responsible for modulating the clearance of *A. fumigatus* from the lungs of immunodeficient [24] and *A. fumigatus*-sensitized mice [23]. Thus, we have been able to examine both the innate and adaptive immune responses employed, which enable us to draw conclusions regarding the impact of chemokines on many facets of asthmatic-type fungal lung disease [25]. The following is a summary of mouse studies that we have completed, which specifically address the role of chemokine receptors in the initiation, amplification, and maintenance of chronic fungal asthma. All of the studies described below involved the use of gene deficient mice and we have observed unique and non-redundant roles for each chemokine receptor in this chronic fungal asthma model.

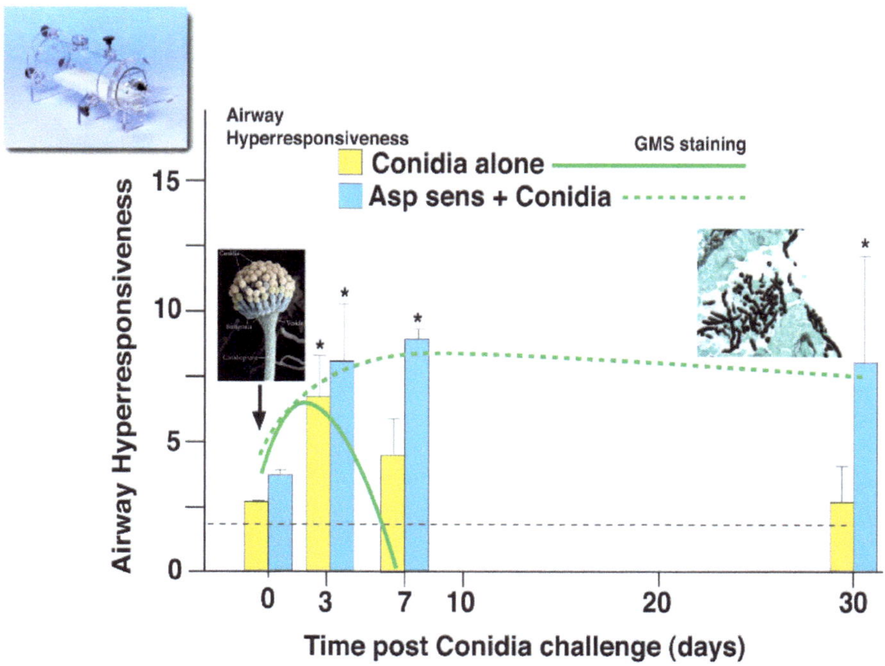

Fig. 1 In our initial characterization of the fungal asthma model, we examined the effect of the intratracheal conidia challenge on changes in airway resistance in non-sensitized mice versus *Aspergillus fumigatus*-sensitized and conidia challenged mice. On a technical note, changes in airway resistance were elicited by intravenously administered methacholine in anesthetized and ventilated mice placed in a Buxco plethysmograph body box (shown in the inset to this Figure). In the group of mice that received conidia alone (*yellow bar*), significantly increased airway hyperreactivity was observed in non-sensitized mice on day 3 but not at any other time after conidia challenge. In contrast, Aspergillus-sensitized and challenged mice (blue bar) exhibited a significant increase in airway hyperresponsiveness at all times after the conidia challenge, up to 30 days after this challenge. Another key observation that arose from these early studies was that in contrast to non-sensitized mice in which fungal material was cleared by day 7 after conidia introduction (*solid green line*), the presence of GMS-positive material or fungus persisted in the lungs of Aspergillus-sensitized and challenged mice (*dashed green line*)

CXCR2

CXCR2 was found to be necessary for the development and persistence of chronic fungal asthma in mice and to play a pivotal role in eosinophil and lymphocyte recruitment [26]. Studies with the CXCR2$^{-/-}$ mouse suggested that CXCR2 is required for the development and maintenance of the characteristic pulmonary features of chronic fungal asthma, but not for clearance of fungal components by phagocytes. Surprisingly, in the absence of CXCR2, signaling neutrophils were

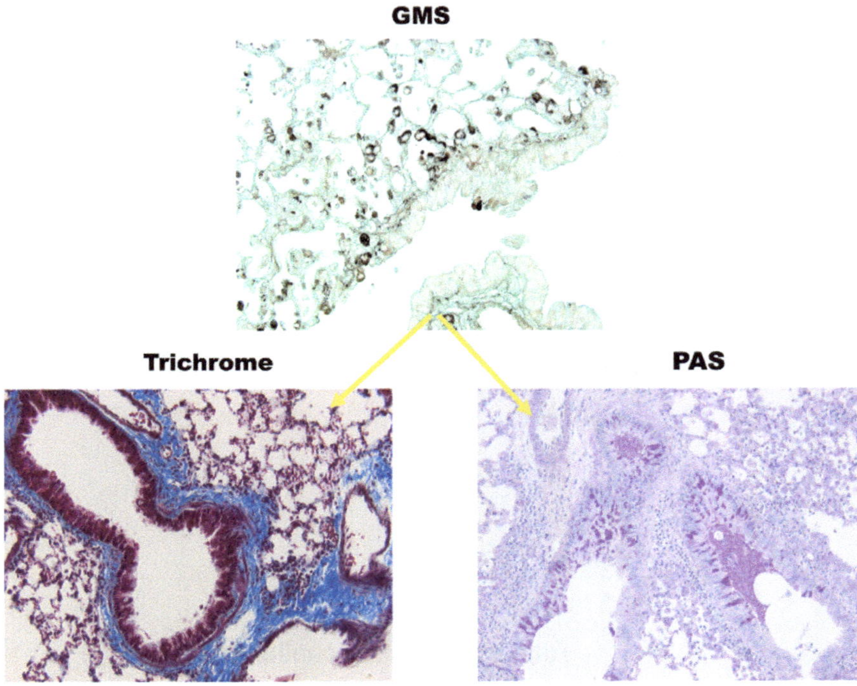

Fig. 2 The accumulation of GMS material, corresponding to fungal material, in the lungs of *Aspergillus fumigatus*-sensitized and conidia challenged mice leads to other chronic changes in the lung, including the accumulation of extracellular matrix around the airways, as revealed by Trichrome Masson staining of extracellular matrix, blue, and the appearance of mucus containing goblet cells in the epithelium of the airways, as revealed by Periodic Acid Schiff (PAS) staining of mucus, magenta

recruited by CXCL9 and CXCL10. A shift towards a Th1-type cytokine environment facilitated the clearance of fungal material by neutrophils and alveolar macrophages in the absence of CXCR2 [26]. The deletion of CXCR2 conferred protection against the damaging remodeling of the airways in response to *A. fumigatus* challenge, but enhancement of the CXCR2 pathway had no clear effect on fungal colonization. These data suggest that CXCR2 contributed to the persistence of asthmatic disease.

CCR1

Intra-tracheal challenge with *A. fumigatus* conidia increased the expression of CCR1, a major receptor for CCL3, CCL5, and CCL6. Genetic deletion of CCR1 dramatically attenuated remodeling processes in response to *A. fumigatus*, with reductions in goblet cell hyperplasia, subepithelial fibrosis, and collagen deposition [27].

These results indicate that CCR1 is a major contributor to the processes of airway remodeling and is involved, but not essential for the development of AHR.

CCR2

$CCR2^{-/-}$ mice exhibited greater airways hyperreactivity compared to wild-type controls with increases in peribronchial and perivascular inflammation, goblet cell hyperplasia and subepithelial fibrosis [28]. This exaggerated asthmatic phenotype in CCR2 gene-deficient mice was attributed to enhanced levels of CCL11 and CCL5, as well as IL-5 and IL-13, together with decreased levels of CXCL1 and reduced neutrophil and monocyte infiltrations in the lung. The lack of neutrophils and monocytes appeared to allow the pulmonary persistence of fungal conidia, consequently prolonging the allergic response in these mice. The deletion of either CCR2 or CCL2 had little effect upon the magnitude of allergic responses to soluble *A. fumigatus* antigens, which further underlines the complexity of the contribution of CCR2 and CCL2 in fungal asthma. Furthermore, these results suggest a distinction in chemokine pathways involved in response to soluble antigen versus live *A. fumigatus* conidia. Further experiments uncovered a dichotomous role of CCL2 in chronic fungal asthma. As a potent chemoattractant, it is required for efficient recruitment of $CCR2^{+ve}$ phagocytes into the airways, suggesting that early CCL2 release might be advantageous in fungal asthma. In contrast, continued presence of CCL2 appears to be deleterious at later time points of this model [29]. Thus, the role of CCR2 and CCL2 in fungal asthma is complex and reflects the multi-faceted effects of this receptor–ligand interaction during chronic disease.

CCR4

Defects in the ability of neutrophils or macrophages to kill *A. fumigatus* result in severe fungal lung diseases, as seen in chronic fungal asthma. $CCR4^{-/-}$ mice exhibited an aggressive anti-fungal response characterized by enhanced neutrophil function and macrophage recruitment [30]. In addition, $CCR4^{-/-}$ mice had a reduction in bronchoalveolar and peribronchial eosinophilia and an attenuated Th2 cytokine response, which might have limited the chronicity of AHR in these mice [30]. Whole lung levels of IL-4 and IL-5 were significantly increased in $CCR4^{-/-}$ mice on day 3 after conidia challenge, whereas IL-4, IL-5, and IL-13 were decreased on day 30 compared to their wild-type counterparts. Levels of the CCR4 agonists CCL22 and CCL17 were significantly elevated on days 3 and 7 after conidia challenge in *A. fumigatus*-sensitized $CCR4^{+/+}$ mice. No differences in collagen deposition or peribronchial fibrosis were found between lungs from CCR4-deficient mice and controls suggesting that CCR4-mediated pathways did not affect airway remodeling.

Despite the lack of involvement of CCR4 in remodeling features during fungal allergic aspergillosis, the rapid clearance of fungal material in the absence of CCR4 makes CCR4 and its ligands, CCL17 and CCL22 attractive targets as pathophysiological and therapeutically relevant players in chronic fungal asthma. These studies revealed a novel immunomodulatory effect of CCR4 on the innate immune response to Aspergillus and suggest that one strategy for attenuating allergic disease might involve bolstering the ability of the innate immune system to eliminate offending environmental pathogens such as mold.

CCR5

Nature actually provides an interesting gene deficiency in humans. The CCR5Δ32 polymorphism renders this chemokine receptor nonfunctional and recent genetic analyses have shown that this polymorphism is associated with reduced asthma susceptibility in children but not adults. [31]. Deletion of CCR5 in mice had a transient effect in reducing inflammation and AHR on days 2, 20, 30, and 40 post-allergen challenge [32]. Furthermore, $CCR5^{-/-}$ mice exhibited significantly less peribronchial T-cell and eosinophil accumulation, as well as goblet cell hyperplasia and peribronchial fibrosis, compared to $CCR5^{+/+}$ mice. Immunoneutralization of CCL5 in sensitized $CCR5^{+/+}$ and $CCR5^{-/-}$ mice for 12 days after the conidia challenge significantly reduced the AHR and peribronchial inflammation in the respective mice [32]. Besides, signaling via CCR5 and CCL5 might act independently to promote AHR, probably mediated via CCR1. Overall, these data indicate that CCR5 signaling is required for the persistence of chronic fungal asthma in mice.

CCR8

A. fumigatus-sensitized and challenged $CCR8^{-/-}$ mice exhibited an enhanced antifungal response on day 7 and a marked remission of many of the features of allergic airway disease on day 14 after the conidia challenge. The remission of allergic airway disease in $CCR8^{-/-}$ mice appeared to be associated with enhanced macrophage activation, increased mDC numbers in the lung, and enhanced *A. fumigatus*-antigen driven IFN-γ and IL-10 in the spleen. The persistence of fungal material in the lungs of allergic mice following conidial exposure has been shown to explain the chronicity of the allergic airway response in this model, as the fungal material supplies a continual allergen exposure. From the present study, histological sections showed that fungal material was cleared from the lungs of $CCR8^{-/-}$ mice whereas considerable fungal material was present in the lungs of the wild type mice on days 7 and 14 post-conidia challenge. Thus, several immune-related protein and cellular elements appeared to combine to enhance the clearance of fungal material from the lungs of mice lacking CCR8.

Strategies for Targeting Chemokine Receptors in Allergic Airway Disease

Clearly, aside from individuals lacking CCR5 due to genetic mutation, the gene deletion approach is simply not feasible in a human population with asthma. This fact has driven research toward the exploration of other targeting strategies directed at blocking or ablating chemokine receptor function. What follows is a short synopsis of various strategies that have shown pre-clinical promise in models of Aspergillus-induced allergic airway disease.

Immunoneutralizing Antibodies

Immunoneutralizing antibody therapeutic approaches hold tremendous promise and several candidates are presently under experimental consideration. Immunoneutralization of the CCR3 ligand CCL11 failed to affect disease parameters in the chronic allergic airways disease model, suggesting that CCL11 has little input in maintenance of established allergic inflammation in experimental fungal asthma [22]. The failure of anti-CCL11 to inhibit chronic fungal asthma appears to be due to the fact that other isoforms of CCL11, namely CCL24 [33], are induced in this model suggesting that these other forms of CCL11 compensate for the absence of CCL11. Further discussion regarding the therapeutic utility in targeting CCR3 is found below.

Small Molecule Antagonists

Because of a lack of species cross-reactivity, it has not always been possible to test small molecule antagonists against human receptors in murine models of allergic airway disease [34]. Nevertheless, a few small molecule drugs with species cross-reactivity have been tested in pre-clinical models and these early studies suggest that chemokine receptor blockage through this approach has tremendous potential. For example, blockade of CCR1 with a receptor antagonist, BX-471, revealed a major role for CCR1 in the development of AHR in genetically intact mice [35]. BX-471 treatment of isolated macrophages inhibited CCL22 release, increased toll like receptor-9 (TLR9), and decreased TLR2 and TLR6 expression in these macrophages [35]. The significance of these alterations in TLR expression is addressed below. Overall, the therapeutic administration of BX-471 abolished all features of established fungal asthma, thereby highlighting the need for further studies to explore the therapeutic potential of CCR1 targeting in clinical asthma. In other studies, the use AMD-3100, a small molecule antagonist directed against CXCR4, effectively blocked the initiation of fungal asthma [36]. Several more small molecule antagonists with activity in murine systems are presently under development, thereby facilitating additional pre-clinical studies directed at targeting chemokine receptors in fungal asthma.

Chimeric Proteins Containing Exotoxins

The recruitment of inflammatory cells into the asthmatic airway is not always completely blocked via an immunoneutralization or small antagonist approach [36]. The persistent presence of inflammatory cells in the airway leads to airway remodeling. One therapeutic approach involves the directed killing of these recruited cells. In the chronic fungal asthma model, simultaneous targeting of CCR5, CCR3, and CCR1 with a chimeric chemokine comprised of RANTES (CCL5) and a truncated Pseudomonas exotoxin (RANTES (CCL5)-PE38) on days 0–15 or 15–30 demonstrated that CCL5 is important in the initiation phase to *A. fumigatus* (i.e. from the time of asthma initiation to day 15 after challenge) [37]. RANTES-PE38 treatment significantly reduced airway inflammation and attenuated AHR, which mimicked the phenotype of CCR4$^{-/-}$ mice. RANTES-PE38 also modulated the expression of CCL17 and CCL22 [37]. This approach was highly effective when administered early, but proved relatively ineffective in established fungal asthma. Another chimeric protein, comprised of IL-13 and the same exotoxin (abbreviated IL13-PE), has shown tremendous preclinical efficacy in established fungal asthma [38,39] supporting the contention that this approach warrants further investigation in asthmatic conditions.

Future Pre-Clinical Research Directions

Given our experimental data showing the modulation of the pulmonary immune response via the targeting of pro-allergic factors described above, such strategies may be appropriate in the context of allergic asthma. The added benefit of modifying the innate immune response within the lung environment may also extend to the elimination of other persistent asthma-inducing agents including pollens, house dust mite, cockroach antigens, and viruses. Altogether, the data obtained from acute and fungal asthma reveal crucial roles for CXCR2, CCR1, CCR2, CCR4, and CCR5 and their ligands in fungal persistence (CXCR2, CCR5), AHR (CCR1, CCR2, CCR4, CCR5), airway remodeling (CCR1), and/or fungal phagocytosis and killing (CCR2, CCR4) in this model. Furthermore, these studies suggest that a CCR4^{+}CCR5^{+} phagocyte population is required for the switch from an early Th1 inflammatory response to Th2-dominated chronic disease, allowing persistence of fungal material. Thus, CCR4 and/or CCR5 and their ligands provide attractive targets to examine and modulate the immune response in ABPA patients among humans. While CCR2, CCR5, and their ligands CCL2 and CCL3 are suggested to suppress fungal clearance, CCR4/CCL17 appears to support or promote fungal growth, a finding confirmed in a model of invasive aspergillosis [40]. Future directions of interest in our laboratory involve the study of additional chemokine receptors in this preclinical model of fungal asthma. CX3CR1, the fractalkine receptor, mediates cell-adhesive and migratory functions in inflammation. This receptor has been localized in bronchial tissues of asthmatic subjects and at least five CX3CR1 single nucleotide polymorphisms have been identified in asthma [41].

Concluding Comments

Of the chemokine receptors explored in the context of experimental fungal asthma, CCR3, CCR4, and CCR8 rank highest on the list of chemokine receptors that justify preclinical and clinical evaluation as therapeutic targets in clinical allergic asthma [34]. CCR3 is prominently expressed on eosinophils and Th2 cells, and small molecule antagonists against this receptor are presently under clinical consideration [19]. CCR4 and CCR8 have been identified on Th2 cells present in adolescent [40] and adult asthma [42]. Small molecule antagonists appear to be the therapeutics of choice in targeting these three chemokine receptors in asthma, but recent pre-clinical advances in targeting CCR3 via a bispecific antibody fragment linking CCR3 to CD300a [43] or an antisense oligodeoxynucleotides targeting CCR3 [44] might provide other equally effective therapeutic strategies. Clinical studies with these and other therapeutic strategies directed against these receptors or the chemokines that bind these receptors are warranted.

References

1. http://www.cdc.gov/asthma/brfss/02/current/tableC1.html.
2. Schaub, B., Lauener, R., and von Mutius, E. 2006. The many faces of the hygiene hypothesis. J Allergy Clin Immunol 117:969–977; quiz 978
3. Yazdanbakhsh, M., Kremsner, P.G., and van Ree, R. 2002. Allergy, parasites, and the hygiene hypothesis. Science 296:490–494
4. Lugauskas, A., Krikstaponis, A., and Sveistyte, L. 2004. Airborne fungi in industrial environments--potential agents of respiratory diseases. Ann Agric Environ Med 11:19–25
5. Green, B.J., Mitakakis, T.Z., and Tovey, E.R. 2003. Allergen detection from 11 fungal species before and after germination. J Allergy Clin Immunol 111:285–289
6. Kauffman, H.F., and van der Heide, S. 2003. Exposure, sensitization, and mechanisms of fungus-induced asthma. Curr Allergy Asthma Rep 3:430–437
7. Engelhart, S., et al. 2003. Impact of portable air filtration units on exposure of haematology-oncology patients to airborne Aspergillus fumigatus spores under field conditions. J Hosp Infect 54:300–304
8. Schwartz, H.J., and Greenberger, P.A. 1991. The prevalence of allergic bronchopulmonary aspergillosis in patients with asthma, determined by serologic and radiologic criteria in patients at risk. J Lab Clin Med 117:138–142

9. Boulet, L.P., et al. 1997. Comparative degree and type of sensitization to common indoor and outdoor allergens in subjects with allergic rhinitis and/or asthma. Clin Exp Allergy 27:52–59
10. Mari, A., et al. 2003. Sensitization to fungi: epidemiology, comparative skin tests, and IgE reactivity of fungal extracts. Clin Exp Allergy 33:1429–1438
11. Black, P.N., Udy, A.A., and Brodie, S.M. 2000. Sensitivity to fungal allergens is a risk factor for life-threatening asthma. Allergy 55:501–504
12. Nelson, H.S., et al. 1999. The relationships among environmental allergen sensitization, allergen exposure, pulmonary function, and bronchial hyperresponsiveness in the Childhood Asthma Management Program. J Allergy Clin Immunol 104:775–785
13. Schuh, J.M., Blease, K., Kunkel, S.L., and Hogaboam, C.M. 2003. Chemokines and cytokines: axis and allies in asthma and allergy. Cytokine Growth Factor Rev 14:503–510
14. Randolph, D.A., et al. 1999. The role of CCR7 in TH1 and TH2 cell localization and delivery of B cell help in vivo. Science 286:2159–2162
15. Cosmi, L., et al. 2001. Chemoattractant receptors expressed on type 2 t cells and their role in disease. Int Arch Allergy Immunol 125:273–279
16. Kallinich, T., et al. 2005. Chemokine-receptor expression on T cells in lung compartments of challenged asthmatic patients. Clin Exp Allergy 35:26–33
17. Ochi, H., et al. 1999. T helper cell type 2 cytokine-mediated comitogenic responses and CCR3 expression during differentiation of human mast cells in vitro. J Exp Med 190:267–280
18. Chantry, D., and Burgess, L.E. 2002. Chemokines in allergy. Curr Drug Targets Inflamm Allergy 1:109–116
19. Garcia, G., Godot, V., and Humbert, M. 2005. New chemokine targets for asthma therapy. Curr Allergy Asthma Rep 5:155–160
20. Kurup, V.P., Raju, R., and Manickam, P. 2005. Profile of gene expression in a murine model of allergic bronchopulmonary aspergillosis. Infect Immun 73:4381–4384
21. Hogaboam, C.M., et al. 1999. Immunomodulatory role of C10 chemokine in a murine model of allergic bronchopulmonary aspergillosis. J Immunol 162:6071–6079
22. Schuh, J.M., Blease, K., Kunkel, S.L., and Hogaboam, C.M. 2002. Eotaxin/CCL11 is involved in acute, but not chronic, allergic airway responses to Aspergillus fumigatus. Am J Physiol Lung Cell Mol Physiol 283:L198–204
23. Hogaboam, C.M., Blease, K., and Schuh, J.M. 2003. Cytokines and chemokines in allergic bronchopulmonary aspergillosis (ABPA) and experimental Aspergillus-induced allergic airway or asthmatic disease. Front Biosci 8:e147–156
24. Mehrad, B., Moore, T.A., and Standiford, T.J. 2000. Macrophage inflammatory protein-1 alpha is a critical mediator of host defense against invasive pulmonary aspergillosis in neutropenic hosts. J Immunol 165:962–968
25. Buckland, K.F., and Hogaboam, C.M. 2006. Cytokine and chemokine responses in fungal allergy. Research Signpost 37:288–308
26. Schuh, J.M., Blease, K., and Hogaboam, C.M. 2002. CXCR2 is necessary for the development and persistence of chronic fungal asthma in mice. J Immunol 168:1447–1456
27. Blease, K., et al. 2000. Airway remodeling is absent in CCR1-/- mice during chronic fungal allergic airway disease. J Immunol 165:1564–1572
28. Blease, K., et al. 2000. Enhanced pulmonary allergic responses to Aspergillus in CCR2-/- mice. J Immunol 165:2603–2611
29. Blease, K., et al. 2001. Antifungal and airway remodeling roles for murine monocyte chemoattractant protein-1/CCL2 during pulmonary exposure to Asperigillus fumigatus conidia. J Immunol 166:1832–1842
30. Schuh, J.M., et al. 2002. Airway hyperresponsiveness, but not airway remodeling, is attenuated during chronic pulmonary allergic responses to Aspergillus in CCR4-/- mice. Faseb J 16:1313–1315
31. Le Souef, P.N. 2006. Variations in genetic influences on the development of asthma throughout childhood, adolescence and early adult life. Curr Opin Allergy Clin Immunol 6:317–322
32. Schuh, J.M., Blease, K., and Hogaboam, C.M. 2002. The role of CC chemokine receptor 5 (CCR5) and RANTES/CCL5 during chronic fungal asthma in mice. Faseb J 16:228–230

33. Buckland, K.F., et al. 2007. Remission of chronic fungal asthma in the absence of CCR8. J Allergy Clin Immunol 119:997–1004
34. Lloyd, C.M., and Rankin, S.M. 2003. Chemokines in allergic airway disease. Curr Opin Pharmacol 3:443–448
35. Carpenter, K.J., et al. 2005. Therapeutic targeting of CCR1 attenuates established chronic fungal asthma in mice. Br J Pharmacol 145:1160–1172
36. Hogaboam, C.M., et al. 2005. The therapeutic potential in targeting CCR5 and CXCR4 receptors in infectious and allergic pulmonary disease. Pharmacol Ther 107:314–328
37. Schuh, J.M., et al. 2003. Intrapulmonary targeting of RANTES/CCL5-responsive cells prevents chronic fungal asthma. Eur J Immunol 33:3080–3090
38. Blease, K., et al. 2001. IL-13 fusion cytotoxin ameliorates chronic fungal-induced allergic airway disease in mice. J Immunol 167:6583–6592
39. Blease, K., et al. 2002. Stat6-deficient mice develop airway hyperresponsiveness and peribronchial fibrosis during chronic fungal asthma. Am J Pathol 160:481–490
40. Carpenter, K.J., and Hogaboam, C.M. 2005. Immunosuppressive effects of CCL17 on pulmonary antifungal responses during pulmonary invasive aspergillosis. Infect Immunol 73:7198–7207
41. Tremblay, K., et al. 2006. Association study between the CX3CR1 gene and asthma. Genes Immun 7:632–639
42. Panina-Bordignon, P., et al. 2001. The C-C chemokine receptors CCR4 and CCR8 identify airway T cells of allergen-challenged atopic asthmatics. J Clin Invest 107:1357–1364
43. Munitz, A., Bachelet, I., and Levi-Schaffer, F. 2006. Reversal of airway inflammation and remodeling in asthma by a bispecific antibody fragment linking CCR3 to CD300a. J Allergy Clin Immunol 118:1082–1089
44. Fortin, M., et al. 2006. Effects of antisense oligodeoxynucleotides targeting CCR3 on the airway response to antigen in rats. Oligonucleotides 16:203–212

Dendritic Cell Vaccines

Martin Thurnher

Introduction

Dendritic cells play a central role in the induction and regulation of immune responses [1,2]. Dendritic cells are at the starting point of virtually each and every immune reaction and are, therefore, critical for the organism to defend itself not only against pathogens but also against malignant, cancerous cells. In both the cases, infection and cancer, the ultimate goal of immunosurveillance is the maintenance of the organism's integrity. Dendritic cells pick up antigens in the periphery and migrate to the regional lymph nodes, where they instruct the activation and survival of helper T cells from various lineages via production of distinct cytokines such IL-12 (T_H1) or IL-23 (T_H17) [3]. The various subsets of the helper T cells (T_H1, T_H2, T_H17) subsequently provide qualitatively support of different kinds to the phagocytic (macrophages), cytotoxic (T and NK cells), and antibody-producing cells (B cells), which are physiologically involved in the different steps of the defense against diverse pathogens or, pathologically, contribute to the development of atopic or autoimmune disease and to the transplant rejection.

Conventional dendritic cell subsets described in humans include both myeloid and plasmacytoid dendritic cells [4]. Myeloid dendritic cells develop from $CD11c^+HLA\text{-}DR^+$ blood precursors and undergo maturation in response to the triggering of toll-like receptors (TLR), a class of pattern recognition receptors that detect microbial products, and in response to inflammatory cytokines and lipids [5]. Dendritic cell maturation is accompanied by an upregulation of major histocompatibility complex (MHC) class II and costimulatory molecules. Plasmacytoid dendritic cells might differentiate either from a common blood dendritic cell precursor or from a committed lymphoid progenitor. They express CD123, CD4, and CD62L and secrete type I interferon in response to viruses and/or TLR9 ligands.

M. Thurnher
Department of Urology, Immunotherapy Unit, Innsbruck Medical University and KMT Center of Excellence in Medicine, Anichstrasse 35, 6020 Innsbruck, Austria
e-mail: martin.thurnher@i-med.ac.at
www.immuntherapie-ibk.at

R. Pawankar et al. (eds.), *Allergy Frontiers: Future Perspectives*,
DOI 10.1007/978-4-431-99365-0_17, © Springer 2010

Dendritic cells are also pivotal in deciding between the development of immunity and tolerance. The immunity-inducing capacity of dendritic cells can be exploited in infectious diseases and cancer [6–8], while the tolerogenic potential of the dendritic cells is important for the treatment of allergy, autoimmune disease including transplant rejection [4].

The outstanding immunogenic or tolerogenic capacity of dendritic cells in vivo is increasingly being harnessed for the development of cellular therapies. The clinical implementation of dendritic cell-based immunotherapy, which began more than ten years ago, represents a paradigm of translational research and a contribution to personalized medicine. After a decade of clinical research with dendritic cell vaccines in cancer patients, which demonstrated the safety of this approach and the capacity of dendritic cells generated in vitro to induce immune and clinical responses in vivo, the next decade may be dedicated to the extension of dendritic cell-based immunotherapy to other diseases including infectious, atopic and autoimmune disease.

Dendritic Cell Vaccines for the Treatment of Cancer

The greatest experience with human dendritic cell vaccination has been obtained in cancer patients with progressive disease [6–8]. The use of dendritic cells is based on the concept of cancer immunosurveillance, originally put forward in Burnet's theory, that the sentinel thymus-dependent cells (T cells) of the body constantly examine the host tissues for nascently transformed cells (i.e. tumor cells) [9]. The last fifteen years have seen a re-emergence of interest in cancer immunosurveillance [10]. Today, a large body of evidence confirms Burnet's assumption that a competent immune system protects the host from the development of neoplasia and that - even in the case of established tumors - the immune system often successfully counteracts the progression of cancer [10].

Infiltration of tumor tissue by immune cells, which is frequently observed in different tumor types including renal cell carcinoma [11–13], has always been considered an indication that the immune system has recognized the growing tumor and somehow interacts with it. Only recently, Galon *et al.* demonstrated in a large cohort of colorectal cancers that type, density, and location of immune cells within the tumor predict the clinical outcome [14]. Likewise, the presence of B7-H1, a molecule that functions as a negative regulator of immunity, in human renal cell carcinoma tissue results in a significant risk of rapid cancer progression and accelerated rates of mortality [15]. B7-H1 appears to function as a tolerogenic determinant in renal cell carcinoma, abrogating the T cell immune responses directed against the otherwise immunogenic tumor.

The discovery that dendritic cells can be cultured in sufficient numbers from abundant circulating precursor cells [16–18] paved way for clinical research. In the majority of trials, monocyte-derived dendritic cells were used whereas in other studies dendritic cells were generated from early bone marrow progenitor cells

[19]. The results of these studies have been published and study data summarized in recent reviews [8].

The clinical trials with dendritic cells performed so far are rather heterogenous. They differ in the source of the dendritic cells (monocyte-derived, bone marrow progenitor-derived, autologous versus allogeneic), in the maturation status (immature versus mature), in the antigen formulation used for the dendritic cell loading (tumor lysate with or without helper antigen, tumor - dendritic cell fusion, tumor RNA transfection) as well as in the use of helper antigen. Comparison and definitive conclusions are, therefore, difficult or impossible.

However, as data accumulate and the follow-up times increase it becomes apparent that the absence of severe side effects in combination with considerable survival times reveal a presentable risk:benefit ratio of dendritic cell vaccines in cancer treatment. In contrast, some previously much-lauded small molecule drugs are now confronted with substantial clinical toxicity in the absence of significant increase in survival times [20].

In our own studies of dendritic cell vaccination on patients with metastatic renal cell carcinoma [21–23], we started from a leukapheresis product generated with the Cobe Spectra cell separator. $CD14^+$ monocytes were then isolated by positive selection using the MACS Technology from Miltenyi Biotec (CD14 Reagent and the CliniMACS Instrument). The purified $CD14^+$ cells (50×10^6 in 50 ml) were subsequently cultured in 162 cm^2 cell culture flasks in AIM-V culture medium containing 1% heat-inactivated human AB plasma, and also in a combination of recombinant human GM-CSF and recombinant human IL-4 to induce differentiation of monocytes towards dendritic cells. On Day 5, immature dendritic cells were harvested and aliquots frozen in liquid nitrogen using a standard protocol (50% AIM-V, 40% human AB plasma, 10% DMSO).

Two days before vaccination, a vial of immature dendritic cells was thawed, cells were counted and 18×10^6 cells were replated in 6-well plates with $1{,}8 \times 10^6$ cells per well in 6 ml of fresh medium containing cytokines as well as 1% heat-inactivated human AB plasma. Tumor antigen was added in the form of tumor lysate (10 µg protein/ml). Keyhole limpet hemocyanin (KLH; 10 µg/ml) was added as a helper antigen, that supports the relatively weak antitumor response, and also as a tracer antigen, that can easily be monitored and thus allow the validation of the dendritic cell vaccine.

Dendritic cell maturation was induced by a combination of TNF-α, IL-1ß, IL-6 and PGE2 [5,21–24]. Although this combination may not be the ultimate cocktail for the maturation of "optimal" dendritic cells, it has nevertheless been extremely reliable for the maturation of $CD83^+$ dendritic cells. Meanwhile, more than 100 patients received a total of more than 500 dendritic cell vaccinations in our Department. Dendritic cell generation in sufficient numbers was successful in all patients, and all final vaccines remained sterile demonstrating the feasibility of the dendritic cell therapy. Administration of dendritic cells (10^7 cells) was partly intranodal (ultrasound-guided) and partly intravenous. Treatment was very well tolerated with delayed-type hypersensitivity (DTH)-like reactions at the injection site and transient, moderate fever as the only side effect, although these effects might even be desirable as they also indicate the inflammatory / immune responses to the vaccine. The great majority of the patients developed immunity against the control antigen KLH, which could be measured by assessing the proliferative and cytokine responses of pre- versus postvaccination peripheral blood mononuclear cells (PBMCs) after stimulation with KLH [21,22,25]. Assessment of the much weaker antitumor immune responses is difficult. Nevertheless, proliferative and cytokine responses against tumor lysate and oncofetal antigen/immature laminin receptor, which is expressed in renal cell carcinoma [26] could be detected in some patients [22,26]. Median overall survival of 94 patients evaluated so far in our Department is 20.1 months. Median overall survival of patients with metastatic renal cell carcinoma in the literature is 13 months [27]. In summary, our data thus confirm the feasibility and tolerability of dendritic cell vaccination and together with the survival data reveal a positive benefit:risk ratio for this treatment modality.

In spite of the promising results from the first clinical trials, several critical parameters still need to be improved and optimized. Variables of dendritic cell immunotherapy, still in discussion, include general approaches to improve clinical cell therapy such as the selection of the right patient for tumor immunotherapy (for instance, cytokine gene polymorphisms) [28], the selection of the right tumor antigens ("hunting a tumor's Achilles heel") and the increase of patient survival by generating T cells that also mediate long-term protection [29]. Additional variables that may improve the dendritic cell therapy, in particular, include the introduction of novel cytokines in dendritic cell differentiation protocols, the development of adjuvants that can boost the efficacy of immunotherapy (toll-like receptor agonists) as well as the improvement of dendritic cell migration in vivo. Finally, a better recognition and evaluation of cell therapy-induced responses is also desirable and may include immune monitoring of lipid-specific T cell responses, in addition to peptide-specific responses, and a better characterization of humoral immune responses.

A generally important issue would be the application of dendritic cell vaccines in minimal residual disease. Usually, vaccines serve as prophylactic treatments that prevent disease. In minimal residual disease, when the tumor burden is reduced by surgical removal of the primary tumor and, possibly, also of the accessible metastases, dendritic cell vaccines may stimulate a relatively intact immune system and may be able to prevent tumor recurrence.

The full understanding of dendritic cell-mediated antitumor immunity will hopefully result in the development of more effective immunotherapeutic approaches to control and/or eliminate human cancers.

Dendritic Cell Vaccines for the Treatment of Allergy?

An increasing part of the population in the Western countries suffers from allergic diseases, which include asthma, allergic rhinitis, atopic dermatitis, and food allergy [30]. Allergic inflammation is induced by dysregulated T_H2 cytokines including

IL-4, IL-5, and IL-13, which enhance IgE production, mucus secretion and eosinophilia. Dendritic cells can actively determine the induction of T_H1 and T_H17, by either producing IL-12, which promotes IFN-γ producing T_H1 cells, or by producing IL-23, which is a key cytokine for the activation and survival of IL-17 producing T_H17 cells [3] (Fig. 1b). In contrast, dendritic cells cannot produce cytokines such

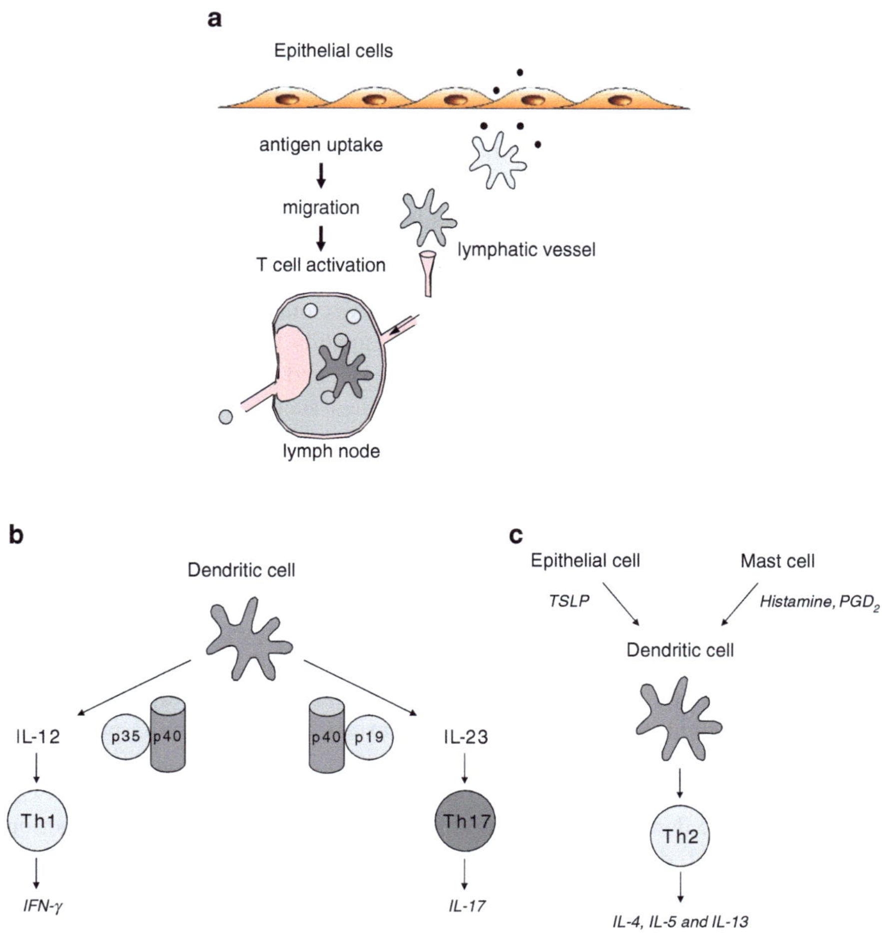

Fig. 1 (**a**) Dendritic cells pick up antigens in the periphery, for instance, at the epithelial barriers, where contact with invading pathogens is likely to occur. Dendritic cells then migrate via lymphatic vessels to the draining lymph nodes and activate antigen-specific T cells, which in turn exit the lymph node again and patrol the body in order to find and eliminate pathogens. (**b**) Dendritic cells instruct the activation of helper T cells, T_H1 and T_H17, by either producing IL-12, which promotes IFN-γ producing T_H1 cells, or by producing IL-23, which is a key cytokine for the activation and survival of IL-17 producing T_H17 cells. Importantly, IL-12 and IL-23 share the non-proprietary p40 subunit. (**c**) Epithelial cell-derived TSLP or mast cell-derived mediators such as histamine or PGD_2 can re-program dendritic cells, which then polarize naïve $CD4^+$ T cells towards T helper cells producing the T_H2 cytokines IL-4, IL-5 and IL-13

as IL-4 that stimulate T_H2 development. Therefore, dendritic cells were initially not implicated in the T_H2-mediated diseases and were considered T_H1-inducing antigen-presenting cells. The discovery of thymic stromal lymphopoietin (TSLP), which is an IL-7-like cytokine, however, bridged the gap and clearly implicated dendritic cells in the development of allergic inflammation. TSLP, which seems to be critical in $CD4^+$ T cell homeostasis and in the positive selection of T_{reg} cells under normal physiological conditions, can be highly expressed by keratinocytes from atopic dermatitis patients [31]. Epithelial cell-derived TSLP potently activates dendritic cells, which produce T_H2-attracting chemokines (CCL17 and CCL22) and TSLP-activated dendritic cells prime naïve T_H cells to produce the T_H2 cytokines IL-4, IL-5, and IL-13 (Fig. 1c) [32–34]. In patients with atopic dermatitis, TSLP expression is associated with Langerhans cell activation and migration in situ, suggesting that TSLP may contribute directly to the activation of Langerhans cells, which may migrate to the draining lymph nodes and prime allergen-specific T_H2 responses [31].

In addition to cytokines, potent bioamines like histamine and members of the eicosanoid family of arachidonic acid derivatives may act on immature dendritic cells to change their T_H cell polarizing capacity [35]. Immature dendritic cells express two active histamine receptors H1 and H2. Histamine potently altered the profile of cytokines and chemokines secreted by dendritic cells. Histamine increased IL-10 and diminished IL-12 production via the H2 receptor. Dendritic cells exposed to histamine polarized naïve $CD4^+$ T cells towards a T_H2 type, while dendritic cells matured in the absence of histamine induced a T_H1 type.

The prostaglandin (PG) series of arachidonic acid metabolites are potent regulators of inflammation [36]. Mast cell–derived prostaglandin D_2 (PGD_2) is a proinflammatory mediator causing vasodilation, bronchoconstriction, and chemoattraction of eosinophils and T_H2 cells. It is found in increased levels in the bronchoalveolar lavage (BAL) fluid of atopic asthmatics and mice with experimentally induced asthma [37]. PGD2 exerts its effects via D prostanoid receptors (DP1 and DP2, the latter also known as CRTH2). In addition, PGD_2 can affect cellular differentiation and function via binding to PPAR-γ. PGD_2 was found to alter the dendritic cell maturation by suppressing the IL-12 production and PGD_2-treated dendritic cells promoted differentiation of naïve T cells towards T_H2 type T cells [38]. Whether PGD_2 could also have anti-inflammatory effects through selective usage of the DP1 or DP2 receptor was unknown until recently. The opportunity to therapeutically attempt airway inflammation with dendritic cells is exemplified by a recent study. In a murine model of airway inflammation, DP1 agonist-treated dendritic cells induced an increase in $Foxp3^+$ $CD4^+$ regulatory T cells that were able to suppress inflammation in an interleukin 10–dependent way [39]. Triggering DP1 on dendritic cells appears to be an important mechanism to induce regulatory T cells and to control the extent of airway inflammation. This pathway could be exploited to develop novel dendritic cell-based treatments for asthma.

Dendritic Cell Vaccines for the Treatment of Autoimmune Disease and the Prevention of Transplant Rejection?

Under normal physiological conditions, dendritic cells are not only in charge of inducing immune responses against invading pathogens, but are also responsible for the maintenance of tolerance against self antigens. Under steady-state conditions, for instance, immature dendritic cells capture apoptotic cells arising from tissue turnover and, upon migration to draining lymph nodes, silence the T cells specific to self antigens. Moreover, thymic dendritic cells exposed to TSLP express costimulatory molecules and MHC class II but release negligible amounts of IL-12p70 and promote the conversion of $CD4^{+}CD25^{-}$ thymocytes into $CD4^{+}CD25^{+}FoxP3^{+}$ T_{reg} cells [40]. Thus, regulatory, tolerogenic dendritic cells prevent autoimmunity and contribute to self tolerance by both inactivating self-reactive T cells and by generating T_{reg} cells. It is this regulatory, tolerogenic potential of dendritic cells that must be exploited for the treatment of autoimmune disease, and in the prevention of transplant rejection. In principle, dendritic cells for clinical application might be generated ex vivo from monocyte populations with good manufacturing practice (GMP)-grade cytokine cocktails containing, for instance, 1α,25-dihydroxyvitamin D_3 that induce the differentiation of tolerogenic dendritic cells. Pharmacologic arrest of dendritic cell maturation or use of genetically engineered dendritic cells expressing immunosuppressive molecules might selectively enhance dendritic cell tolerogenicity. Along this line, transfection of dendritic cells with a gene construct encoding a modified CTLA4 molecule results in deficient expression of CD80/CD86 and induction of T-cell anergy and might represent an attractive means of inducing and restoring tolerance in autoimmune diseases. Blockade of the CD40-CD154 (CD40 ligand) signaling pathway might act synergistically with dendritic cell therapy, thus promoting the survival of transplanted organs. Pharmacologic treatment of dendritic cells that prevents full maturation might also contribute to the maintenance of transplantation tolerance through the promotion of T_{reg}-cell differentiation. Simultaneous enhancement of tolerogenic dendritic cells and stimulation of T_{reg} cells might be a desirable approach to induce transplantation tolerance [4].

Conclusions

Collectively, basic findings on dendritic cell development and function nurtures optimism in the clinical translation of immunogenic and tolerogenic dendritic cells to human immune-mediated diseases. The exact controlling and timing of dendritic cell effector functions will be prerequisite for safe and efficacious dendritic cell-based therapies in the near future. Unfortunately, individual, tailor-made, cell-based therapies do not fit the concepts of the big pharmaceutical industry, which usually promotes one-fits-all concepts based on small molecules. The further development of such promising cell therapies should, therefore, also be in the common public interest and supported by distinguished translational research programs.

Figdor and colleagues have recently proposed minimum quality criteria for the design of clinical trials with dendritic cells as well as quality criteria for the dendritic cell vaccine providing useful guidelines for future trials [7]. Following these guidelines would also allow comparison of different trials. Steinman and Mellman previously emphasized that immunotherapy - to be successful – requires a broadening of basic research in humans. Fundamental changes in infrastructure, funding mechanisms and eventually the culture of the scientific community are required to bring immunology to medicine [41]. Although currently restricted to cancer patients, the analysis of the human immune system should also help to improve therapies of other disorders associated with immune dysfunction. There is probably no biomedical discipline that has a greater potential for affecting human health than studies of the immune system.

Acknowledgements I thank my colleagues Nikolaus Romani, Reinhold Ramoner, Andrea Rahm, Hubert Gander and Nicolai Leonhartsberger for helpful comments and apologize to other colleagues whose studies could not be cited because of space restrictions.

References

1. Steinman, R. M. 1991. The dendritic cell system and its role in immunogenicity. Annu Rev Immunol 9:271.
2. Banchereau, J., and R. M. Steinman. 1998. Dendritic cells and the control of immunity. Nature 392:245.
3. Reiner, S. L. 2007. Development in motion: helper T cells at work. Cell 129:33.
4. Rutella, S., S. Danese, and G. Leone. 2006. Tolerogenic dendritic cells: cytokine modulation comes of age. Blood 108:1435.
5. Rieser, C., G. Bock, H. Klocker, G. Bartsch, and M. Thurnher. 1997. Prostaglandin E2 and tumor necrosis factor alpha cooperate to activate human dendritic cells: synergistic activation of interleukin 12 production. J Exp Med 186:1603.
6. Banchereau, J., and A. K. Palucka. 2005. Dendritic cells as therapeutic vaccines against cancer. Nat Rev Immunol 5:296.
7. Figdor, C. G., I. J. de Vries, W. J. Lesterhuis, and C. J. Melief. 2004. Dendritic cell immunotherapy: mapping the way. Nat Med 10:475.
8. Schuler, G., B. Schuler-Thurner, and R. M. Steinman. 2003. The use of dendritic cells in cancer immunotherapy. Curr Opin Immunol 15:138.
9. Burnet, F. M. 1970. The concept of immunological surveillance. Prog Exp Tumor Res 13:1
10. Dunn, G. P., L. J. Old, and R. D. Schreiber. 2004. The immunobiology of cancer immunosurveillance and immunoediting. Immunity 21:137.
11. Thurnher, M., C. Radmayr, R. Ramoner, S. Ebner, G. Bock, H. Klocker, N. Romani, and G. Bartsch. 1996. Human renal-cell carcinoma tissue contains dendritic cells. Int J Cancer 68:1.
12. Radmayr, C., G. Bock, A. Hobisch, H. Klocker, G. Bartsch, and M. Thurnher. 1995. Dendritic antigen-presenting cells from the peripheral blood of renal-cell-carcinoma patients. Int J Cancer 63:627.
13. Thurnher, M., C. Radmayr, A. Hobisch, G. Bock, N. Romani, G. Bartsch, and H. Klocker. 1995. Tumor-infiltrating T lymphocytes from renal-cell carcinoma express B7-1 (CD80): T-cell expansion by T-T cell co-stimulation. Int J Cancer 62:559.

14. Galon, J., A. Costes, F. Sanchez-Cabo, A. Kirilovsky, B. Mlecnik, C. Lagorce-Pages, M. Tosolini, M. Camus, A. Berger, P. Wind, F. Zinzindohoue, P. Bruneval, P. H. Cugnenc, Z. Trajanoski, W. H. Fridman, and F. Pages. 2006. Type, density, and location of immune cells within human colorectal tumors predict clinical outcome. Science 313:1960.
15. Thompson, R. H., S. M. Kuntz, B. C. Leibovich, H. Dong, C. M. Lohse, W. S. Webster, S. Sengupta, I. Frank, A. S. Parker, H. Zincke, M. L. Blute, T. J. Sebo, J. C. Cheville, and E. D. Kwon. 2006. Tumor B7-H1 is associated with poor prognosis in renal cell carcinoma patients with long-term follow-up. Cancer Res 66:3381.
16. Romani, N., S. Gruner, D. Brang, E. Kampgen, A. Lenz, B. Trockenbacher, G. Konwalinka, P. O. Fritsch, R. M. Steinman, and G. Schuler. 1994. Proliferating dendritic cell progenitors in human blood. J Exp Med 180:83.
17. Sallusto, F., and A. Lanzavecchia. 1994. Efficient presentation of soluble antigen by cultured human dendritic cells is maintained by granulocyte/macrophage colony-stimulating factor plus interleukin 4 and downregulated by tumor necrosis factor alpha. J Exp Med 179:1109.
18. Caux, C., C. Dezutter-Dambuyant, D. Schmitt, and J. Banchereau. 1992. GM-CSF and TNF-alpha cooperate in the generation of dendritic Langerhans cells. Nature 360:258.
19. Banchereau, J., A. K. Palucka, M. Dhodapkar, S. Burkeholder, N. Taquet, A. Rolland, S. Taquet, S. Coquery, K. M. Wittkowski, N. Bhardwaj, L. Pineiro, R. Steinman, and J. Fay. 2001. Immune and clinical responses in patients with metastatic melanoma to CD34(+) progenitor-derived dendritic cell vaccine. Cancer Res 61:6451.
20. Brugarolas, J. 2007. Renal-cell carcinoma--molecular pathways and therapies. N Engl J Med 356:185.
21. Holtl, L., C. Rieser, C. Papesh, R. Ramoner, G. Bartsch, and M. Thurnher. 1998. CD83+ blood dendritic cells as a vaccine for immunotherapy of metastatic renal-cell cancer. Lancet 352:1358.
22. Holtl, L., C. Zelle-Rieser, H. Gander, C. Papesh, R. Ramoner, G. Bartsch, H. Rogatsch, A. L. Barsoum, J. H. Coggin, Jr., and M. Thurnher. 2002. Immunotherapy of metastatic renal cell carcinoma with tumor lysate-pulsed autologous dendritic cells. Clin Cancer Res 8:3369.
23. Holtl, L., R. Ramoner, C. Zelle-Rieser, H. Gander, T. Putz, C. Papesh, W. Nussbaumer, C. Falkensammer, G. Bartsch, and M. Thurnher. 2004. Allogeneic dendritic cell vaccination against metastatic renal cell carcinoma with or without cyclophosphamide. Cancer Immunol Immunother.
24. Jonuleit, H., U. Kuhn, G. Muller, K. Steinbrink, L. Paragnik, E. Schmitt, J. Knop, and A. H. Enk. 1997. Pro-inflammatory cytokines and prostaglandins induce maturation of potent immunostimulatory dendritic cells under fetal calf serum-free conditions. Eur J Immunol 27:3135.
25. Rieser, C., R. Ramoner, L. Holtl, H. Rogatsch, C. Papesh, A. Stenzl, G. Bartsch, and M. Thurnher. 1999. Mature dendritic cells induce T-helper type-1-dominant immune responses in patients with metastatic renal cell carcinoma. Urol Int 63:151.
26. Zelle-Rieser, C., A. L. Barsoum, F. Sallusto, R. Ramoner, J. W. Rohrer, L. Holtl, G. Bartsch, J. J. Coggin, and M. Thurnher. 2001. Expression and immunogenicity of oncofetal antigen-immature laminin receptor in human renal cell carcinoma. J Urol 165:1705.
27. Cohen, H. T., and F. J. McGovern. 2005. Renal-cell carcinoma. N Engl J Med 353:2477.
28. Kleinrath, T., C. Gassner, P. Lackner, M. Thurnher, and R. Ramoner. 2007. Interleukin-4 promoter polymorphisms: a genetic prognostic factor for survival in metastatic renal cell carcinoma. J Clin Oncol 25:845.
29. Lanzavecchia, A., and F. Sallusto. 2005. Understanding the generation and function of memory T cell subsets. Curr Opin Immunol 17:326.
30. Kay, A. B. 2001. Allergy and allergic diseases. First of two parts. N Engl J Med 344:30.
31. Ziegler, S. F., and Y. J. Liu. 2006. Thymic stromal lymphopoietin in normal and pathogenic T cell development and function. Nat Immunol 7:709.
32. Soumelis, V., P. A. Reche, H. Kanzler, W. Yuan, G. Edward, B. Homey, M. Gilliet, S. Ho, S. Antonenko, A. Lauerma, K. Smith, D. Gorman, S. Zurawski, J. Abrams, S. Menon, T. McClanahan, R. de Waal-Malefyt Rd, F. Bazan, R. A. Kastelein, and Y. J. Liu. 2002. Human epithelial cells trigger dendritic cell mediated allergic inflammation by producing TSLP. Nat Immunol 3:673.

33. Zhou, B., M. R. Comeau, T. De Smedt, H. D. Liggitt, M. E. Dahl, D. B. Lewis, D. Gyarmati, T. Aye, D. J. Campbell, and S. F. Ziegler. 2005. Thymic stromal lymphopoietin as a key initiator of allergic airway inflammation in mice. Nat Immunol 6:1047.
34. Ebner, S., V. A. Nguyen, M. Forstner, Y. H. Wang, D. Wolfram, Y. J. Liu, and N. Romani. 2007. Thymic stromal lymphopoietin converts human epidermal Langerhans cells into antigen-presenting cells that induce proallergic T cells. J Allergy Clin Immunol 119:982.
35. Mazzoni, A., H. A. Young, J. H. Spitzer, A. Visintin, and D. M. Segal. 2001. Histamine regulates cytokine production in maturing dendritic cells, resulting in altered T cell polarization. J Clin Invest 108:1865.
36. Thurnher, M. 2007. Lipids in dendritic cell biology: messengers, effectors, and antigens. J Leukoc Biol 81:154.
37. Liu, M. C., E. R. Bleecker, L. M. Lichtenstein, A. Kagey-Sobotka, Y. Niv, T. L. McLemore, S. Permutt, D. Proud, and W. C. Hubbard. 1990. Evidence for elevated levels of histamine, prostaglandin D2, and other bronchoconstricting prostaglandins in the airways of subjects with mild asthma. Am Rev Respir Dis 142:126.
38. Gosset, P., F. Bureau, V. Angeli, M. Pichavant, C. Faveeuw, A. B. Tonnel, and F. Trottein. 2003. Prostaglandin D2 affects the maturation of human monocyte-derived dendritic cells: consequence on the polarization of naive Th cells. J Immunol 170:4943.
39. Hammad, H., M. Kool, T. Soullie, S. Narumiya, F. Trottein, H. C. Hoogsteden, and B. N. Lambrecht. 2007. Activation of the D prostanoid 1 receptor suppresses asthma by modulation of lung dendritic cell function and induction of regulatory T cells. J Exp Med 204:357.
40. Watanabe, N., Y. H. Wang, H. K. Lee, T. Ito, W. Cao, and Y. J. Liu. 2005. Hassall's corpuscles instruct dendritic cells to induce CD4+CD25+ regulatory T cells in human thymus. Nature 436:1181.
41. Steinman, R. M., and I. Mellman. 2004. Immunotherapy: bewitched, bothered, and bewildered no more. Science 305:197.

The Use of Microbes and Their Products in Allergy Prevention and Therapy

Paolo Maria Matricardi

Introduction

The immune system requires continuous contact with microorganisms in order to develop properly. Animals grown in germ-free environment (gnotobiotic animals) are not only deficient in effective immune response to pathogens [1], but also lack immune tolerance, thus over-expressing the "pro-allergic" T helper type 2 (Th2)-biased immune response to orally delivered antigen [2]. Results of these and other similar studies provided biological plausibility to the "hygiene hypothesis," proposing that the increasing incidence rates of allergic diseases in the Western societies can be explained with improved sanitary and lifestyle conditions, and reduced cross-infections within young families [3]. In its simplest iteration, increasing hygienic living conditions, the increasing use of antibiotic and sterile food preparations resulted in the separation of the immune system from positive microbial exposure early in life, especially those stimulating the gastrointestinal-associated lymphoid tissue [4, 5]. A reduced microbial stimulation caused an increased expression of the T helper type 2-polarized immune response towards allergens [4, 6] and reduced activities of anti-inflammatory networks, including T regulatory cells and their cytokines (e.g., TGF-β, IL-10), suppressing both Th1- and Th2-mediated immune disorders [7] (Fig. 1). T regulatory cells are generated from naïve T cells principally at the mucosal sites after encounter with antigen and under the direction of dendritic cells (DCs) with an exceptional, semi-mature activation status (MHC class-II^{hi}, CD86^{hi}, CD40^{low}). Antigen-mediated induction of regulatory T cells by dendritic cells is mediated by a set of so-called toll-like receptors (TLRs) in the presence of immunosuppressive cytokines, IL-10 and TGF-β, secreted by dendritic cells [8]. Regulatory mechanism of the immune system, in response to microbial stimulation, received therefore a great deal of attention. Mouse models of asthma have been treated with different kinds of microbial or parasite products

P.M. Matricardi
Department of Pediatric Pneumology and Immunology, Charité – Universitätsmedizin, Augustenburger Platz 1, D-13353 Berlin, Germany
e-mail: paolo.matricardi@charite.de

R. Pawankar et al. (eds.), *Allergy Frontiers: Future Perspectives*,
DOI 10.1007/978-4-431-99365-0_18, © Springer 2010

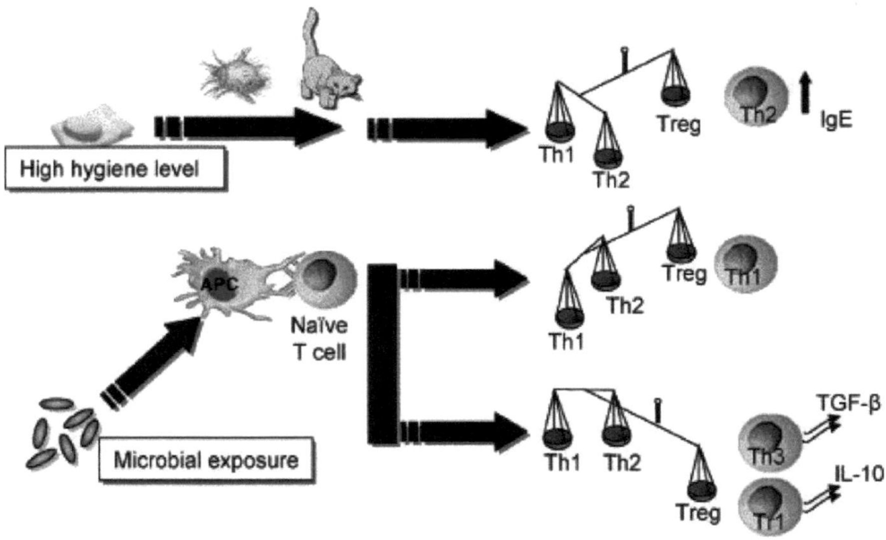

Fig. 1 According to current mechanistic explanations of the hygiene hypothesis, exposure to microorganisms (decreased hygiene) during early age is important for the development of a balanced immune system. Increased hygiene leads to an uncontrolled T helper type 2 immune response to allergens, resulting in atopic diseases. In contrast, repeated microbial pressure promotes T helper type 1 immune responses or results in the upregulation of regulatory mechanisms, which counterbalance pathologic immune response to allergens (reprinted with permission from [69])

Table 1 Bacterial and parasite products used against allergy in humans

1. Mycobacteria
2. Lactobacilli and other probiotics
3. Oligodeoxyribonucleotides (ODN)
4. Others: Bacterial extracts, LPS-derived molecules, Engineered bacteria, Oligodeoxynucleotides

to prevent the development of allergic sensitization or to suppress the allergic inflammation. A central, common feature of all these studies is the attempt to properly stimulate the Toll-like receptors on cells of the innate immune system (e.g., dendritic cells) to produce cytokines directing naïve T cells into desired T cell subtypes (e.g., Th1, Th3, Tr1, etc.). Many of these approaches find a parallel in attempts to prevent or treat allergic diseases in humans [9]. Most of the recent data concern the use of mycobacteria, lactobacilli and other probiotics, and olygodeoxynucleotides. Other approaches include the use of bacterial extracts (lysates), LPS derivatives (MPL), engineered bacteria (e.g., *E. coli* producing peanut allergens), and helminthic products (Table 1). Aim of this review is to summarize the current knowledge about the use of bacteria and parasites or their products as new therapeutic strategies for the treatment of allergic disorders in humans.

Mycobacteria

Background

The hypothesis that mycobacteria protect humans from the development of allergic sensitization and allergic diseases [6] received support from a pioneer study among 867 Japanese children, all immunized with BCG: responders to tuberculin had lower serum levels of total IgE and TH2 cytokines (IL-4, IL-10, and IL-13), higher serum levels of IFN-γ, and lower prevalence of atopy and atopic diseases when compared to tuberculin non-responder subjects [10]. Hence, it was proposed that children with strong tuberculin responses were protected from atopy by a higher natural exposure to environmental mycobacteria. This epidemiological observation was not replicated in different settings and populations [11], and hence, it is doubtful if the traditional BCG vaccination can revert the immunological dysregulation which may underlie the allergy epidemic [12]. However, many other strong arguments supported the initial hypothesis [13]. Thus, non-pathogenic mycobacteria, such as BCG and *Mycobacterium vaccae*, were investigated as preventive or therapeutic tools against experimental asthma in rodents and allergic diseases in human patients.

Experimental Evidence

Both BCG and *M. vaccae* have been proved to be extremely effective in treating asthma in mouse models, and the mechanisms of their action have been identified. Perhaps the most convincing experiment is the one showing the treatment with a killed *M. vaccae* suspension (SRP 299) that block allergic inflammation in a mouse model of asthma by inducing allergen-specific $CD4^{+}CD45RB^{Lo}$ regulatory T cells and in IL-10 and TGF-β dependent way [14]. Similarly, subcutaneous injections of SRP 299 soon after birth were able to delay the onset of spontaneous dermatitis in NC/Nga Mice and to ameliorate its clinical course, with a significant reduction in the scratching behavior [15]. Lastly, intra-gastric administration of SRP 299 inhibited pulmonary allergic inflammation in a mouse model of asthma [16], indicating that stimulation of the gastrointestinal-associated immune system and related lymphonodes can affect the allergic immune response in the lung, as previously hypothesized [5].

Bacillus Calmette-Guerin was shown to hinder the IgE/IgG1 antibody responses, airway hyperresponsiveness, eosinophilic influx into the airway, IL-4 and IL-5 levels in bronchoalveolar lavage (BAL) fluid, in high IgE responder Balb/c mice, when administered 2 weeks before the allergen (ovalbumin) [17]. BCG intranasal infection, preceding the allergen challenge in sensitized mice, inhibited airway eosinophilia in an IFN-γ dependent manner [18]. The subcutaneous injection of heat-killed BCG suppressed the serum total IgE [19] and allergic inflammation [20] in a mouse model of allergic asthma.

Trials in Humans

Both *M. vaccae* and BCG have been used to treat the allergic diseases in humans. Significant reduction in the extent of eczematous changes was observed in children (age 5–18years) with atopic dermatitis 3 months after a single intradermal dose of a preparation of killed *M. vaccae* (SRL-172) (–48%, 95%CI 32–65%, p=0.001) but not in those receiving placebo (–4%, 95%CI –29 to 22%) [21]. A similar effect was not observed in AD patients younger than 5 years [15] and in a third, larger trial in 5–16 years old AD patients [22].

Intradermal injections of heat-killed *M. vaccae* (HKMV) (0.5 mg), or delipidated deglycolipidated *M. vaccae* (DDMV) (0.05 mg) were not better than placebo in the treatment of 42 patients with stable moderately severe asthma sensitized to house dust mites [23]. Intranasal administration of DDMV did not reduce the asthma severity in adult patients with established disease [24]. However, the observation that *M. vaccae* by gavage was as effective as s.c. injection in significantly reducing the severity of pulmonary allergic inflammation in a mouse model [16] raises exciting new possibilities to test the same approach in humans.

Observational studies investigating the putative allergy and asthma protective effect of early BCG immunization provided conflicting results (reviewed in [11, 12]). Total and allergen-specific serum IgE levels decreased significantly in 20 adult allergic patients after BCG vaccination [25], no control group, however, was examined in this study. Medication-, and not symptom-scores decreased significantly in a trial on adult patients with moderate-to-severe asthma [26], a result which was reinforced through a second BCG immunization performed a year later [27]. Conversely, repeated intradermal injections of heat-inactivated BCG in adults with asthma did not induce any clinical improvement, and the trial had to be interrupted because of severe local reactions [28].

Perspectives

Clinical studies on the efficacy of intradermal BCG or *M. vaccae* are still in a preliminary phase and the trials completed so far have not fulfilled the theoretical expectations, showing little efficacy in eczema and no efficacy in asthma. Different administration routes and schedules are being discussed on the basis of more recent data in animal models.

Probiotics

Background

According to FAO and WHO, the term "probiotics" is referred to "Live microorganisms which when administered in adequate amounts confer a health benefit on the host" (Joint FAO/WHO Working Group, 2002); however, several other definitions have been proposed and changed subsequently over time [29]. The most commonly used probiotics are lactobacilli and bifidobacteria, but enterococci and *E. coli* have also been proposed in the light of the above definition. Probiotics have been investigated as a therapy for a broad array of diseases, including cancer, inflammatory bowel diseases, diarrhea, lactose intolerance, allergies, hypercholesterolemia, dental caries, vaginal infections, etc.; some of these promoted for their claimed health benefits, including "keeping healthy" or "immune support."

The rationale for the use of probiotics in allergy prevention and therapy was largely based on the observation in small cross-sectional or birth cohort studies that early intestinal colonization with *Bifidobacterium spp.* or *Lactobacillus spp.* were associated with a reduced risk of allergy development [30–32]. The hygiene hypothesis was also utilized as a rationale to "invent" the probiotic functional food for patients with allergic disease [33]. By contrast, a large and comprehensive, multi-centre birth cohort study of the pattern of acquisition of commensal bowel microbiota in infancy could not demonstrate that the microbiota of children developing atopic eczema or atopy lacked any key groups of faecal bacteria, including lactobacilli, bifidobacteria, enterococci, and *E.coli* [34].

Trials in Humans

Probiotics have been used in trials to evaluate their preventive or therapeutic efficacy against allergic diseases. Initial studies were promising, but they have been criticized for their insufficient design and other weaknesses in data handling or data interpretation [35]. The evidence provided was then considered insufficient to advise the use of probiotics for primary prevention or therapy of allergies, and this approach was considered an experimental one by a Task Force of EAACI [9], the GINA group [36], and individual opinion leaders [37]. Since then, further trials using probiotics for the prevention or therapy of allergic diseases have been published. A Finnish intervention trial in over 900 infants demonstrated that probiotic treatment containing *Lactobacillus rhamnosus GG* (LGG) and three other probiotic strains had no effect on the incidence of allergic diseases by age 2 but significantly prevented eczema, especially atopic eczema [38]. By contrast, an Australian intervention trial in over 170 Australian infants demonstrated that early probiotic supplementation with *L. acidophilus* did not reduce the risk of AD in high risk infants, but was associated with increased allergen sensitization in infants receiving probiotics [39]. A combination of *L. rhamnosus* and *L. reuteri* did not improve the

SCORAD index of AD patients significantly compared to placebo; nevertheless, the treatment was considered "beneficial" on the basis of the patients' subjective evaluation during intervention [40]. No differences were observed in infants with AEDS and suspected cow milk allergy which were treated with LGG, compared to placebo [41]. No therapeutic effect was observed in a DBPC trial of LGG in German infants with moderate atopic dermatitis [42]. There was no significant improvement of the SCORAD values between the placebo and treatment group in a trial studying the effect of *L. fermentum* in Australian infants with atopic dermatitis [43]. Finally, no clinical or immunological effect of LGG was observed in Dutch infants with atopic dermatitis, compared to placebo [44]. A case report showed that contamination of probiotic preparations with milk allergens can cause anaphylaxis in children with cow's milk allergy [45]; the same report alerted that two out of three probiotics widely used in France contain significant amount of beta-lactoglobulin.

Perspectives

The evidence from observational studies that naturally acquired lactobacilli and bifidobacteria do not protect European children from the development of atopic eczema weakens the rationale supporting the use of probiotics in the prevention of atopic dermatitis. With the exception of a Finnish study on the prevention of atopic dermatitis, all the trials on the use of probiotics in the prevention or therapy of atopic dermatitis published after 2003 do not support the hypothesis, that probiotics are useful in allergy prevention and therapy. Recent literature, therefore, reinforced the negative conclusions drawn by the EAACI Task Force, the GINA group and individual opinion leaders on the basis of trials published before 2003. Prevention and therapy of allergies should be considered an unapproved indication for probiotics. Presently, market claims accompanying supplement forms of probiotics are limited to somewhat vague structure-function claims such as "supports a healthy intestinal flora," "fortifying the immune system," and are a long way from claims that many believe should be permitted.

Olygodeoxynucleotides

Background

Bacterial and viral genomic DNA is enriched, compared to that of mammals, in unmethylated sequences of cytosine and guanine (CpG motifs) [46]. These motifs are recognized by the innate immune system through the Toll-like-Receptor-9 (this being one of the mechanisms identifying the presence of bacteria) [47]. For therapeutic applications, TLR9 can be stimulated with synthetic oligodeoxynucleotides containing one or more unmethylated CpG dinucleotides (CpG ODN). Among resting immune cells, TLR9 is expressed in humans only among B lymphocytes and plasmacytoid DCs (pDCs) [48] while in mouse it is expressed also by monocytes, and myeloid DC. This difference in the TLR9 distribution is important as it explains why it is extremely difficult to predict the effects of TLR9 activation in humans by extrapolating the results obtained with mice.

Experimental Evidence

DNA sequences containing CpG motifs have been synthesized and successfully used to prevent or treat asthma in animal models or as adjuvants to prevent or reverse specific allergic sensitization in murine models of allergy [49]. Immunization using ISS-ODN as an adjuvant resulted effectively in rodent models of allergic disease, including anaphylaxis [50], asthma [49], and allergic conjunctivitis [51]. Mice sensitized to an allergen but treated with ISS-ODN alone (as an immunomodulating agent) had attenuated hypersensitivity responses to subsequent allergen challenge [49]. ISS-ODN were effective as corticosteroids in the prevention of the immediate phase hypersensitivity response of allergic conjunctivitis, more effective than corticosteroids used in the prevention of the late phase inflammatory responses observed in murine models of allergic conjunctivitis and asthma [49].

TLR-9 stimulation affects the human immune system also, its effects include secretion of IFN-inducible chemokines and cytokines, pro- (IL-6, TNFα) as well as anti-inflammatory cytokines (IL-10, IL-1RA); induction of IgG isotype switching and antibody secretion, and suppression of IgE antibody production and differentiation of TH1 cells [52]. The resultant effect of TLR9 activation in humans is to induce TH1-biased cellular and humoral effector functions of innate and adaptive immunity [52]. The anti-allergic effects of CpG ODN have also been seen in humans. Synthetic phosphorothioate ODN were able to induce B cell proliferation and shift the in vitro differentiation of Dermatophagoides pteronyssinus group 1-specific hCD4+ T cells from atopic donors into Th1 phenotype [53]. ISS-ODN also led to a significant increase of IFN-γ production by NK cells through an IL-12-dependent mechanism and increased the mRNA expression of IL-12 and IL-18 in hPBMC and monocyte-derived dendritic cells, both in atopic and non-atopic individuals. In hPBMC from atopic patients, stimulation with ISS-ODN led to a considerable increase of the polyclonal IgG and IgM synthesis while the production of total IgE was suppressed. ISS-ODN also induced a significant increase of IgG and IgM, specific for allergens, to which the patients were sensitized whereas allergen-specific IgE levels remained unchanged [54]. In a phase 1 trial involving 19 patients with ragweed allergy, the administration of the same AIC preparation with a similar, 6 weeks/6 s.c. injection protocol produced a re-direction in the T cell response against Amb a 1 from Th2 to Th1 [55]. It has also been shown that immunotherapy with AIC decreases the nasal inflammatory response after challenge in vivo [56].

Trials

A conjugate of a CpG ODN to a portion of the ragweed allergen (Amb a 1) was created, which provided evidence of safety and immunogenicity in phase I trials (AIC) [57]. Subsequently, a randomized, double-blind, placebo-controlled phase 2 trial of AIC was completed in a small trial involving 25 adults allergic to ragweed [58]. Patients received six weekly injections of the AIC or placebo vaccine before the first ragweed season and were monitored during the next two ragweed seasons. No pattern of vaccine-associated systemic reactions or clinically significant laboratory abnormalities were observed during the study period (3 years). During the first ragweed season, the AIC group had better peak-season rhinitis scores on the visual-analogue scale (p=0.006), peak-season daily nasal symptom diary scores (p=0.02), and midseason overall quality-of-life scores (p=0.05) than the placebo group. AIC induced a transient increase in Amb a 1-specific IgG antibody but suppressed the seasonal increase in Amb a 1-specific IgE antibody. A reduction in the number of interleukin-4-positive basophils in AIC-treated patients correlated with lower rhinitis visual-analogue scores (r=0.49, p=0.03). Clinical benefits of AIC were again observed in the subsequent ragweed season, with improvements over placebo in peak-season rhinitis visual-analogue scores (p=0.02) and peak-season daily nasal symptom diary scores (p=0.02). The seasonal specific IgE antibody response was again suppressed, with no significant change in IgE antibody titer during the ragweed season (p=0.19). The authors concluded that a 6-week regimen of the AIC vaccine appeared to offer long-term clinical efficacy in the treatment of ragweed allergic rhinitis [58].

After this preliminary study, a much larger, multi-centre Phase 2/3 clinical trial of AIC was started in adults with ragweed allergic rhinitis [59]. This trial involved 462 subjects, aged 18–55 years, with moderate to severe ragweed allergy (hay fever). Prior to the 2004 ragweed season, subjects received six weekly doses of either placebo or increasing doses of up to 30 μg of AIC (1.2, 3, 6, 15, 21, and 30 μg), in a two-to-one randomization. Prior to the 2005 ragweed season, one half of the AIC-treated subjects received two additional booster shots (3 and 30 μg, respectively, in 1 week interval) , while the other half of the group treated in the first season with AIC received placebo injections; the group treated with placebo in 2004 received again placebo injections prior to the 2005 season. A total nasal symptom score was measured using four parameters (congestion, sneezing, itching, and runny nose), each rated on a four-point scale. Patients treated with AIC prior to the 2004 season experienced a statistically significant reduction in total nasal symptom scores (TNSS) during the peak season period compared to placebo-treated patients (p=0.045). The safety profile of AIC was favorable as severe adverse effects were observed in 4.2% of AIC-treated subjects and in 5.3% of patients receiving placebo. The authors concluded that AIC can be safely administered to ragweed allergic adults and that this preparation is associated with a trend towards improved ragweed hay fever symptoms during the first season [59].

Perspectives

The results derived on the use of AIC in the therapy of ragweed allergy are of interest but, given the study design proposed, it is not possible to differentiate the proportion of the observed improvement due to the allergen component and that due to the adjuvant component per se [60]. The effect shown by the larger, multi-centre trial [59] are of lower magnitude and, again, it will not be possible to discriminate how much of this result can be attributed to the adjuvant used.

Other Approaches

MPL

A detoxified derivative of lipopolysaccharide (monophosphoryl-lipid-A, MPL) has been used as an adjuvant combined with inhalant allergens [61]. This vaccine resulted effectively in phase III trials among adults with asthma or allergic rhinitis [61, 62]. As the control group of these studies was treated with placebo (and not with the same preparation in the absence of MPL), it is not possible to know if and how much of the effect can be attributed to MPL itself, as suggested by in vitro studies [63].

Helminths

Based on the concept that helminths strongly stimulate the T-regulatory cells, the regular administration of larvae of *Trichuris suis* has been successfully used to treat an immune disorder, such as inflammatory bowel disease, associated with a dis-regulation of the immune response at intestinal level [64]. A similar experimental approach has been successfully tested in animal models of allergy and asthma [65]. Trials using *Necator americanus* have been planned in volunteers with asthma or food allergies, but no data are yet available [66].

Engineered Bacteria

A quite original and novel approach to specific immunotherapy of allergy has been attempted by generating engineered (mutated) peanut proteins (modified (m) Ara h1, mAra h2, mAra h3) in which IgE-binding epitopes have been altered by a critical amino acid to eliminate, or drastically reduce, the IgE binding to the protein, and therefore, to reduce the risk of eliciting allergic reactions. Because these engineered peanut proteins were generated in *E. coli*, a mixture of heat-killed *E. coli* producing the modified peanut proteins was administered rectally to peanut allergic C3H/HeJ mice. This treatment induced long-term down-regulation of peanut hypersensitivity, which might be secondary to decreased antigen-specific Th2 and increased Th1 and T regulatory cytokine production [67].

Conclusions

A large number of new molecules and preparations have been tested for the prevention or treatment of allergic diseases. Unfortunately, the outcomes of many of these attempts are quite discouraging, while some approaches (CpG ODN) seem more promising. The reason for disappointing effects may be the lack of clear understanding of all the events preceding and causing allergic diseases. All the new therapeutic strategies in allergy target the immune system and have been tested in adults. IgE-mediated allergic diseases start with an immune dysfunction predisposing to IgE-mediated sensitivity, requiring an end-organ related dysfunction and exposure to appropriate environmental factors which facilitate the expression of these genetic inclinations. Targeting only the immune system might not be enough as immune dysfunction might be only one of the features defining allergy. Successful prevention or cure might also require identification and treatment of the end-organ dysfunctions. Furthermore, preventative or curative therapeutic strategies based on microbial products may need to be initiated very early in life, before the occurrence of the irreversible changes linked to chronic allergic inflammation. It is evident that until we identify the causes of allergy, we will not be able to design products with a high rate of success [68].

References

1. Nicaise P, Gleizes A, Sandre C, et al. 1998. Influence of intestinal microflora on murine bone marrow and spleen macrophage precursors. Scand J Immunol 48, 585–591
2. Sudo N, Sawamura S, Tanaka K, Kubo C, Koga Y, 1997. The requirement of intestinal bacterial flora for the development of an IgE production system fully susceptible to oral tolerance induction. J Immunol 159, 1739–1745
3. Strachan DP, 1989. Hay fever, hygiene and household size. Br Med J 299, 1259–1260
4. Holt PG, 1995. Environmental factors and primary T-cell sensitisation to inhalant allergens in infancy: reappraisal of the role of infections and air pollution. Pediatr Allergy Immunol 6, 1–10
5. Matricardi PM, 1997. Infections preventing atopy: facts and new questions. Allergy 52, 879–882
6. Romagnani S, 1994. Regulation of the development of type 2 T-helper cells in allergy. Curr Opin Immunol 6, 838–846
7. Yazdanbakhsh M, Kremsner PG, van Ree R, 2002. Allergy, parasites and the hygiene hypothesis. Science 296, 490–494
8. Mills KH, McGuirk P, 2004. Antigen-specific regulatory T cells--their induction and role in infection. Semin Immunol 16, 107–117

9. EAACI Task Force 7, 2003. Microbial products in allergy prevention and therapy. Allergy 58, 461–471
10. Shirakawa T, Enomoto T, Shimazu S, Hopkin JM, 1997. The inverse association between tuberculin responses and atopic disorder. Science 275, 77–79
11. Matricardi PM, Yazdanbakhsh M, 2003. Mycobacteria and atopy, 6 years later: a fascinating, still unfinished, business. Clin Exp Allergy 33, 717–720
12. Gruber C, Paul KP, 2002. Tuberculin reactivity and allergy. Allergy 57, 277–280
13. Rook GA, Stanford JL, 1998. Give us this day our daily germs. Immunol Today 19, 113–116
14. Zuany-Amorim C, Sawicka E, Manlius C, Le Moine A, Brunet LR, Kemeny DM, Bowen G, Rook G, Walker C, 2002. Suppression of airway eosinophilia by killed Mycobacterium vaccae-induced allergen-specific regulatory T-cells. Nat Med 8, 625–629
15. Arkwright PD, David TJ, 2003. Effect of Mycobacterium vaccae on atopic dermatitis in children of different ages. Br J Dermatol 149, 1029–1034
16. Hunt JR, Martinelli R, Adams VC, Rook GA, Brunet LR, 2005. Intragastric administration of Mycobacterium vaccae inhibits severe pulmonary allergic inflammation in a mouse model. Clin Exp Allergy 35, 685–690
17. Herz U, Gerhold K, Gruber C, Braun A, Wahn U, Renz H, Paul K, 1998. BCG infection suppresses allergic sensitization and development of increased airway reactivity in an animal model. J Allergy Clin Immunol 102, 867–874
18. Erb KJ, Holloway JW, Sobeck A, Moll H, Le Gros G, 1998. Infection of mice with Mycobacterium bovis-Bacillus Calmette-Guerin (BCG) suppresses allergen-induced airway eosinophilia. J Exp Med 187, 561–189
19. Tukenmez F, Bahceciler NN, Barlan IB, Basaran MM, 1999. Effect of pre-immunization by killed Mycobacterium bovis and vaccae on immunoglobulin E response in ovalbumin-sensitized newborn mice. Pediatr Allergy Immunol 10, 107–111
20. Ozdemir C, Akkoc T, Bahceciler NN, Kucukercan D, Barlan IB, Basaran MM, 2003. Impact of Mycobacterium vaccae immunization on lung histopathology in a murine model of chronic asthma. Clin Exp Allergy 33, 266–270
21. Arkwright PD, David TJ, 2001. Intradermal administration of a killed Mycobacterium vaccae suspension (SRL 172) is associated with improvement in atopic dermatitis in children with moderate-to-severe disease. J Allergy Clin Immunol 107, 531–534
22. Berth-Jones J, Arkwright PD, Marasovic D, Savani N, Aldridge CR, Leech SN, Morgan C, Clark SM, Ogilvie S, Chopra S, Harper JI, Smith CH, Rook GA, Friedmann PS, 2006. Killed Mycobacterium vaccae suspension in children with moderate-to-severe atopic dermatitis: a randomized, double-blind, placebo-controlled trial. Clin Exp Allergy 36, 1115–1121
23. Shirtcliffe PM, Easthope SE, Cheng S, Weatherall M, Tan PL, Le Gros G, Beasley R, 2001. The effect of delipidated deglycolipidated (DDMV) and heat-killed Mycobacterium vaccae in asthma.Am J Respir Crit Care Med 163, 1410–1414
24. Shirtcliffe PM, Goldkorn A, Weatherall M, Tan PL, Beasley R, 2003. Pilot study of the safety and effect of intranasal delipidated acid-treated Mycobacterium vaccae in adult asthma. Respirology 8, 497–503
25. Cavallo GP, Elia M, Giordano D, Baldi C, Cammarota R, 2002. Decrease of specific and total IgE levels in allergic patients after BCG vaccination: preliminary report. Arch Otolaryngol Head Neck Surg 128, 1058–1060
26. Choi IS, Koh YI, 2002. Therapeutic effects of BCG vaccination in adult asthmatic patients: a randomized, controlled trial. Ann Allergy Asthma Immunol 88, 584–591
27. Choi IS, Koh YI, 2003. Effects of BCG revaccination on asthma. Allergy 58, 1114–1116
28. Shirtcliffe PM, Easthope SE, Weatherall M, Beasley R, 2004. Effect of repeated intradermal injections of heat-inactivated Mycobacterium bovis bacillus Calmette-Guerin in adult asthma. Clin Exp Allergy 34, 207–212
29. Schrezenmeier J, de Vrese M, 2001. Probiotics, prebiotics, and synbiotics – approaching a definition. Am J Clin Nutr 73, 361S–364S
30. Kalliomaki M, Kirjavainen P, Eerola E, Kero P, Salminen S, Isolauri E, 2001. Distinct patterns of neonatal gut microflora in infants in whom atopy was and was not developing. J Allergy Clin Immunol 107, 129–134

31. Watanabe S, Narisawa Y, Arase S, Okamatsu H, Ikenaga T, Tajiri Y, Kumemura M, 2003. Differences in fecal microflora between patients with atopic dermatitis and healthy control subjects. J Allergy Clin Immunol 111, 587–591
32. Sepp E, Julge K, Mikelsaar M, Bjorksten B, 2005. Intestinal microbiota and immunoglobulin E responses in 5-year-old Estonian children. Clin Exp Allergy 35, 1141–1146
33. Laiho K, Ouwehand A, Salminen S, Isolauri E, 2002. Inventing probiotic functional foods for patients with allergic disease. Ann Allergy Asthma Immunol 89(6 Suppl 1), 75–82
34. Adlerberth I, Strachan DP, Matricardi PM, Ahrné S, Orfei L, Åberg N, Perkin MR, Tripodi S, Hesselmar B, Saalman H, Coates AR, Bonnano CL, Panetta V, Wold AE 2007. Gut microbiota and development of atopic eczema in three European birth cohorts. J Allergy Clin Immunol 120:343–350
35. Matricardi PM, 2002. Probiotics against allergy: data, doubts, and perspectives. Allergy 57, 185–187
36. Global Strategy for Asthma Management and Prevention. Washington DC: National Institutes of Health, National Heart, Lung, and Blood Institute, 2002: NIH Publication No. 02-3659, p.99
37. Flohr C, Pascoe D, Williams HC, 2005. Atopic dermatitis and the hygiene hypothesis: too clean to be true? Br J Dermatol 152, 202–216
38. Kukkonen K, Savilahti E, Haahtela T, Juntunen-Backman K, Korpela R, Poussa T, Tuure T, Kuitunen M, 2007. Probiotics and prebiotic galacto-oligosaccharides in the prevention of allergic diseases: a randomized, double-blind, placebo-controlled trial. J Allergy Clin Immunol 119, 192–198
39. Taylor AL, Dunstan JA, Prescott SL, 2007. Probiotic supplementation for the first 6 months of life fails to reduce the risk of atopic dermatitis and increases the risk of allergen sensitization in high-risk children: a randomized controlled trial. J Allergy Clin Immunol 119, 184–191
40. Rosenfeldt V, Benfeldt E, Nielsen SD, Michaelsen KF, Jeppesen DL, Valerius A, Paerregaard A, 2003. Effect of probiotic Lactobacillus strains in children with atopic dermatitis. J Allergy Clin Immunol 111, 389–395
41. Viljanen M, Savilahti E, Haahtela T, Juntunen-Backman K, Korpela R, Poussa T, Tuure T, Kuitunen M, 2005. Probiotics in the treatment of atopic eczema/dermatitis syndrome in infants: a double-blind placebo-controlled trial. Allergy 60, 494–500
42. Grüber C, Wendt M, Lau S, Kulig M, Wahn U, Werfel T, Niggemann B, 2005. Randomized placebo-controlled trial of Lactobacillus rhamnosus GG as treatment of mild to moderate atopic dermatitis in infancy. J Allergy Clin Immunol 117, S239
43. Weston S, Halbert A, Richmond P, Prescott SL, 2005. Effects of probiotics on atopic dermatitis: a randomised controlled trial. Arch Dis Child 90, 892–897
44. Brouwer ML, Wolt-Plompen SA, Dubois AE, van der Heide S, Jansen DF, Hoijer MA, Kauffman HF, Duiverman EJ, 2006. No effects of probiotics on atopic dermatitis in infancy: a randomized placebo-controlled trial. Clin Exp Allergy 36(7), 899–906
45. Lee TT, Morisset M, Astier C, Moneret-Vautrin DA, Cordebar V, Beaudouin E, Codreanu F, Bihain BE, Kanny G, 2007. Contamination of probiotic preparations with milk allergens can cause anaphylaxis in children with cow's milk allergy. J Allergy Clin Immunol 119, 746–747
46. Raz E, Tighe H, Sato Y, Corr M, Dudler JA, Roman M, et al. 1996. Preferential induction of a Th1 immune response and inhibition of specific IgE antibody formation by plasmid DNA immunization. Proc Natl Acad Sci U S A 93, 5141–5145
47. Krieg AM, 2002. CpG motifs in bacterial DNA and their immune effects. Annu Rev Immunol 20, 709–760
48. Iwasaki A, Medzhitov R, 2004. Toll-like receptor control of the adaptive immune responses. Nat Immunol 5, 987–995
49. Horner AA, Van Uden JH, Zubeldia JM, Broide D, Raz E, 2001. DNA-based immunotherapeutics for the treatment of allergic disease. Immunology Reviews 179, 102–118
50. Horner AA, Nguyen MD, Ronaghy A, Cinman N, Verbeek S, Raz E, 2000. DNA-based vaccination reduces the risk of lethal anaphylactic hypersensitivity in mice. J Allergy Clin Immunol 106, 349–356

51. Magone MT, Chan CC, Beck L, Whitcup SM, Raz E, 2000. Systemic or mucosal administration of immunostimulatory DNA inhibits early and late phases of murine allergic conjunctivitis. Eur J Immunol 30, 1841–1850
52. Krieg AM, 2006. Therapeutic potential of Toll-like receptor 9 activation. Nat Rev Drug Discov 5, 471–484
53. Parronchi P, Brugnolo F, Annunziato F, Manuelli C, Sampognaro S, Mavilia C, Romagnani S, Maggi E, 1999. Phosphorothioate oligodeoxynucleotides promote the in vitro development of human allergen-specific CD4+ T cells into Th1 effectors. J Immunol 163, 5946–5953
54. Bohle B, Jahn-Schmid B, Maurer D, Kraft D, Ebner C, 1999. Oligodeoxynucleotides containing CpG motifs induce IL-12, IL-18 and IFN-gamma production in cells from allergic individuals and inhibit IgE synthesis in vitro. Eur J Immunol 29, 2344–2353
55. Simons FE, Shikishima Y, Van Nest G, Eiden JJ, HayGlass KT, 2004. Selective immune redirection in humans with ragweed allergy by injecting Amb a1 linked to immunostimulatory DNA. J Allergy Clin Immunol 113, 1144–1151
56. Tulic MK, Fiset PO, Christodoulopoulos P, Vaillancourt P, Desrosiers M, Lavigne F, Eiden J, Hamid Q, 2004. Amb a 1-immunostimulatory oligodeoxynucleotide conjugate immunotherapy decreases the nasal inflammatory response. J Allergy Clin Immunol 113, 235–241
57. Tighe H, Takabayashi K, Schwartz D, Van Nest G, Tuck S, Eiden JJ, et al. 2000. Conjugation of immunostimulatory DNA to the short ragweed allergen amb a 1 enhances its immunogenicity and reduces its allergenicity. J Allergy Clin Immunol 106, 124–134
58. Creticos PS, Schroeder JT, Hamilton RG, Balcer-Whaley SL, Khattignavong AP, Lindblad R, Li H, Coffman R, Seyfert V, Eiden JJ, Broide D, 2006. Immune tolerance network group. Immunotherapy with a ragweed-toll-like receptor 9 agonist vaccine for allergic rhinitis. N Engl J Med 355, 1445–1455
59. Busse W, Gross G, Korenblat P, Nayak N, Tarpay M, Levitt D, 2006. Phase 2/3 study of the novel vaccine Amb a 1 immunostimulatory oligodeoxyribonucleotide conjugate AIC in ragweed allergic adults. J Allergy Clin Immunol 117, S88–S89
60. Seymour SM, Chowdhury BA, 2007. Immunotherapy with a ragweed vaccine. N Engl J Med 356, 86
61. Drachenberg KJ, Wheeler AW, Stuebner P, Horak F, 2001. A well-tolerated grass pollen specific allergy vaccine containing a novel adjuvant, Monophosphoryl Lipid A reduces allergic symptoms after only four preseasonal injections. Allergy 56, 498–505
62. von Baehr V, Hermes A, von Baehr R, Scherf HP, Volk HD, Fischer von Weikersthal-Drachenberg KJ, Woroniecki S, 2005. Allergoid-specific T-cell reaction as a measure of the immunological response to specific immunotherapy (SIT) with a Th1-adjuvanted allergy vaccine. J Investig Allergol Clin Immunol 15, 234–241
63. Puggioni F, Durham SR, Francis JN, 2005. Monophosphoryl lipid A (MPL) promotes allergen-induced immune deviation in favour of Th1 responses. Allergy 60, 678–684
64. Weinstock J, Summers RW, Elliott DE, Urban JF Jr, Thompson RA, Weinstock JV, 2005. Trichuris suis therapy for active ulcerative colitis: a randomized controlled trial. Gastroenterology 128, 825–832
65. Wilson MS, Taylor MD, Balic A, Finney CA, Lamb JR, Maizels RM, 2005. Suppression of allergic airway inflammation by helminth-induced regulatory T cells. J Exp Med 202, 1199–1212
66. Falcone FH, Pritchard DI, 2005. Parasite role and reversal: worms on trial. Trends in Parasitol 21, 157–160
67. Li XM, Srivastava K, Grishin A, Huang CK, Schofield B, Burks W, Sampson HA, 2003. Persistent protective effect of heat-killed Escherichia coli producing "engineered," recombinant peanut proteins in a murine model of peanut allergy. J Allergy Clin Immunol 112, 159–167
68. Matricardi PM, Bonini S, 2000. Mimicking microbial 'education' of the immune system: a strategy to revert the epidemic trend of atopy and allergic asthma? Respir Res 1, 129–132
69. Feleszko W, Jaworska J, Hamelmann E, 2006. Toll-like receptors – novel targets in allergic airway disease (probiotics, friends and relatives). Eur J Pharmacol 533(1–3), 308–318

Targeting Insulin-Like Growth Factor-I in Allergen-Induced Airway Inflammation and Remodeling

Ken Ohta, Hiroyuki Nagase, and Naomi Yamashita

Introduction

Airway inflammation and airway remodeling are major characteristics of asthma [1,2]. When we perform bronchial biopsy in asthmatic patients and observe a specimen under the microscope, we can notice the thickening of the region adjacent to the basement membrane as well as desquamation of airway epithelial cells and accumulation of various inflammatory cells including eosinophils. The thickening of the region adjacent to the basement membrane is a part of the process called *airway remodeling*. Airway remodeling in asthma is the predecessor of various structural changes, such as airway wall thickening (AWT), subepithelial fibrosis, mucus metaplasia, and smooth muscle cell hypertrophy and hyperplasia, which are manifestations of the irreversible pathology of severe asthma [1,2].

During subepithelial fibrosis, the fibroblast is activated and collagen synthesis increases. Several cytokines are involved in fibroblastic proliferation. Among those, platelet-derived growth factor (PDGF) and fibronectin function as competence factors which push fibroblasts from G0 to G1 phase, while insulin-like growth factor-I (IGF-I), which used to be called as alveolar macrophage-derived growth factor (AMDGF), is a progression factor acting on fibroblasts from G1 phase to mitosis in the cell cycle and to synthesize collagen. [3,4]. We previously reported that PDGF plays a critical role in remodeling in asthma [5]. Neutralizing antibody to PDGF-B inhibited both diesel exhaust particulate (DEP)-induced AWT and hyperresponsiveness to acetylcholine (Ach), suggesting that AWT, which is a result of airway remodeling,

K. Ohta (✉), H. Nagase, and N. Yamashita
Division of Respiratory Medicine and Allergology, Department of Medicine, Teikyo University School of Medicine, 2-11-1 Kaga, Itabashi-Ku, Tokyo 173-8665, Japan
e-mail: kenohta@med.teikyo-u.ac.jp

N. Yamashita
Present address: Department of Pharmacology, Research Institute of Pharmaceutical Science, Musashino University, 1-1-20 Shin-machi, Nishitokyo-Shi, Tokyo, Japan

R. Pawankar et al. (eds.), *Allergy Frontiers: Future Perspectives*,
DOI 10.1007/978-4-431-99365-0_19, © Springer 2010

is at least in part directly involved in airway hyperresponsiveness. Although the involvement of IGF-I in remodeling in asthma is also suggested [6,7], the functional involvement of IGF-I in the pathogenesis of asthma must be elucidated.

What is IGF-I?

Among IGFs, IGF-I is a single-chain polypeptide that has a high degree of homology to insulin and acts in the manner of endocrines [8]. It is produced in the liver and released into the blood as the complex with the IGF-binding protein (IGFBP). The serum level of IGF-I is mainly controlled by growth hormone (GH). IGFBP consists of six subtypes, i.e. from IGFBP-1 to IGFBP-6, and 75% of IGF-I binds to IGFBP-3, which is synthesized in the liver in a GH-dependent manner. The function of IGF-I is modified by IGFBP-3 and degradation enzyme for IGFBP-3. IGF-I is involved in suppression of apoptosis as well as differentiation and proliferation in various cells. In fact, IGF-I knockout mice have shown the delay of development during the embryo stage and impairment of weight gain after birth. In addition, IGF-I is known to have some effects on immune cells, such as inducing T-cell proliferation and preventing T-cell apoptosis [9,10]. As mentioned earlier, IGF-I is a progression factor acting on fibroblasts from G1 phase to mitosis in the cell cycle and to synthesize collagen [3,4]. Based on this fact, we investigated the role of IGF-I in airway inflammation and remodeling in asthma [11]. We would like to overview what we found through the experiments, which have already been published in the [11].

The Role of IGF-I in a Murine Model of Asthma

Murine Model of Asthma

Specific pathogen-free male A/J mice (10–12 weeks old), which have native airway hyperresponsiveness to acetylcholine (ACh), were purchased from SLC (Shizuoka, Japan). The mice were initially immunized four times with 10 μg OVA + 2 mg alum on days 0, 28, 35, and 49. After immunization with the four injections, enzyme-linked immunosorbent assay (ELISA) titers of OVA-specific IgE were significantly elevated following inhalation of 20 mg/ml OVA for 10 min every other day from day 49 to day 63, as previously reported [12]. Importantly, we were able to show the pivotal role of granulocyte-macrophage colony-stimulating factor (GM-CSF) in the previous study by using neutralizing antibody to.GM-CSF [12]. So, the use of neutralizing antibodies to IGF-I in our murine asthma model is reliable to reveal the functional involvement of IGF-I in asthma. Neutralizing antibody for murine IGF-I was kindly provided by Dr. Jui-Lan Su [13]. This antibody was originally made against human IGF-I but is fully cross-reactive with murine IGF-I [13]. The mice were divided into four groups for administration of inhaled challenge: (1) 0.9 M NaCl, (2) OVA + sham control mouse IgG (4 mg/mouse in 0.9 M NaCl), (3) OVA + anti-IGF-I (4 mg/mouse in 0.9 M NaCl), (4) OVA + anti-IGF-I (0.4 mg/mouse in 0.9 M NaCl) . The antibodies were administered using osmotic pumps (Alzet Minipump), which continuously released its contents for 2 weeks.

Synthesis of IGF-I is Observed in OVA-Challenged Mice

By means of western blot analysis, IGF-I synthesis was found to be elevated after OVA inhalation in our murine model [11]. Mouse sera and bronchoalveolar lavage fluids (BALF) were first precleared using protein A columns (Pharmacia Biotech, Wilstrom, Sweden) followed by incubation with goat anti-IGF-I (Becton Dickinson) and protein G Microbeads (Miltenyi Biotec, Gladbach, Germany) for 30 min. Subsequently, immunoprecipitates were separated in the magnetic field of an mMACS separator. The immunoprecipitates were eluted with sodium dodecyl sulfate (SDS) sample buffer, after which they were separated by SDS-PAGE (sodium dodecyl sulfate-polyacrylamide gel electrophoresis) and electrotransferred onto Hybond-P membranes (Amersham Pharmacia Biotech, Inc., Piscataway, NJ). Membranes were then blocked in buffer containing 4% bovine serum albumin (BSA), and incubated first with rabbit anti-IGF-I (Chemicon), and then with horseradish peroxidase-conjugated F $(ab')_2$ donkey anti-rabbit antibody (1:2,000) (Amersham Pharmacia Biotech, Inc.) The immunoblotted proteins were visualized using an enhanced chemiluminescence (ECL) kit from Amersham Pharmacia Biotech, Inc. IGF-I protein was detected in both serum and BALF samples obtained from OVA-sensitized mice (Fig. 1a). The majority of IGF-I positive cells were macrophages and airway epithelial cells

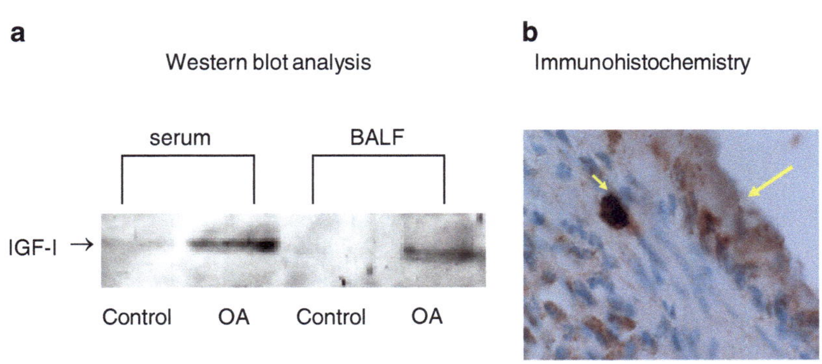

Fig. 1 Expression of IGF-I mRNA and protein (**a**) western blot analysis of IGF-I. IGF-I protein was detected in both serum and BALF. (**b**) Histological analysis of IGF-I protein expression. Positive cells are indicated by arrows. (Original magnification: ×400)

(Fig. 1b). Inhalation of OVA resulted in detection of mRNA expression for IGF-I in lung tissue at 3–24 h, and IGF-I mRNA and TGF-β were detected from the total lung lysate at 24 h after the last OVA inhalation [11].

IGF-I Neutralization Inhibits Airway Hyperresponsiveness and Inflammation

Inhitory Effect on Airway Hyperresposiveness

The effect of murine IGF-I neutralizing antibody on airway response to Ach was tested by administering the antibody continuously for 2 weeks using an osmotic pump [11]. Airway responsiveness to Ach was assessed at 24 h after the last exposure to ovalbumin (OA) by measuring airway resistance (Raw) with a body plethysmograph box (Buxo Electronics, Inc., Troy, NY) under general anesthesia and controlled ventilation, as reported previously, after 24 h of the last OVA inhalation [13]. Increasing doses of ACh (1.25–5.0 mg/ml) were administered by ultra-nebulization for 3 min. Data are expressed as [(*Raw after inhalation of ACh/Raw before inhalation*) × 100 (%)].

Baseline airway resistance was the same in both OVA-treated and nontreated mice. After the inhalation of 1.25–5.0 mg/ml ACh, OVA-treated mice exhibited higher Raw than controls (Fig. 2). Airway response following doses of 1.25, 2.5 and 5 mg/ml of Ach was significantly inhibited in the mice treated with anti-IGF-I antibody (Fig. 2).

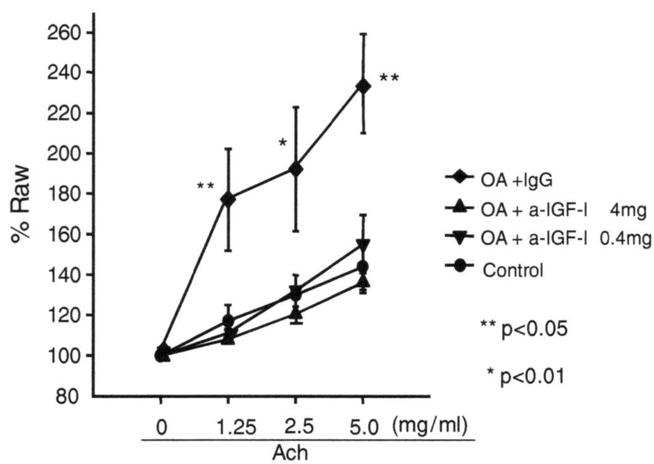

Fig. 2 Effects of neutralization of IGF-I on bronchoconstriction induced with acetylcholine (Ach) inhalation. IGF-I neutralizing antibody was administered by an osmotic pump for 2 weeks during OVA inhalation. The indicated concentrations of Ach were inhaled for 3 min. Raw was measured using whole-body plethysmograph as described in Materials and Methods. Data are expressed as %Raw, i.e. (*Raw after inhalation of ACh/Raw before inhalation*) ×100 (%). The data shown are the mean ± SEM for six mice

After measuring airway responsiveness, we performed bronchoalveolar lavage (BAL), fixation of the lung tissue with formalin, and extraction of mRNA for further investigation.

Inhitory Effect on Airway Inflammation

Airway inflammation was analyzed by BALF cell analysis. Following OVA inhalation, the number of cells in BALF increased, mainly due to an increase in eosinophils (Fig. 3). In mice treated with both OVA and anti-IGF-I, the increment in BALF cell numbers was significantly inhibited (Fig. 3).

In order to identify the effects of anti-IGF-I on the eosinophil-related cytokine, we examined the level of IL-5 by ELISA. As shown in Fig. 4, the level of IL-5 is not influenced by treatment with anti-IGF-I antibody.

Histopathological Improvement is Observed by IGF-I Neutralization

The inflammation and airway remodeling that occurred after OVA inhalation were histologically evaluated [11]. The lungs fixed with 20% formalin were fully inflated using 10 cm H_2O pressure for hematoxylin-eosin (HE) and elastica van Gieson

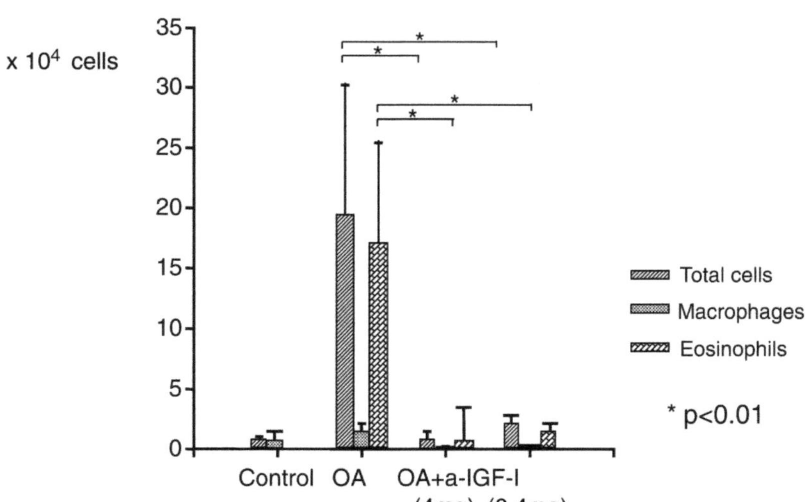

Fig. 3 Cellular analysis in BALF of mice intubated for BAL with a total of 5 mL of saline (0.9 M NaCl). Cells were pelleted from the lavage fluid, resuspended in 1 mL of saline, and placed on glass slides for counting and fixation using Cytospin. Slides were then stained with Diff Quik, and cell differentiation was assessed microscopically. The data shown are mean ± SEM of six mice

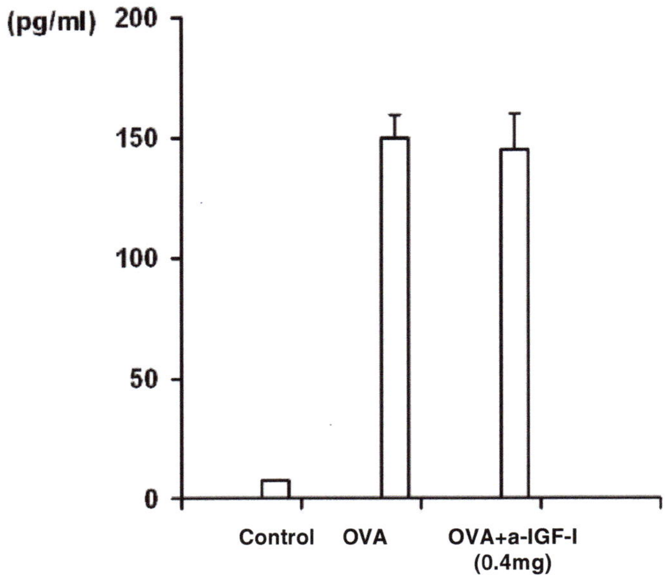

Fig. 4 Effect of IGF-I neutralizing antibody on IL-5 production. The levels of IL-5 in the BALF supernatants were examined using ELISA Quantikine kit (R&D System, Inc., Minneapolis, MN). Each bar consists of mean ± SEM from five samples

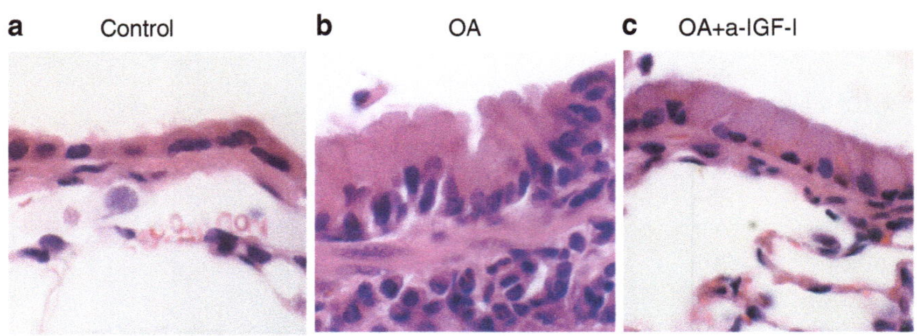

Fig. 5 Effect of IGF-I neutralizing antibody on the histological characteristics of lung tissue. Sections of lung were stained with HE. (**a**) Control untreated mouse; (**b**) OVA inhalation and sham IgG-treated mouse; (**c**) OVA inhalation and anti-IGF-I treated mouse. Original magnification: ×400

(EVG) staining. Thickening beneath the basement membrane was analyzed using an image analyzer and standardized. The AWT index was calculated as external perimeter minus inner perimeter divided by the inner perimeter [5]. HE staining disclosed that airway inflammation was attenuated by the administration of anti-IGF-I (Fig. 5c vs. b). EVG staining clearly showed that the lung tissue obtained from mice treated with OVA had both thickening of the airway wall and deposition of pink-stained elastic fibers, and the administration of anti-IGF-I antibody decreased the amounts of elastic fibers beneath the epithelial cells (Fig. 6c vs. b). When the AWT index was calculated, anti-IGF-I treatment significantly decreased the AWT index (Fig. 7a). Moreover, we measured the hydroxyproline content of the lung as a parameter for tissue fibrosis by the previously described method [5] to assess airway remodeling involving subepithelial fibrosis (Fig. 7b). As in the case

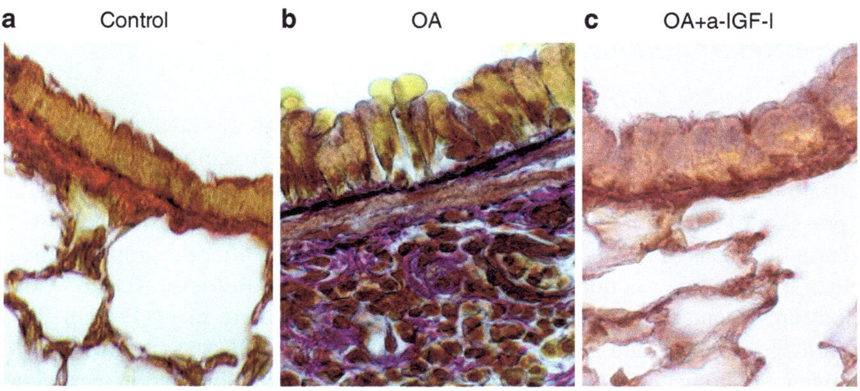

Fig. 6 Effect of IGF-I neutralizing antibody on the histological characteristics of lung tissue. Sections of lung were stained with elastica van Gieson (EVG). (**a**) Control untreated mouse; (**b**) OVA inhalation and sham IgG-treated mouse; (**c**) OVA inhalation and anti-IGF-I treated mouse. Original magnification: ×400

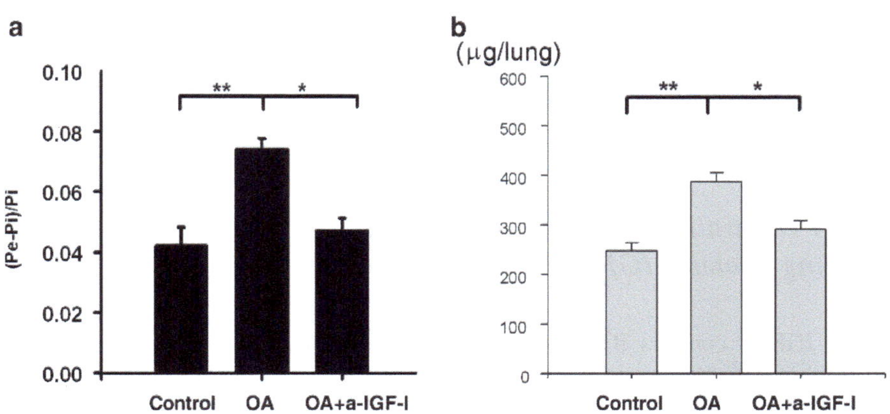

Fig. 7 Analysis of airway wall thickness (**a**) and hydroxyproline content (**b**) in the lung. (**a**) The sample stained with elastica van Gieson (EVG) was analyzed using an image analyzer. The airway wall thickening index was calculated as the external perimeter minus internal perimeter divided by the internal perimeter of bronchioles. Data are means ± SEM of six bronchioles from at least three different sites in eight mice. $^{*}P<0.05$, $^{**}P<0.01$ (**b**) Total lung was freeze-dried and measured for weight. The hydroxyproline content was measured as described in Materials and Methods. Control, mice with intranasal administration of saline only; OVA, mice treated with OVA + sham IgG; OVA + aIGF-I, mice treated with both OVA and anti-IGF-I. Data are means ± SEM of six mice. $^{*}P<0.05$, $^{**}P<0.01$

of the AWT index, the increase of hydroxyproline content of the lung in OVA-treated mice was inhibited by IGF-I neutralization. Importantly, treatment with nonspecific IgG instead of anti-IGF-I did not change either the AWT index or hydroxyproline content of the lung, confirming that neutralization of IGF-I is involved in the inhibitory effects of anti-IGF-I antibody.

Expression of ICAM-1 Protein as well as mRNA is Reduced by IGF-I Neutralization

Recruitment of inflammatory cells at the site of the airway was attenuated by IGF-I neutralization in addition to reduction in deposition of extracellular matrix (ECM) beneath the basement membrane. Inasmuch as IGF-I has been reported to regulate expression of adhesion molecules [14,15], we explored the expression of ICAM-I protein by means of immunohistochemistry [11] . Briefly, after deparaffination and rehydration, tissue sections were treated with Target Retrieval (Dako, Corp., Glodtrup, Denmark) at 95°C, blocked at room temperature using Protein Block Serum-Free (Dako), and incubated with either anti-ICAM-1 or control rabbit IgG. Antigen–antibody complexes were detected using a streptavidin–biotin–peroxidase technique (Immunotech, Cedex, France), and visualized colorimetrically after conversion of the 3-Amino-9-ethylcarbazole (AEC) peroxidase substrate. The expression of ICAM-1 protein was observed in the endothelium and epithelium after OVA inhalation, and was reduced in the group treated with anti-IGF-I antibody. We quantified ICAM-1 mRNA expression in the lung. Results are shown as ratios of quantities of cytokine to b-actin mRNA. Primers were synthesized by Nihon Gene Research Lab., Inc. (Sendai, Japan), and the amplified products were also electrophoresed on 2% agarose gels. We found that mRNA expression of ICAM-1 was significantly reduced by neutralization of IGF-I (Fig. 8).

IGF-I Neutralization Decreased mRNA Expression of IGF Binding Protein (IGFBP)

Since IGFBP controls IGF-I activity and, conversely, IGF-I influences IGFBP expression [16–18], we examined mRNA expression of IGFBP-3. Lungs of mice were frozen in liquid nitrogen immediately after excision and were used for RNA extraction. Each lung tissue was moved quickly into 1 ml ISOGEN (Nippon Gene Co., Ltd., Tokyo, Japan). Lung tissue was homogenized and total RNA was extracted, using a modified acid guanidium–phenol–chloroform method, and cDNA was synthesized and amplified using a GeneAmp PCR system 9700 (Applied Biosystems, Foster City, CA). The mRNA levels of IGFBP-3 were quantified by real-time polymerase chain reaction (PCR) using the Light Cycler-Fast Start DNA Master SYBR Green I kit (Roche Diagnostics, Mannheim, Germany) for amplification

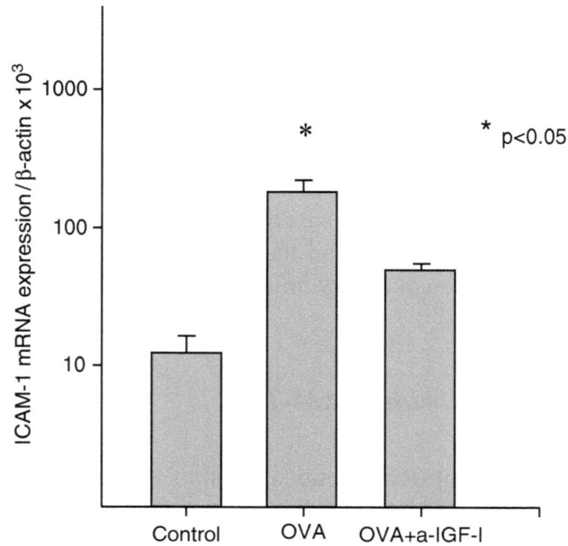

Fig. 8 Analysis of ICAM-1 expression ICAM-1 mRNA expression quantified using real-time PCR. Results are shown as ratios of quantities of cytokine to β-actin mRNA. Data show mean ± SEM of four lungs. $*P<0.05$

of cDNA. An increase of IGFBP-3 mRNA expression following OVA inhalation was observed and the increase was significantly suppressed by neutralization of IGF-I with the antibody [11].

Discussion

We have shown that the administration of anti-IGF-I to our murine model of asthma resulted in suppression of airway hyperresponsiveness to Ach, airway inflammation, and airway wall thickening, which is a part of the process called remodeling. These anti-inflammatory effects were partly attributed to suppression of expression of adhesion molecules [11].

IGF-I and Airway Remodeling

Neutralization of IGF-I inhibited subepithelial fibrosis, which is a part of airway remodeling, making asthma intractable [2,19,20]. Subepithelial fibrosis is brought about by deposition of collagen and laminin, which are secreted by myofibroblasts and fibroblasts at the layer beneath the basement membrane so-called lamina reticularis [21,22]. We have previously reported that subepithelial fibrosis could directly induce airway hyperresponsiveness [5], which is consistent with previous reports [23–25]. Consequently, the attenuation of airway responsiveness to ACh by IGF-I neutralization could be ascribed to diminution of subepithelial fibrosis. On the same line, treatment with anti-TGF-β antibody also suppressed airway remodeling, but what is different from anti-IGF-I is that anti-TGF-β did not affect airway inflammation [26]. From these data, we could speculate that anti-IGF-I suppresses airway remodeling by direct effect on the process of airway remodeling and by indirect effect via inhibition of airway inflammation.

Association of IGF-I with ICAM-1

The mechanism of how anti-IGF-I antibody inhibits airway inflammation could be downregulation of Th2 cytokines and chemokines, or adhesion molecules involved in recruitment of inflammatory cells, and induction of apoptosis in inflammatory cells. Lymphocytes, monocytes, neutrophils, endothelial cells, and smooth muscle cells express IGF-1 receptors [8]. IGF-I has various functions on immune competent cells. We have found that anti-IGF-I treatment did not change the level of IL-5 (Fig. 4) primarily derived from Th2 cells, suggesting that it is unlikely that anti-IGF-I inhibited inflammation via suppressive effect on production of Th2 cytokines. Since we observed a decease in ICAM-1 expression after neutralization of IGF-I, inhibition of inflammatory response by treatment with anti-IGF-I antibody is probably through suppression of adhesion molecules. This hypothesis is supported by the fact that IGF-I is associated with ICAM-1 gene expression [17,18], and that administration of IGF-I directly increases ICAM-1 expression on endothelial cells in a dose-dependent manner [17]. Importantly, the neutralization of ICAM-1 inhibited eosinophil migration to the airway in a monkey model for asthma [27]. Consequently, the anti-inflammatory effects by IGF-I neutralization could be at least in part due to the attenuation of ICAM-1 expression. Moreover, since IGF-I prevents apoptosis, and inhibition of IGF-I has been reported to induce apoptosis in inflammatory cells [10,28], we can predict that anti-IGF-I antibody resulted in induction of apoptosis in the cells involved in airway inflammation in our murine asthma model. This possibility is now under investigation.

IGF-I and IGFBP-3

We also considered a possibility that modulation of IGFBP-3 with anti-IGF-I antibody is involved in decrement of subepithelial fibrosis, since a deposition of interstitial matrix in idiopathic pulmonary fibrosis is accompanied by a spontaneous increase of both IGF-I and IGFBP-3 synthesis [29–32]. When we studied IGFBP-3 mRNA expression in the lung tissue, we found that IGFBP-3 mRNA increased in mice that inhaled OVA and decreased after IGF-I neutralization [11], suggesting that anti-IGF-I treatment could inhibit deposition of the ECM augmented by IGF-I through downregulation of IGFBP-3 biosynthesis.

Modulation of IGF-I Axis

Our data support the possibility that modulation of the IGF-I axis, i.e. consisting of IGF-I, IGF-I receptor (IGF-IR) and IGF-I binding protein (IGFBP), modifies allergic inflammation and remodeling in asthma [33,34]. The strategy to modulate the IGF-I axis is not only the use of anti-IGF-I neutralizing antibody but also neutralization of IGF-IR and IGFBP, which has been successful in the research for cancer [35,36] and neurogenic diseases [37]. In addition, modulation of intracellular signal transduction for IGF-I has been reported to suppress the action of IGF-I [38,39].

Conclusions

In conclusion, IGF-I, which is a progression factor for fibroblasts, could be involved in airway remodeling and inflammation as well as airway hyperresponsiveness in asthma. To inhibit function of IGF-I by some means such as administration of a neutralizing antibody could be a new strategy to treat asthma.

References

1. Holgate, S. T., (2002) Airway inflammation and remodeling in asthma: current concepts. Biotechnol 22, 179–89
2. Busse, W. W. and Rosenwasser, L. J., Mechanisms of asthma.(2003) J Allergy Clin Immunol 111, S799–804
3. Bitterman, P. B., Wewers, M. D., Rennard, S. I., Adelberg, S. and Crystal, R. G. (1986) Modulation of alveolar macrophage-driven fibroblast proliferation by alternative macrophage mediators. J Clin Invest 77, 700–8
4. Rennard, S. I., Bitterman, P. B., Ozaki, T., Rom, W. N. and Crystal, R. G. (1988) Colchicine suppresses the release of fibroblast growth factors from alveolar macrophages in vitro. The basis of a possible therapeutic approach ot the fibrotic disorders. Am Rev Respir Dis 137, 181–5
5. Yamashita, N., Sekine, K., Miyasaka, T., Kawashima, R., Nakajima, Y., Nakano, J., Yamamoto, T., Horiuchi, T., Hirai, K. and Ohta, K (2001) Platelet-derived growth factor is involved in the augmentation of airway responsiveness through remodeling of airways in diesel exhaust particulate-treated mice. J Allergy Clin Immunol 107, 135–42
6. Zhang, S., Smartt, H., Holgate, S. T. and Roche, W. R. (1999) Growth factors secreted by bronchial epithelial cells control myofibroblast proliferation: an in vitro co-culture model of airway remodeling in asthma. Lab Invest 79, 395–405
7. Hoshino, M., Nakamura, Y., Sim, J. J., Yamashiro, Y., Uchida, K., Hosaka, K. and Isogai, S. (1998) Inhaled corticosteroid reduced lamina reticularis of the basement membrane by modulation

of insulin-like growth factor (IGF)-I expression in bronchial asthma. Clin Exp Allergy 28, 568–77
8. LeRoith, D., Clemmons, D., Nissley, P. and Rechler, M. M. (1992) NIH conference. Insulin-like growth factors in health and disease. Ann Intern Med 116, 854–62
9. Galvan, V., Logvinova, A., Sperandio, S., Ichijo, H. and Bredesen, D. E. (2003) Type 1 insulin-like growth factor receptor (IGF-IR) signaling inhibits apoptosis signal-regulating kinase 1 (ASK1). ,J Biol Chem 278, 13325–32
10. Butt, A. J., Firth, S. M. and Baxter, R. C. (1999) The IGF axis and programmed cell death. Immunol Cell Biol 77, 256–62
11. Yamashita N, Tashimo H, Ishida H, Matsuo Y, Arai H, Nagase H, Adachi T, Ohta K. (2005) Role of insulin-like growth factor-I in allergen-induced airway inflammation and remodeling. Cell Immunol 235, 85–9
12. Yamashita, N., Tashimo, H., Ishida, H., Kaneko, F., Nakano, J., Kato, H., Hirai, K., Horiuchi, T. and Ohta, K. (2002) Attenuation of airway hyperresponsiveness in a murine asthma model by neutralization of granulocyte-macrophage colony-stimulating factor (GM-CSF). Cell Immunol 219, 92–7
13. Su JL, Stimpson S, Edwards C, Arnold V, Burgess S, Lin P (1997) Neutralizating IGF-1 monoclonal antibody with cross-species reactivity. Hybridoma 16:513–518
14. Balaram, S. K., Agrawal, D. K., Allen, R. T., Kuszynski, C. A. and Edwards, J. D. (1997) Cell adhesion molecules and insulin-like growth factor-1 in vascular disease. J Vasc Surg 25, 866–76
15. Lovett-Racke, A. E., Bittner, P., Cross, A. H., Carlino, J. A. and Racke, M. K. (1998) Regulation of experimental autoimmune encephalomyelitis with insulin-like growth factor (IGF-1) and IGF-1/IGF-binding protein-3 complex (IGF-1/IGFBP3). J Clin Invest 101, 1797–804
16. Sivaprasad, U., Fleming, J., Verma, P. S., Hogan, K. A., Desury, G. and Cohick, W. S. (2004) Stimulation of insulin-like growth factor (IGF) binding protein-3 synthesis by IGF-I and transforming growth factor-alpha is mediated by both phosphatidylinositol-3 kinase and mitogen-activated protein kinase pathways in mammary epithelial cells. Endocrinology 145, 4213–21
17. Pilewski, J. M., Liu, L., Henry, A. C., Knauer, A. V. and Feghali-Bostwick, C. A. (2005) Insulin-like growth factor binding proteins 3 and 5 are overexpressed in idiopathic pulmonary fibrosis and contribute to extracellular matrix deposition. Am J Pathol 166, 399–407
18. Fleming, J. M., Leibowitz, B. J., Kerr, D. E. and Cohick, W. S. (2005) IGF-I differentially regulates IGF-binding protein expression in primary mammary fibroblasts and epithelial cells. J Endocrinol 186, 165–78
19. Vignola, A. M., Gagliardo, R., Siena, A., Chiappara, G., Bonsignore, M. R. (2001) Bousquet, J. and Bonsignore, G., Airway remodeling in the pathogenesis of asthma. Curr Allergy Asthma Rep 1, 108–15
20. Busse, W., Elias, J., Sheppard, D. and Banks-Schlegel, S. (1999) Airway remodeling and repair. Am J Respir Crit Care Med 160, 1035–42
21. Laitinen, A., Altraja, A., Kampe, M., Linden, M., Virtanen, I. and Laitinen, L. A. (1997) Tenascin is increased in airway basement membrane of asthmatics and decreased by an inhaled steroid. Am J Respir Crit Care Med 156, 951–8
22. Altraja, A., Laitinen, A., Virtanen, I., Kampe, M., Simonsson, B. G., Karlsson, S. E., Hakansson, L., Venge, P., Sillastu, H. and Laitinen, L. A. (1996) Expression of laminins in the airways in various types of asthmatic patients: a morphometric study. Am J Respir Cell Mol Biol 15, 482–8
23. Wiggs, B. R., Bosken, C., Pare, P. D., James, A. and Hogg, J. C. (1992) A model of airway narrowing in asthma and in chronic obstructive pulmonary disease. Am Rev Respir Dis 145, 1251–8
24. Chetta, A., Foresi, A., Del Donno, M., Consigli, G. F., Bertorelli, G., Pesci, A., Barbee, R. A. and Olivieri, D. (1996) Bronchial responsiveness to distilled water and methacholine and its relationship to inflammation and remodeling of the airways in asthma. Am J Respir Crit Care Med 153, 910–7

25. Boulet, L. P., Laviolette, M., Turcotte, H., Cartier, A., Dugas, M., Malo, J. L. and Boutet, M. (1997) Bronchial subepithelial fibrosis correlates with airway responsiveness to methacholine. Chest 112, 45–52
26. McMillan, S. J., Xanthou, G. and Lloyd, C. M. (2005) Manipulation of allergen-induced airway remodeling by treatment with anti-TGF-beta antibody: effect on the Smad signaling pathway. J Immunol 174, 5774–80
27. Wegner, C. D., Gundel, R. H., Reilly, P., Haynes, N., Letts, L. G. and Rothlein, R. (1990) Intercellular adhesion molecule-1 (ICAM-1) in the pathogenesis of asthma. Science 247, 456–9
28. Jones, J. I. and Clemmons, D. R. (1995) Insulin-like growth factors and their binding proteins: biological actions. Endocr Rev 16, 3–34
29. Krein, P. M. and Winston, B. W. (2002) Roles for insulin-like growth factor I and transforming growth factor-beta in fibrotic lung disease. Chest 122, 289S–93S
30. Aston, C., Jagirdar, J., Lee, T. C., Hur, T., Hintz, R. L. and Rom, W. N. (1995) Enhanced insulin-like growth factor molecules in idiopathic pulmonary fibrosis. Am J Respir Crit Care Med 151, 1597–603
31. Homma, S., Nagaoka, I., Abe, H., Takahashi, K., Seyama, K., Nukiwa, T. and Kira, S. (1995) Localization of platelet-derived growth factor and insulin-like growth factor I in the fibrotic lung. Am J Respir Crit Care Med 152, 2084–9
32. Pala, L., Giannini, S., Rosi, E., Cresci, B., Scano, G., Mohan, S., Duranti, R. and Rotella, C. M. (2001) Direct measurement of IGF-I and IGFBP-3 in bronchoalveolar lavage fluid from idiopathic pulmonary fibrosis. J Endocrinol Invest 24, 856–64
33. Noveral, J. P., Bhala, A., Hintz, R. L., Grunstein, M. M. and Cohen, P. (1994) Insulin-like growth factor axis in airway smooth muscle cells. Am J Physiol 267, L761–5
34. Cohen, P., Rajah, R., Rosenbloom, J. and Herrick, D. J. (2000) IGFBP-3 mediates TGF-beta1-induced cell growth in human airway smooth muscle cells. Am J Physiol Lung Cell Mol Physiol 278, L545–51
35. Hailey, J., Maxwell, E., Koukouras, K., Bishop, W. R., Pachter, J. A. and Wang, Y. (2002) Neutralizing anti-insulin-like growth factor receptor 1 antibodies inhibit receptor function and induce receptor degradation in tumor cells. Mol Cancer Ther 1, 1349–53
36. Shen, W. H., Zhou, J. H., Broussard, S. R., Freund, G. G., Dantzer, R. and Kelley, K. W. (2002) Proinflammatory cytokines block growth of breast cancer cells by impairing signals from a growth factor receptor. Cancer Res 62, 4746–56
37. Streppel, M., Azzolin, N., Dohm, S., Guntinas-Lichius, O., Haas, C., Grothe, C., Wevers, A., Neiss, W. F. and Angelov, D. N. (2002) Focal application of neutralizing antibodies to soluble neurotrophic factors reduces collateral axonal branching after peripheral nerve lesion. Eur J Neurosci 15, 1327–42
38. Kiley, S. C., Thornhill, B. A., Tang, S. S., Ingelfinger, J. R. and Chevalier, R. L. (2003) Growth factor-mediated phosphorylation of proapoptotic BAD reduces tubule cell death in vitro and in vivo. Kidney Int 63, 33–42
39. Tu W, Cheung PT, Lau YL. (2000) Insulin-like growth factor 1 promotes cord blood T cell maturation and inhibits its spontaneous and phytohemagglutinin-induced apoptosis through different mechanisms. J Immunol 165:1331–1336
40. Ohta K, Yamashita N, Tajima M, Miyasaka T, Nakano J, Nakajima M, Ishii A, Horiuchi T, Mano K, Miyamoto T. (1999) Diesel exhaust particulates induces airway hyperresponsiveness in a murine model: essential role of GM-CSF. J Allergy Clin Immunol 104:1024–1230

Exosomes: Naturally Occurring Minimal Antigen-Presenting Units

Elodie Segura and Clotilde Théry

Introduction

Exosomes were first described as involved in the shedding of transferrin receptors during reticulocyte maturation [1]. Exosomes are small membrane vesicles (diameter 50–100 nm) that form within late endocytic compartments by invagination of the limiting membrane into the lumen. Internal vesicles accumulate in those compartments, named multi-vesicular bodies (MVBs), and are released in the extracellular medium by fusion of the limiting membrane with the plasma membrane (Fig. 1). As a consequence of this formation mechanism, membrane orientation of exosomes is similar to that of the whole cell: extracellular domains of transmembrane molecules are exposed at the surface of exosomes and a small amount of cytosol from the secreting cell is trapped into the lumen (Fig. 1).

Exosomes have been purified from in vitro cultures of various cell types (see supplemental table in [2] for references): reticulocytes, mast cells, dendritic cells (DCs), platelets, B lymphocytes, T lymphocytes, tumour cells, intestinal epithelial cells (IEC), Schwann cells, and more recently microglia [3], neurons [4] and fibroblasts [5]. But exosomes have also been purified from several body fluids, suggesting that exosome secretion is a naturally occurring phenomenon: in human serum [6], broncho-alveolar fluid [7], urine [8], tumoural effusions [9,10], epididymal fluid [11].

Much attention has been drawn to exosomes since the discovery that exosomes from B cells and DCs could activate T cells and induce immune responses [12,13]. In this review[1], where we summarise the recent data on exosomes as "minimal antigen-presenting units", we will focus on exosomes secreted by antigen-presenting cells (APC) (cells that can express major histocompatibility complex (MHC) class II molecules), namely exosomes from DCs and B cells (where expression of

---

E. Segura and C. Théry (✉)
Institut Curie, Centre de Recherche, 26 rue d'Ulm, 75245 Paris Cedex 05, France
INSERM U932, 26 rue d'Ulm, 75245 Paris Cedex 05, France
e-mail: clotilde.thery@curie.fr

[1] This review was written in June 2007 and updated in December 2007. Please, note that a vast amount of new data has been published in 2008 and 2009, but will not be discussed here. For a more recent update, see Thery et al. [61].

R. Pawankar et al. (eds.), *Allergy Frontiers: Future Perspectives*,
DOI 10.1007/978-4-431-99365-0_20, © Springer 2010

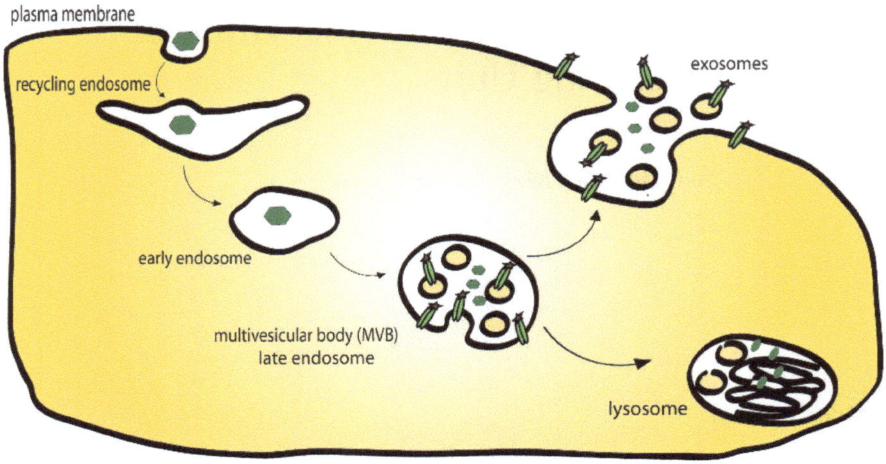

Fig. 1 *Exosome formation*. Exosomes form in late endocytic compartments by invagination of the limiting membrane of MVBs. Internal vesicles are secreted upon fusion of the limiting membrane of MVBs with the plasma membrane, and then called "exosomes." Note that the membrane orientation of exosomes is similar to that of the whole cell. Extracellular domains of transmembrane molecules point towards the lumen of MVBs, but are exposed at the surface of exosomes as a consequence of their formation by invagination of the limiting membrane. During this process, cytosol from the secreting cell is trapped into the lumen of exosomes

MHC class II is constitutive), as well as mastocytes and IEC (where MHC class II expression can be induced by cytokines).

Exosome Characterization

Principles of Exosome Isolation

Exosomes can be isolated from the supernatant of cells cultured in vitro or from physiological fluids by differential ultracentrifugation (for detailed protocols, see [14]). As culture medium can contain exosomes and vesicles from serum, it is necessary to culture cells either in a serum-free medium, or in a culture medium that has been pre-depleted from contaminating vesicles. A standard purification procedure includes centrifugations at increasing speed to eliminate large cell debris and aggregates, followed by ultracentrifugation at 100,000*g* to pellet exosomes, which can then be stored at −80°C. To increase purity, a further purification step can be performed by ultracentrifugation on a sucrose gradient; contaminating non-membranous material sediments at the bottom of the gradient, while exosomes float at their characteristic density. However, these techniques do not allow separation of exosomes from viruses that could be present in the medium, and have the same density as exosomes. A good manufacturing procedure (GMP) for purification of clinical grade exosomes has also been described [15] and involves diafiltration of the medium containing exosomes (500 kDa membrane) and ultracentrifugation on a 30% sucrose/deuterium oxide (D_2O) density cushion. Sucrose can then be removed from exosome preparations by diafiltration. Finally, exosomes can be isolated for phenotypic characterization from cell-free supernatants by using latex or magnetic beads that have been coated with antibodies against abundant exosome surface molecules, such as MHC class II molecules [15,16].

Biophysical Properties of Exosomes

Since they correspond to the internal vesicles of MVBs, exosomes have specific structural and morphological properties: they are limited by a bilipidic layer and characterised by their small diameter (50–100 nm) and a cup-shaped morphology in electron microscopy [12]. Floatation on a sucrose gradient has defined their density as lying between 1.13 and 1.19 g/mL, depending on the producing cell type [12,17].

To qualify as "exosomes", vesicles isolated from fluids or supernatants must meet these criteria, and one should be careful not to assimilate other types of vesicles with exosomes. For instance, "exosome-like" vesicles secreted by endothelial cells, and bearing type I tumour necrosis factor receptor, are smaller (20–50 nm), lighter (1.1 g/mL on sucrose gradient) and are pelleted at higher speed ultracentrifugation than exosomes [18]. It is not clear whether "tolerosomes" purified from serum of antigen-fed mice are exosomes or not, given their small size (40 nm) and the lack of extensive characterization [19]. Finally, exosomes are different from larger membrane vesicles (150–300 nm in diameter) shed from the plasma membrane rather than from internal endocytic compartments, such as "microvesicles" shed by activated platelets [20], or "ectosomes" shed by neutrophils [21]. The term "microvesicle", however, has been used by some authors to designate vesicles of 50–100 nm in diameter, bearing late endosome markers and originating from the MVBs of T cells [22] of several tumour cell lines [23], or purified from the plasma of patients with melanoma [24]: these microvesicles are probably exosomes, although their density on sucrose gradients was not reported. Conversely, vesicles enriched in late endosome markers and of less than 100 nm diameter (i.e. similar to exosomes), but budding at the plasma membrane of T-cell lines, have also been called "exosomes" [25], although this use is not accepted by other authors. A unified terminology on secreted vesicles is thus not yet achieved in the literature.

Exosome Composition

The few studies that have investigated the lipid composition of exosomes indicate that it is quite similar to the composition of parental cell plasma membrane [26,27]; however, exosome membrane is enriched in sphingomyelin [26,27], and phosphatidyl serine (PS) is exposed at the surface of DC-derived exosomes [28]. Although they expose PS at their surface, probably due to the absence of lipid translocase like apoptotic and dead cells, exosomes are clearly distinct from membrane vesicles released by dying cells in terms of protein composition and density [29].

Exosomes are also enriched in molecules associated with lipid rafts (specialised membrane micro-domains that are enriched in cholesterol and sphingolipids) such as flotillin-1, stomatin, prohibitin [2,30,31]. Enrichment in raft components confers raft-like properties to exosomes: for instance, partial resistance to detergents [31] and enrichment in glycosylphosphatidyinositol (GPI) anchored proteins, such as CD55 and CD59 [32], which could protect B-lymphocyte-derived exosomes from destruction by complement.

The protein composition of exosomes has been analysed by various techniques: western blot, fluorescence-activated cell sorting (FACS) analysis on exosome-coated beads or proteomic analysis (summarised in [2]). These studies have shown that exosomes contain a defined set of cellular proteins: some are common to exosomes from any cell type and others are cell-specific (Fig. 2). Exosomes bear transmembrane molecules such as MHC class I molecules, integrins (CD11a, CD11b, CD18), tetraspan molecules (CD9, CD63, CD81, CD82), GPI-anchored molecules (CD55, CD59), surface peptidases (CD13, CD26) and, in their lumen, molecules associated with the internal side of membranes: clathrin, annexins, GTPases of the Rab family proteins. Exosomes also contain cytosolic proteins:

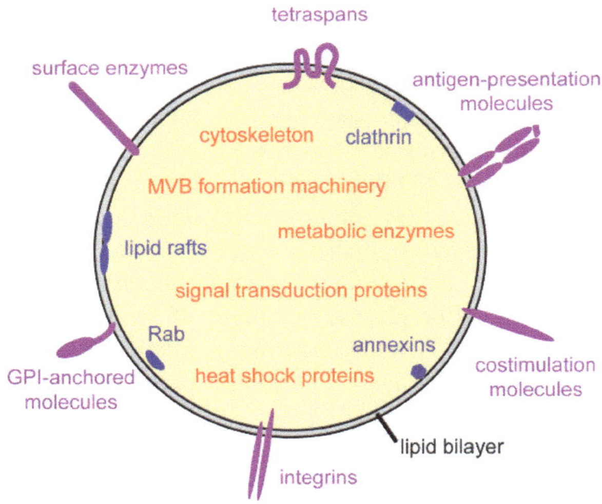

Fig. 2 Schematic representation of an exosome from an antigen-presenting cell. Exosomes are limited by a lipid bilayer (*black/grey*) and contain cytosol from the producing cell (*yellow*), and various components are represented here in their physical location in exosomes: exposed at the outer face of the limiting membrane (*purple*), associated to the inner (cytosolic) face of the membrane (*blue*) or in the lumen (*red*)

cytoskeleton proteins (myosin, tubulin, actin and actin-binding molecules), signal transduction molecules (protein kinases, heterodimeric G proteins, 14-3-3 proteins), chaperone molecules (heat shock protein (hsp) molecules, cyclophilin A) and metabolic enzymes (GAPDH, M2 pyruvate kinase).

An important feature of exosomes secreted by APCs is that they also bear molecules involved in antigen presentation (MHC class I and II molecules, CD1) and T-cell stimulation (CD86, ICAM-1). Exosome protein composition reflects that of the secreting cells and therefore exosomes display molecules that are specific of cell types: B-cell receptor on B-cell-derived exosomes, CD11c (a specific marker of DCs) on DC-derived exosomes, A33 antigen (a molecule essentially restricted to intestinal epithelium) in IEC-derived exosomes. Exosome molecular composition may also vary according to the activation state of the secreting cells. Exosomes secreted by IEC exposed to interferon-γ (IFN-γ) display more MHC class II molecules than those from non-treated IEC [33]. Exosomes from B cells exposed to heat stress are enriched in hsp molecules [34]. Exosomes from DCs exposed to a maturation stimulus are enriched in molecules that are up-regulated during DC maturation: MHC class II molecules, CD86, ICAM-1 [2].

Consistent with the endocytic origin of exosomes, proteins found in exosomes are exclusively from the plasma membrane, cytosol or endocytic compartments. Moreover, proteins involved in the formation of MVBs are found in exosomes (tsg101, Alix). The absence on exosomes of abundant membrane proteins, such as Fc receptors for DCs, and presence in exosomes of molecules that are not expressed at the cell surface (LAMP-2) [29] further demonstrate that exosomes are not mere plasma membrane fragments.

Exosomes and Antigen Presentation

Activation of CD4 T Cells

In APCs, exosomes form in compartments where MHC class II molecules accumulate and, therefore, APC-derived exosomes bear abundant MHC class II molecules. In a pioneer study, Raposo et al. showed that exosomes from Epstein–Barr virus (EBV) transformed B cells incubated with an antigen (hsp65) bear MHC class II-peptide complexes and can stimulate in vitro hsp65-specific CD4 T-cell clones [12]. Exosomes secreted by a mast cell line engineered to bear a single MHC–peptide complex can induce in vitro activation of a CD4 T-cell line expressing the cognate T-cell receptor (TCR) [35]. Exosomes derived from male DCs or female DCs pulsed with MHC class II-restricted male antigen H-Y can activate H-Y-specific naive CD4 T cells, both in vitro (when incubated with recipient DCs) and in vivo, showing that DC-derived exosomes can display antigen from endogenous and exogenous origin [36]. When incubated with MHC class II-deficient recipient DCs (which cannot activate T cells in the presence of the specific peptide), exosomes secreted by H-Y-pulsed DCs could induce CD4 T-cell proliferation, showing that exosomes bear functional pre-formed MHC class II-peptide complexes that can be directly used by recipient cells to activate antigen-specific CD4 T cells [36].

Proteins present in exosomes, either constitutively or after loading of exosome-secreting cells with a soluble protein, could also represent a source of exogenous antigen for DCs. For instance, exosomes secreted by DCs of H-2^d haplotype are degraded into endocytic compartments of recipient DCs of H-2^b haplotype, followed by presentation on endogenous MHC class II molecules of peptides derived from exosome-born MHC class II molecules [28]. Exosomes secreted by mast cells incubated with ovalbumin (OVA) can be up-taken and processed by DCs, which generate MHC class II–OVA peptide complexes able to activate OVA-specific T cells [37].

Finally, exosomes secreted by MHC class II-expressing IEC pulsed with a MHC II-binding human serum albumin (HSA) peptide are captured in vitro by recipient DCs, which use them to generate complexes between the HSA peptide and their own MHC class II molecules [38]. In this setting, MHC class II–peptide complexes on IEC-derived exosomes are not used as such by DCs to activate T cells, but they allow transfer of peptide to endogenous MHC class II molecules. In this work, however, free peptide, i.e. not bound to MHC, could also be present in the exosome preparation.

Activation of CD8 T Cells

Exosomes also bear MHC class I molecules that can be used for CD8 T-cell activation. The first evidence for exosome-induced CD8 T-cell activation came from the finding that exosomes derived from tumour peptides-pulsed DCs can trigger rejection of established tumours in a mouse model [13]. This rejection was no longer observed in nude mice (i.e. lacking T cells), which indicated that this response was T-cell-dependant. In vitro, DC-derived exosomes bearing MHC class I molecule–peptide complexes could induce activation of CD8 cytotoxic T lymphocytes (CTL) clones, even when incubated with MHC class I-deficient DCs, showing that exosomes bear functional MHC class I–peptide complexes [39,40]. In vivo, DC-derived MHC class I–peptide bearing exosomes could only induce CD8 T-cell activation when injected with adjuvants, such as mature DCs, or toll-like receptor ligands (CpG oligodeoxynucleotides, or pIC) [41].

Since all cell types express MHC class I molecules, exosomes from non-APCs also bear MHC class I molecules that could induce CD8 T-cell activation. It has been shown that exosomes from murine mammary adenocarcinoma could induce in vitro and in vivo T-cell activation leading to protection against tumour challenge [42]. In the same study, the authors showed that exosomes from melanoma cells could induce IFN-γ production by specific CTL clones in vitro, but only when incubated with DCs. Therefore tumour-derived exosomes cannot directly activate T cell but need to be re-captured by APCs. However tumour-derived exosomes of irrelevant MHC class I haplotype could efficiently induce CTL activation, suggesting that tumour-derived exosomes mainly transfer to DCs tumour antigens that are processed and presented on endogenous MHC molecules [42].

Direct or Indirect T-Cell Activation?

Exosomes from APCs display MHC molecule–peptide complexes and co-stimulatory molecules, and represent therefore potential cell-free T-cell-stimulating units. Whether exosomes can directly stimulate T cells remains controversial. In vitro, H-Y-pulsed DC-derived exosomes incubated with antigen-specific naive CD4 T cells could only induce T-cell proliferation when DCs, but not B cells or macrophages, were added in the culture [36]. Only mature DC-derived exosomes could also be presented by B cells [2]. In another study, DC-derived exosomes could only induce IFN-γ production by CD8 CTL clones when incubated with DCs, but not fibroblasts or macrophages [40]. These results suggest that T-cell activation through exosome-born MHC–peptide complexes requires re-capture by APCs for presentation to T cells.

By contrast, B-cell-derived exosomes bearing MHC class II–peptide complexes could directly activate CD4 T-cell clones when incubated together [12]. Mast cell-derived exosomes bearing MHC class II–peptide complexes could also directly activate specific CD4 T cells when coated on latex beads, but T-cell activation was much stronger when these exosomes were incubated with recipient DCs [35]. Similarly, exosomes from Drosophila APCs transfected with murine MHC class I and co-stimulatory molecules could directly stimulate IFN-γ production by specific CD8 T cells [43], but T-cell stimulation was more efficient when exosomes were incubated with DCs. Finally, immobilised antigen-bearing exosomes from DCs could stimulate IFN-γ production by autologous CD8 T cells from human peripheral blood [44].

Under some circumstances, exosomes can thus directly stimulate T cells, but re-capture by DCs seems to trigger better T-cell stimulation. Exosomes, as "natural" antigen-presenting units, are probably less efficient to activate CD8 T cells than artificially generated vesicles bearing high amounts of MHC and co-stimulatory molecules: for instance "immunosomes" released by cells transfected with viral gag-pol cDNA plus GPI-anchored T-cell-activation proteins [45], or membrane vesicles obtained from sonicated cytokine-treated DCs [46], activate naïve CD8 T cells directly. Results obtained with exosome-coated beads or immobilised exosomes suggest that concentration of exosome-born MHC molecule–peptide complexes at the surface of DCs could be an important factor, lowering the threshold for T-cell activation. The observation that co-stimulatory molecules CD80 and CD86 are not essential on DC-derived exosomes, since exosomes deficient for both molecules were as efficient as wild-type exosomes for naive CD4 T cells activation [2], but important on recipient DCs supports the idea that DCs are also important for delivering co-stimulatory signals to T cells via ligation with co-stimulatory molecules or even cytokines. It is also possible that exosomes could directly activate effector or memory T cells but would need recipient DCs for efficient activation of naïve T cells.

Exosomes can therefore transfer antigenic material to APCs – antigen, transmembrane or contained in their lumen – which requires processing and presentation on endogenous MHC molecules and functional pre-formed MHC–peptide complexes that can directly be used for T-cell stimulation. In particular, DC-derived exosomes allow transfer of information between different DCs and could be involved in amplification of immune responses, transferring MHC–peptide complexes from DCs that have been exposed to an antigen or other DCs that have not been in contact with the same antigen.

Outcome of Exosome-Induced Immune Responses

A number of studies have shown that exosomes can not only induce activation and proliferation of T cells, but can also induce effector T-cell differentiation and subsequent immune responses. DC-derived exosomes bearing MHC class I–tumour peptide complexes can induce the rejection of established tumours [13], although exosomes secreted by immature DCs only allow efficient tumour rejection when co-injected with chemical adjuvants (CpG oligodeoxynucleotides, or pIC) [41], or mature DCs [40]. Injection of exosomes from MHC class II-restricted H-Y antigen-pulsed DCs leads to fast male skin graft rejection by female recipient mice, showing in vivo priming and effector differentiation of activated CD4 T cells [2]. However, this effect could only be seen when mature DC-derived exosomes (which bear high levels of MHC class II and ICAM-1 molecules) were injected. Exosomes secreted by *Toxoplasma gondii* antigen-pulsed DCs can elicit humoral responses to the pathogen, with induction of IgM and IgG, IFN-γ production by splenocytes and strong protection against acute infection with *Toxoplasma gondii* [47]. In vivo injection of exosomes secreted by diphtheria toxin (DT)-pulsed DCs triggers specific humoral responses and induction of type 1 (IgG2b and IgG2a) DT-specific antibodies [48]. Exosomes secreted by IFN-γ exposed OVA-pulsed IEC can also induce OVA-specific humoral immune responses [33].

Exosomes have also been studied in the context of immune tolerance. In a heart allograft model, in which donor blood cells transfusion prior to the graft can induce tolerance, it has been shown that pre-treatment of rats with DC-derived exosomes of the same haplotype as donor animals could induce prolonged or infinite graft survival [49]. In exosome-treated animals, proliferation of donor antigen-specific CD4 T cells was impaired, suggesting a tolerogenic effect of exosomes. When exosomes are injected after transplantation, they can still prolong graft survival but do not induce tolerance [50].

In a rheumatoid arthritis model, in which local adenoviral-mediated gene transfer of IL-10 to a single joint can suppress disease in both treated and untreated contralateral joints, the potential effect of exosomes has been investigated.

Injection of exosomes secreted by IL-10-treated DCs or by DCs transduced with an adenovirus expressing IL-10 could suppress delayed-type hypersensitivity (DTH) to an antigen (keyhole lympet hemocyanine) in injected and contralateral footpads [51]. However, in this study it was not clear whether this suppressive effect is antigen-specific. In the same model, exosomes secreted by Fas-L expressing DCs can suppress DTH in treated and untreated paws [52]. DTH suppression could no longer be observed in Fas-deficient mice, suggesting a role for Fas/Fas-L interaction in this effect, and was antigen-specific.

In vivo, exosomes can thus trigger either priming or tolerance. The factors determining the fate of exosome-induced responses could be administration route, dose of transferred antigen and in vivo micro-environment, but also the activation state of producing cells. Indeed, DCs are found in the organism in different states of activation defined by their surface phenotype: upon maturation, DCs up-regulate MHC class II molecules and co-stimulatory molecules such as CD40 and CD86. DCs are key initiators of in vivo priming of effector cells, but DCs can also induce peripheral tolerance. It seems that exosomes secreted by tolerogenic DCs, either immature DCs [49], IL-10 producing DCs [51] or Fas-L expressing DCs [52], retained this tolerogenic property. By contrast, exosomes from mature DCs are more potent at stimulating in vitro CD4 T cells [2] and CD8 T cells [44], and only mature DC-derived exosomes can induce fast CD4 T-cell-mediated skin graft rejection [2]. Exosomes from mature DCs were also more efficient at inducing in vivo primary antibody responses against DT as compared to immature-DC derived exosomes [48]. These considerations are especially important when designing therapeutic strategies involving exosomes.

Exosomes as Therapeutic Agents

Advantages of Exosomes for Immunotherapy

Pioneer work performed in a murine model [13] prompted the evaluation of using exosomes in anti-cancer immunotherapy assays. Exosomes secreted by DCs incubated with peptides eluted from the surface of tumour cell lines when injected in mice bearing established tumours [13] induced a striking delay of tumour growth and eradication of the tumour in 60% of recipient mice. Prevention of tumour growth was not observed with exosomes bearing control peptides eluted from spleen cells. It also required a functional adaptive immune system in the host mice, thus suggesting that exosomes bearing MHC–tumour peptide complexes induced in vivo the activation of tumour peptide-specific T lymphocytes, which could destroy the tumour.

This observation suggested that exosomes could be used in clinical anti-cancer immunotherapy settings as an alternative to protocols using DCs loaded with various forms of tumour-derived antigens in vaccination strategies. In these protocols, DCs were generated in vitro from the patient's blood-derived monocytes, exposed to a source of tumour antigens and frozen in aliquots. The potential caveats of this setting were that the percentage of live DCs after thawing up was difficult to control and the behaviour of DCs after in vivo injection was also unknown: they could become mature upon encountering inflammatory stimuli at different time points or location after injection, thereby potentially modifying the array of MHC-bound peptides displayed at their surface. They could also die before, during or after injection. In this context, using defined "minimal antigen-presenting units" such as exosomes, which are not susceptible to modifications of their intrinsic antigen-presenting capacities by the environmental conditions, instead of "versatile" DCs, seems a potential improvement in the protocol.

Phase I Trials of Exosomes in Cancer

Two phase I clinical trials have been performed from 2000 to 2003, on patients bearing advanced stages of melanoma [53] or non-small-cell lung carcinoma [54] expressing the MAGE tumour antigen. In both trials, DCs were generated in vitro from monocytes of the patients, and the GMP procedure was used to purify exosomes from the cell supernatant. Before exosome production, DCs were incubated with MHC class II-binding MAGE-derived peptides (and/or other MHC class II-binding peptides such as tetanus toxoid, or CMV, to activate recall helper responses). Exosomes bearing MHC class I-tumour peptides were obtained initially by loading DCs with the MAGE-derived MHC class I-binding peptides, but another procedure, in which purified exosomes were incubated in acidic conditions with MHC class I-binding MAGE-derived peptides, was used for half of the patients. Loading of MHC class I peptides on purified exosomes, rather than on the DCs before exosome production, had been shown to lead to increased amounts of MHC class I–peptide complexes on the exosomes [39]. Exosomes bearing both MHC class II- and MHC class I–peptide complexes specific for the MAGE tumour antigen were injected subcutaneously weekly for 4 weeks in patients. These studies proved the feasibility of producing GMP exosomes from each patient and the non-toxicity of exosomes, the only side effects being mild localised reactions at the site of injection and some fever in a few patients. The clinical outcomes were encouraging but not optimal: in the melanoma trial, three out of six patients vaccinated with the highest dose of exosomes obtained by the most efficient MHC class I loading method presented a temporary stabilisation of the disease, while in the lung carcinoma trial, 3 out of 11 patients saw stabilisation of their disease for 10–12 months.

Potential Improvements of Future Immunotherapy Protocols

The relatively limited clinical effects of exosomes in these first two clinical trials can be at least partly explained by the very advanced stages of the diseases in human patients, as compared to the experimental situation in pre-clinical studies involving mice. Variabilities in the protocol used to load exosomal MHC class I molecules with tumour peptides between the first and the last patients can also contribute to the low level of clinical outcomes observed. Several pre-clinical studies published after the onset of the phase I trials could, however, suggest ways of improving the efficacy of exosome vaccines. In particular, several studies have shown recently that exosomes secreted by mature DCs are more efficient that exosomes from immature DCs at inducing immune responses, and are probably the only ones able to induce T-cell priming (see above) [2,44,48]. Inducing DC maturation before exosome production would most likely improve their immune efficacy, although it remains to be shown whether clinically accepted DC maturation treatments (such as CpG and pIC) also lead to secretion of exosomes with increased T-cell-priming efficiency, as does LPS, the TLR4 ligand used in most studies.

Similarly, the reported observation that immature DC-derived exosomes can only trigger tumour rejection in mice when co-injected with TLR3 or TLR9 ligands [41], suggests that including clinically accepted adjuvants with the exosome vaccines could also be envisaged.

Finally, the induction of CD4+ CD25+ regulatory T cells (Treg) by tumours themselves can potentially reduce the efficiency of immunotherapy protocols. Another pre-clinical study by the group of L. Zitvogel has thus been performed to evaluate the effect of inhibiting regulatory T cells together with the exosome vaccine in mice bearing MART1-expressing B16F10 melanoma [55]. This work shows that blunting Treg activation without affecting effector T cells, by injecting low doses of cyclophosphamide together with exosome and TLR3 ligands, increased significantly the number of MART1-specific CTLs and led to reduced tumour growth in treated mice. Anti-regulatory T-cell treatments are being tested in clinical immunotherapeutic settings, and should also be considered for future exosome-based vaccine trials.

Therapeutic Use of Exosomes and Tolerance

Since exosomes secreted by tumour cells carry tumour antigens, which they can transfer to DCs to allow CD8 T-cell activation [9,42], their use in anti-cancer immunotherapy was also potentially interesting. More recent reports, however, have pointed at tolerogenic mechanisms induced by some tumour-derived exosomes. Exosomes secreted by melanoma and colorectal carcinoma cell lines bear the pro-apoptotic molecule FasL, which induces T-cell death in vitro [23,24] and induce in vitro differentiation of DCs endowed with T-cell-suppressive activity [56]. Exosomes secreted by murine [57] and human [58] breast carcinoma cell lines, as well as mesothelioma cell lines, inhibit natural killer cell functions in vitro, and thus promote tumour growth in vivo [57]. By contrast, we have recently shown that in vivo secretion by tumours of exosomes bearing a model antigen allows induction of efficient anti-tumour immune responses, ultimately leading to delay in tumour growth [59]. Thus, balance between pro-immune and potential inhibitory functions of tumour-derived exosomes may depend on the tumour, and will have to be taken into account for future use of tumour exosomes in anti-cancer immunotherapy.

On the other hand, tolerogenic effects of exosomes could be used in pathologies where dampening of the immune response has to be induced. Such potential applications include induction of donor-specific tolerance favouring graft survival in allo-transplantation [50] or anti-inflammatory effects of exosomes from modified DCs in arthritis [51,52].

Finally, the roles of exosomes in allergies have been very scarcely analysed so far. Exosomes have been described in human broncho-alveolar lavages [7], and very promising results have been recently published: intranasal injection in naïve mice of exosomes purified from the broncho-alveolar fluid of mice tolerized to an allergen reduce IgE responses to this allergen [60]. These observations therefore suggest new leads to follow for people interested in asthma and airways allergies.

Acknowledgements This work was supported by INSERM, Institut Curie, Fondation pour la Recherche Médicale, European Community Grant #512074.

References

1. Johnstone RM, Adam M, Hammond JR, Orr L, Turbide C (1987) Vesicle formation during reticulocyte maturation. Association of plasma membrane activities with released vesicles (exosomes). J Biol Chem 262:9412–9420.
2. Segura E, Nicco C, Lombard B, Veron P, Raposo G, Batteux F, Amigorena S, Thery C (2005) ICAM-1 on exosomes from mature dendritic cells is critical for efficient naive T-cell priming. Blood 106:216–223.
3. Potolicchio I, Carven GJ, Xu X, Stipp C, Riese RJ, Stern LJ, Santambrogio L (2005) Proteomic analysis of microglia-derived exosomes: metabolic role of the aminopeptidase CD13 in neuropeptide catabolism. J Immunol 175:2237–2243.
4. Faure J, Lachenal G, Court M, Hirrlinger J, Chatellard-Causse C, Blot B, Grange J, Schoehn G, Goldberg Y, Boyer V et al. (2006) Exosomes are released by cultured cortical neurones. Mol Cell Neurosci 31:642–648.
5. Zhang HG, Liu C, Su K, Yu S, Zhang L, Zhang S, Wang J, Cao X, Grizzle W, Kimberly RP (2006) A membrane form of TNF-alpha presented by exosomes delays T cell activation-induced cell death. J Immunol 176:7385–7393.
6. Caby MP, Lankar D, Vincendeau-Scherrer C, Raposo G, Bonnerot C (2005) Exosomal-like vesicles are present in human blood plasma. Int Immunol 17:879–887.
7. Admyre C, Grunewald J, Thyberg J, Gripenback S, Tornling G, Eklund A, Scheynius A, Gabrielsson S (2003) Exosomes with major histocompatibility complex class II and co-stimulatory molecules are present in human BAL fluid. Eur Respir J 22:578–583.
8. Pisitkun T, Shen RF, Knepper MA (2004) Identification and proteomic profiling of exosomes in human urine. Proc Natl Acad Sci U S A 101:13368–13373.
9. Andre F, Schartz NE, Movassagh M, Flament C, Pautier P, Morice P, Pomel C, Lhomme C, Escudier B, Le Chevalier T et al. (2002) Malignant effusions and immunogenic tumour-derived exosomes. Lancet 360:295–305.
10. Bard MP, Hegmans JP, Hemmes A, Luider TM, Willemsen R, Severijnen LA, van Meerbeeck JP, Burgers SA, Hoogsteden HC, Lambrecht BN (2004) Proteomic analysis of exosomes isolated from human malignant pleural effusions. Am J Respir Cell Mol Biol 31:114–121.
11. Gatti JL, Metayer S, Belghazi M, Dacheux F, Dacheux JL (2005) Identification, proteomic profiling, and origin of ram epididymal fluid exosome-like vesicles. Biol Reprod 72:1452–1465.

12. Raposo G, Nijman HW, Stoorvogel W, Liejendekker R, Harding CV, Melief CJ, Geuze HJ (1996) B lymphocytes secrete antigen-presenting vesicles. J Exp Med 183:1161–1172.
13. Zitvogel L, Regnault A, Lozier A, Wolfers J, Flament C, Tenza D, Ricciardi-Castagnoli P, Raposo G, Amigorena S (1998) Eradication of established murine tumours using a novel cell-free vaccine: dendritic cell-derived exosomes. Nat Med 4:594–600.
14. Thery C, Clayton A, Amigorena S, Raposo G (2006) Isolation and Characterization of Exosomes from Cell Culture Supernatants and Biological Fluids. In: Curr Protoc Cell Biol. Edited by Wiley J, and s, vol. 1 Part 3, 3.22.01-29.
15. Lamparski HG, Metha-Damani A, Yao JY, Patel S, Hsu DH, Ruegg C, Le Pecq JB (2002) Production and characterization of clinical grade exosomes derived from dendritic cells. J Immunol Methods 270:211–226.
16. Clayton A, Court J, Navabi H, Adams M, Mason MD, Hobot JA, Newman GR, Jasani B (2001) Analysis of antigen presenting cell derived exosomes, based on immuno-magnetic isolation and flow cytometry. J Immunol Methods 247:163–174.
17. Thery C, Regnault A, Garin J, Wolfers J, Zitvogel L, Ricciardi-Castagnoli P, Raposo G, Amigorena S (1999) Molecular characterization of dendritic cell-derived exosomes. Selective accumulation of the heat shock protein hsc73. J Cell Biol 147:599–610.
18. Hawari FI, Rouhani FN, Cui X, Yu ZX, Buckley C, Kaler M, Levine SJ (2004) Release of full-length 55-kDa TNF receptor 1 in exosome-like vesicles: a mechanism for generation of soluble cytokine receptors. Proc Natl Acad Sci U S A 101:1297–1302.
19. Karlsson M, Lundin S, Dahlgren U, Kahu H, Pettersson I, Telemo E (2001) "Tolerosomes" are produced by intestinal epithelial cells. Eur J Immunol 31:2892–2900.
20. Heijnen HF, Schiel AE, Fijnheer R, Geuze HJ, Sixma JJ (1999) Activated platelets release two types of membrane vesicles: microvesicles by surface shedding and exosomes derived from exocytosis of multivesicular bodies and alpha-granules. Blood 94:3791–3799.
21. Hess C, Sadallah S, Hefti A, Landmann R, Schifferli JA (1999) Ectosomes released by human neutrophils are specialized functional units. J Immunol 163:4564–4573.
22. Monleon I, Martinez-Lorenzo MJ, Monteagudo L, Lasierra P, Taules M, Iturralde M, Pineiro A, Larrad L, Alava MA, Naval J et al. (2001) Differential secretion of Fas ligand- or APO2 ligand/TNF-related apoptosis-inducing ligand-carrying microvesicles during activation-induced death of human T cells. J Immunol 167:6736–6744.
23. Andreola G, Rivoltini L, Castelli C, Huber V, Perego P, Deho P, Squarcina P, Accornero P, Lozupone F, Lugini L et al. (2002) Induction of lymphocyte apoptosis by tumour cell secretion of FasL-bearing microvesicles. J Exp Med 195:1303–1316.
24. Huber V, Fais S, Iero M, Lugini L, Canese P, Squarcina P, Zaccheddu A, Colone M, Arancia G, Gentile M et al. (2005) Human colorectal cancer cells induce T-cell death through release of proapoptotic microvesicles: role in immune escape. Gastroenterology 128:1796–1804.
25. Booth AM, Fang Y, Fallon JK, Yang JM, Hildreth JE, Gould SJ (2006) Exosomes and HIV Gag bud from endosome-like domains of the T cell plasma membrane. J Cell Biol 172:923–935.
26. Laulagnier K, Motta C, Hamdi S, Roy S, Fauvelle F, Pageaux JF, Kobayashi T, Salles JP, Perret B, Bonnerot C et al. (2004) Mast cell- and dendritic cell-derived exosomes display a specific lipid composition and an unusual membrane organization. Biochem J 380:161–171.
27. Wubbolts R, Leckie RS, Veenhuizen PT, Schwarzmann G, Mobius W, Hoernschemeyer J, Slot JW, Geuze HJ, Stoorvogel W (2003) Proteomic and biochemical analyses of human B cell-derived exosomes. Potential implications for their function and multivesicular body formation. J Biol Chem 278:10963–10972.
28. Morelli AE, Larregina AT, Shufesky WJ, Sullivan ML, Stolz DB, Papworth GD, Zahorchak AF, Logar AJ, Wang Z, Watkins SC et al. (2004) Endocytosis, intracellular sorting, and processing of exosomes by dendritic cells. Blood 104:3257–3266.
29. Thery C, Boussac M, Veron P, Ricciardi-Castagnoli P, Raposo G, Garin J, Amigorena S (2001) Proteomic analysis of dendritic cell-derived exosomes: a secreted subcellular compartment distinct from apoptotic vesicles. J Immunol 166:7309–7318.
30. Mobius W, van Donselaar E, Ohno-Iwashita Y, Shimada Y, Heijnen HF, Slot JW, Geuze HJ (2003) Recycling compartments and the internal vesicles of multivesicular bodies harbor most of the cholesterol found in the endocytic pathway. Traffic 4:222–231.

31. de Gassart A, Geminard C, Fevrier B, Raposo G, Vidal M (2003) Lipid raft-associated protein sorting in exosomes. Blood 102:4336–4344.
32. Clayton A, Harris CL, Court J, Mason MD, Morgan BP (2003) Antigen-presenting cell exosomes are protected from complement-mediated lysis by expression of CD55 and CD59. Eur J Immunol 33:522–531.
33. Van Niel G, Mallegol J, Bevilacqua C, Candalh C, Brugiere S, Tomaskovic-Crook E, Heath JK, Cerf-Bensussan N, Heyman M (2003) Intestinal epithelial exosomes carry MHC class II/ peptides able to inform the immune system in mice. Gut 52:1690–1697.
34. Clayton A, Turkes A, Navabi H, Mason MD, Tabi Z (2005) Induction of heat shock proteins in B-cell exosomes. J Cell Sci 118:3631–3638.
35. Vincent-Schneider H, Stumptner-Cuvelette P, Lankar D, Pain S, Raposo G, Benaroch P, Bonnerot C (2002) Exosomes bearing HLA-DR1 molecules need dendritic cells to efficiently stimulate specific T cells. Int Immunol 14:713–722.
36. Thery C, Duban L, Segura E, Veron P, Lantz O, Amigorena S (2002) Indirect activation of naive CD4+ T cells by dendritic cell-derived exosomes. Nat Immunol 3:1156–1162.
37. Skokos D, Botros HG, Demeure C, Morin J, Peronet R, Birkenmeier G, Boudaly S, Mecheri S (2003) Mast cell-derived exosomes induce phenotypic and functional maturation of dendritic cells and elicit specific immune responses in vivo. J Immunol 170:3037–3045.
38. Mallegol J, Van Niel G, Lebreton C, Lepelletier Y, Candalh C, Dugave C, Heath JK, Raposo G, Cerf-Bensussan N, Heyman M (2007) T84-Intestinal Epithelial Exosomes Bear MHC Class II/Peptide Complexes Potentiating Antigen Presentation by Dendritic Cells. Gastroenterology 132:1866–1876.
39. Hsu DH, Paz P, Villaflor G, Rivas A, Mehta-Damani A, Angevin E, Zitvogel L, Le Pecq JB (2003) Exosomes as a tumour vaccine: enhancing potency through direct loading of antigenic peptides. J Immunother 26:440–450.
40. Andre F, Chaput N, Schartz NE, Flament C, Aubert N, Bernard J, Lemonnier F, Raposo G, Escudier B, Hsu DH et al. (2004) Exosomes as potent cell-free peptide-based vaccine. I. Dendritic cell-derived exosomes transfer functional MHC class I/peptide complexes to dendritic cells. J Immunol 172:2126–2136.
41. Chaput N, Schartz NE, Andre F, Taieb J, Novault S, Bonnaventure P, Aubert N, Bernard J, Lemonnier F, Merad M et al. (2004) Exosomes as potent cell-free peptide-based vaccine. II. Exosomes in CpG adjuvants efficiently prime naive Tc1 lymphocytes leading to tumour rejection. J Immunol 172:2137–2146.
42. Wolfers J, Lozier A, Raposo G, Regnault A, Thery C, Masurier C, Flament C, Pouzieux S, Faure F, Tursz T et al. (2001) Tumour-derived exosomes are a source of shared tumour rejection antigens for CTL cross-priming. Nat Med 7:297–303.
43. Hwang I, Shen X, Sprent J (2003) Direct stimulation of naive T cells by membrane vesicles from antigen-presenting cells: distinct roles for CD54 and B7 molecules. Proc Natl Acad Sci U S A 100:6670–6675.
44. Admyre C, Johansson SM, Paulie S, Gabrielsson S (2006) Direct exosome stimulation of peripheral humanT cells detected by ELISPOT. Eur J Immunol.
45. Derdak SV, Kueng HJ, Leb VM, Neunkirchner A, Schmetterer KG, Bielek E, Majdic O, Knapp W, Seed B, Pickl WF (2006) Direct stimulation of T lymphocytes by immunosomes: virus-like particles decorated with T cell receptor/CD3 ligands plus costimulatory molecules. Proc Natl Acad Sci U S A 103:13144–13149.
46. Kovar M, Boyman O, Shen X, Hwang I, Kohler R, Sprent J (2006) Direct stimulation of T cells by membrane vesicles from antigen-presenting cells. Proc Natl Acad Sci U S A 103:11671–11676.
47. Aline F, Bout D, Amigorena S, Roingeard P, Dimier-Poisson I (2004) *Toxoplasma gondii* antigen-pulsed-dendritic cell-derived exosomes induce a protective immune response against *T. gondii* infection. Infect Immun 72:4127–4137.
48. Colino J, Snapper CM (2006) Exosomes from bone marrow dendritic cells pulsed with diphtheria toxoid preferentially induce type 1 antigen-specific IgG responses in naive recipients in the absence of free antigen. J Immunol 177:3757–3762.

49. Peche H, Heslan M, Usal C, Amigorena S, Cuturi MC (2003) Presentation of donor major histocompatibility complex antigens by bone marrow dendritic cell-derived exosomes modulates allograft rejection. Transplantation 76:1503–1510.
50. Peche H, Renaudin K, Beriou G, Merieau E, Amigorena S, Cuturi MC (2006) Induction of tolerance by exosomes and short-term immunosuppression in a fully MHC-mismatched rat cardiac allograft model. Am J Transplant 6:1541–1550.
51. Kim SH, Lechman ER, Bianco N, Menon R, Keravala A, Nash J, Mi Z, Watkins SC, Gambotto A, Robbins PD (2005) Exosomes derived from IL-10-treated dendritic cells can suppress inflammation and collagen-induced arthritis. J Immunol 174:6440–6448.
52. Kim SH, Bianco N, Menon R, Lechman ER, Shufesky WJ, Morelli AE, Robbins PD (2006) Exosomes derived from genetically modified DC expressing FasL are anti-inflammatory and immunosuppressive. Mol Ther 13:289–300.
53. Escudier B, Dorval T, Chaput N, Andre F, Caby MP, Novault S, Flament C, Leboulaire C, Borg C, Amigorena S et al. (2005) Vaccination of metastatic melanoma patients with autologous dendritic cell (DC) derived-exosomes: results of thefirst phase I clinical trial. J Transl Med 3:10.
54. Morse MA, Garst J, Osada T, Khan S, Hobeika A, Clay TM, Valente N, Shreeniwas R, Sutton MA, Delcayre A et al. (2005) A phase I study of dexosome immunotherapy in patients with advanced non-small cell lung cancer. J Transl Med 3:9.
55. Taieb J, Chaput N, Schartz N, Roux S, Novault S, Menard C, Ghiringhelli F, Terme M, Carpentier AF, Darrasse-Jese G et al. (2006) Chemoimmunotherapy of tumours: cyclophosphamide synergizes with exosome based vaccines. J Immunol 176:2722–2729.
56. Valenti R, Huber V, Filipazzi P, Pilla L, Sovena G, Villa A, Corbelli A, Fais S, Parmiani G, Rivoltini L (2006) Human tumour-released microvesicles promote the differentiation of myeloid cells with transforming growth factor-beta-mediated suppressive activity on T lymphocytes. Cancer Res 66:9290–9298.
57. Liu C, Yu S, Zinn K, Wang J, Zhang L, Jia Y, Kappes JC, Barnes S, Kimberly RP, Grizzle WE et al. (2006) Murine mammary carcinoma exosomes promote tumour growth by suppression of NK cell function. J Immunol 176:1375–1385.
58. Clayton A, Tabi Z (2005) Exosomes and the MICA-NKG2D system in cancer. Blood Cells Mol Dis 34:206–213.
59. Zeelenberg IS, Ostrowski M, Krumeich S, Bobrie A, Jancic C, Boissonnas A, Delcayre A, Le Pecq JB, Combadière B, Amigorena S, Théry C (2008) Targeting tumour antigens to secreted membrane vesicles in vivo induces efficient anti-tumour immune responses. Cancer Res 68:1228–1235.
60. Prado N, Marazuela EG, Segura E, Fernandez-Garcia H, Villalba M, Thery C, Rodriguez R, Batanero E (2008) Exosomes from bronchoalveolar fluid of tolerized mice prevent allergic reaction. J Immunol 181(2):1519–1525.
61. Théry C, Ostrowski M, and Segura E, (2009) Membrane vesicles as conveyors of immune responses. Nature Rev Immunol 9:581–593.

Index

FSC
www.fsc.org
MIX
Papier aus verantwortungsvollen Quellen
Paper from responsible sources
FSC® C105338

If you have any concerns about our products,
you can contact us on
ProductSafety@springernature.com

In case Publisher is established outside the EU,
the EU authorized representative is:
Springer Nature Customer Service Center GmbH
Europaplatz 3, 69115 Heidelberg, Germany

Printed by Libri Plureos GmbH
in Hamburg, Germany